ATLAS OF EYE SURGERY

AND RELATED ANATOMY

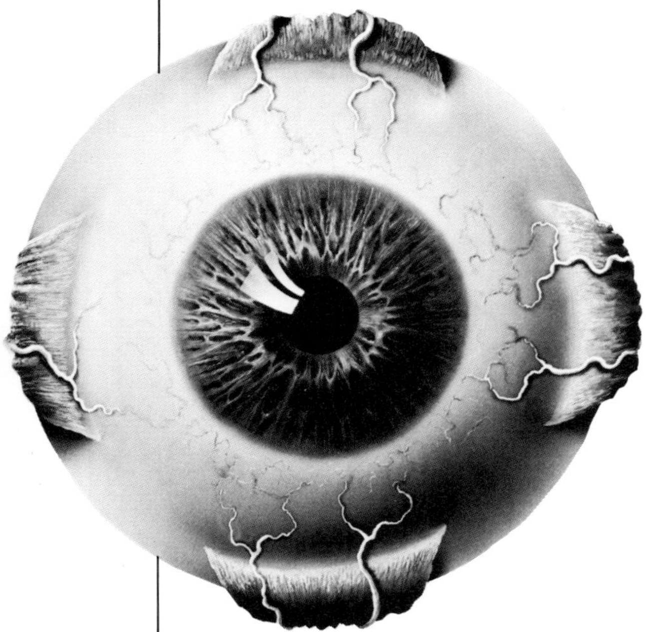

ATLAS OF EYE SURGERY

AND RELATED ANATOMY

Edited by

Frederick H. Davidorf, M.D.

Director of the Retina Service
Associate Professor
Department of Ophthalmology
Ohio State University College of Medicine
Columbus, Ohio

Illustrated by

Donald A. Keller, B.A., P.B.C.

Medical Illustrator
Department of Ophthalmology
Ohio State University College of Medicine
Columbus, Ohio

450 illustrations

published by

OPHTHALMOLOGY ILLUSTRATED

A DIVISION OF KELLER PUBLISHING CO.
P.O. BOX 2566 COLUMBUS, OHIO 43215

Photographs and/or 35-mm slides of the original artwork are available upon request.

KELLER PUBLISHING CO.
P.O. Box 2566
Columbus, Ohio 43215

Library of Congress Catalogue No. 78-61339
Distributed in countries other than the United States exclusively by Appleton-Century Crofts, a division of Prentice-Hall, Inc., and its agents.

Book design and layout by
Donald A. Keller
Photography by
R. Michael Clark

CONTRIBUTING AUTHORS

Department of Ophthalmology
Ohio State University College of Medicine
Columbus, Ohio

JOHN A. BURNS, M.D.
Co-director of the Oculoplastic Surgery Service
Clinical Associate Professor of Ophthalmology

FREDERICK H. DAVIDORF, M.D.
Director of the Retina Service
Associate Professor of Ophthalmology

WILLIAM H. HAVENER, M.D.
Professor and Chairperson
Department of Ophthalmology

FREDERICK M. KAPETANSKY, M.D.
Director of the Glaucoma Service
Associate Professor of Ophthalmology

RICHARD H. KEATES, M.D.
Director of the Corneal Service
Professor of Ophthalmology

RICHARD G. LEMBACH, M.D.
Director of the Contact Lens Service
Assistant Professor of Ophthalmology

ROBERT B. O'DAIR, M.D.
Co-director of the Oculoplastic Surgery Service
Clinical Associate Professor of Ophthalmology

GARY L. ROGERS, M.D.
Director of the Pediatric Ophthalmology Out-patient Service
Clinical Assistant Professor of Ophthalmology

JAMES A. SAVAGE, M.D.
Chief Resident of the Department of Ophthalmology
Clinical Instructor of Ophthalmology

RICHARD E. SIMMONS, M.D.
Attending Physician of the Pediatric Ophthalmology Service
Clinical Assistant Professor of Ophthalmology

FOREWORD

The classic textbooks from which we learned our ophthalmic surgery served this purpose well. However, the relentless progress of time has passed them by. Trabeculectomy, anterior vitrectomy, posterior vitrectomy, phacoemulsification, pseudophakos, radial silicone sponge, fascia lata circle for retinal detachment, microsurgery, 10-0 nylon—all of these are words no surgeon had heard when I was a resident.

With the development of all these intricate procedures, techniques, and skills, no one surgeon is a master of every operation as in the past. Of necessity, a comprehensive surgical atlas now requires the cooperation of a number of subspecialists, each contributing the knowledge unique to his particular field. Fortunately, our Department of Ophthalmology includes men such as Drs. Burns, Davidorf, Kapetansky, Keates, Lembach, O'Dair, Rogers, Savage, and Simmons who were able to contribute this specialized knowledge to the Atlas.

Equally important (since one picture is worth a thousand words) a skilled medical artist, Mr. Donald Keller, had recently joined our Department when Dr. Davidorf became interested in providing such a new and comprehensive ophthalmic surgery atlas. Indeed, the very availability of an expert artist may well have been the stimulus for preparation of the book.

Of course, resources alone do not produce books—only a persistent author can do so. Dr. Frederick Davidorf has become such an author. By virtue of several years of work, he has managed to coordinate the wisdom and the words and the pictures from many persons into the production of this Atlas.

It's really a very special book. It has absolutely superb detailed drawings illustrating every step of the procedures, which in turn are described in meticulously clear and vivid detail. Even if you've never seen a trabeculectomy before, you CAN DO the procedure after you read the chapter. That's the final test of quality teaching.

The Atlas passes the test. Read it. You'll like it.

William H. Havener, M.D.

PREFACE

It has been suggested that surgery is difficult to learn and impossible to teach. This process has been further complicated by the revolutionary change in eye surgery in recent years which has resulted in numerous technologic advancements. These include the development of microsurgical techniques, mechanical devices for removing cataracts and vitreous opacities, small caliber, nonreactive but durable suture, silicone polymers for retinal surgery and countless other instruments and materials, all of which have significantly increased the options available to the practicing ophthalmologist.

When available, the written word describing the application of these developments in ophthalmic surgery is scattered throughout professional journals and in segmented textbooks. This observation brought us to the conclusion that a definite need exists for a comprehensive atlas of eye surgery.

The cumulative experience and willingness of our staff members to participate in a project of this magnitude is one of the primary factors which prompted our decision to produce THE ATLAS OF EYE SURGERY AND RELATED ANATOMY. The academic environment created by our department chairman, William H. Havener, M.D., provided a further stimulus for this endeavor. However, our unique ophthalmologist-medical illustrator working relationship was the principle motivating factor in the decision to pursue a project of this magnitude.

If a medical illustrator attempts to depict a surgical procedure in a series of progressive steps without the assistance of a surgeon, the results, predictably, are aesthetically pleasing but most assuredly inaccurate. Similarly, if a surgeon attempts to graphically display his methods in a series of logical steps, the results would be accurate, but probably decipherable only to himself. Our belief is that the more detailed and accurate the illustrations the greater the benefits to be derived.

It follows, then, that the accuracy and ultimate success of a visually oriented work such as this depend on a mutual respect and understanding of the two disciplines. Endless hours of discussion, involving the modification, exchange and refinement of ideas, have evolved into *what we believe* to be an ideal working relationship. Hopefully, this unity of ideals between ophthalmic surgeon and medical illustrator has produced an indispensable volume for the resident in ophthalmology and a valuable resource for the more accomplished ophthalmic surgeon.

For practical reasons we have limited the discussion of preoperative and postoperative considerations. Our intentions are not to present all possible methods for the solution of a particular surgical problem. On the contrary, the surgical techniques and the opinions expressed are based on personal experience and are, therefore, intentionally biased. No claim of originality is made, and special conditions may dictate modifications of any of the approaches described.

In their formative years, residents are understandably vague about the precise anatomy involved in eye surgery. They need no reminder, however, that they are dealing with one of the most specialized and intrinsically complicated organs of the human body. For this reason we have elected to precede each major division of this book with a series of concise anatomic illustrations and accompanying text.

It has been said that a book's worth is measured by the results it provokes. Our hope is that we have provided a stimulus which will enable the reader to deal more effectively with the surgical problems in ophthalmology, some of which were considered untreatable until just a few years ago.

This preface would be only partially complete if we did not express our gratitude to our wives, Brenda and June, whose seemingly endless patience prevailed throughout the process of making our dream a reality. A special note of appreciation is extended to R. Michael Clark for his tolerance and photographic skills and to Esther Weiss for her editorial assistance. Numerous other people have made their talents available and assisted in the production of this book, for which we are grateful.

Frederick H. Davidorf
Donald A. Keller

ACKNOWLEDGMENTS

An endeavor such as the writing of a surgical atlas is not possible without the contributions of many people. Although not all who were a part of this gratifying experience can be named here, we wish to give special thanks to the many authors whose works have served as a reference for our project. Special thanks are given to the works of Jorg A. Alvarado, Crowell Beard, Alston Callahan, William H. Havener, Eugene M. Helveston, Michael J. Hogan, Norman S. Jaffe, Lester Jones, Edward Pernkopf, Gunter Von Noorden, Eugene Wolff, and Lorenz F. Zimmerman.

The excellent illustrations of Suzanne De Pasquale, Sally Gloeckner Jennings, Leon Schlosberg, and Joan Esperson Weddell must also be acknowledged as they were of invaluable assistance in the preparation of the Atlas. Additionally, recognition is given to those members of the Association of Medical Illustrators whose drawings have been a source of inspiration.

Gratitude is expressed to Ruth Davis for compiling the index. Also, we would like to thank (Stat) Pat Nida for her typing and proofreading contributions and Kathy Werling for her exceptional work in the preparation of microscopic specimens. In addition we wish to recognize Anna Bory, Stella Lawrence, Ann Steinemann, and Lena Warrick who worked tirelessly and contributed many hours toward the completion of this text.

Several of our colleagues at the University whose expertise could not be included in this text nevertheless have devoted much of their time and given their encouragement to this project. Accordingly, we wish to thank Drs. James Andrews, Hans Bredemeyer, Robert Bruce, Elson Craig, Martin Lubow, and Torrence Makley.

Finally, recognition must be given to all of the referring physicians, for it is they who have supplied the wealth of patients that has allowed the authors to become expert in their particular fields. To all of these persons and to the many more who could not be individually named, we extend our sincerest appreciation for turning our dream into a reality.

Frederick H. Davidorf
Donald A. Keller

TABLE OF CONTENTS

CHAPTER VI

EXTRAOCULAR MUSCLE SURGERY

CHAPTER VII

EYELID SURGERY

CHAPTER VIII

LACRIMAL SURGERY

CHAPTER IX

This book is
dedicated to

WILLIAM H. HAVENER
who provided an environment
which made this book possible

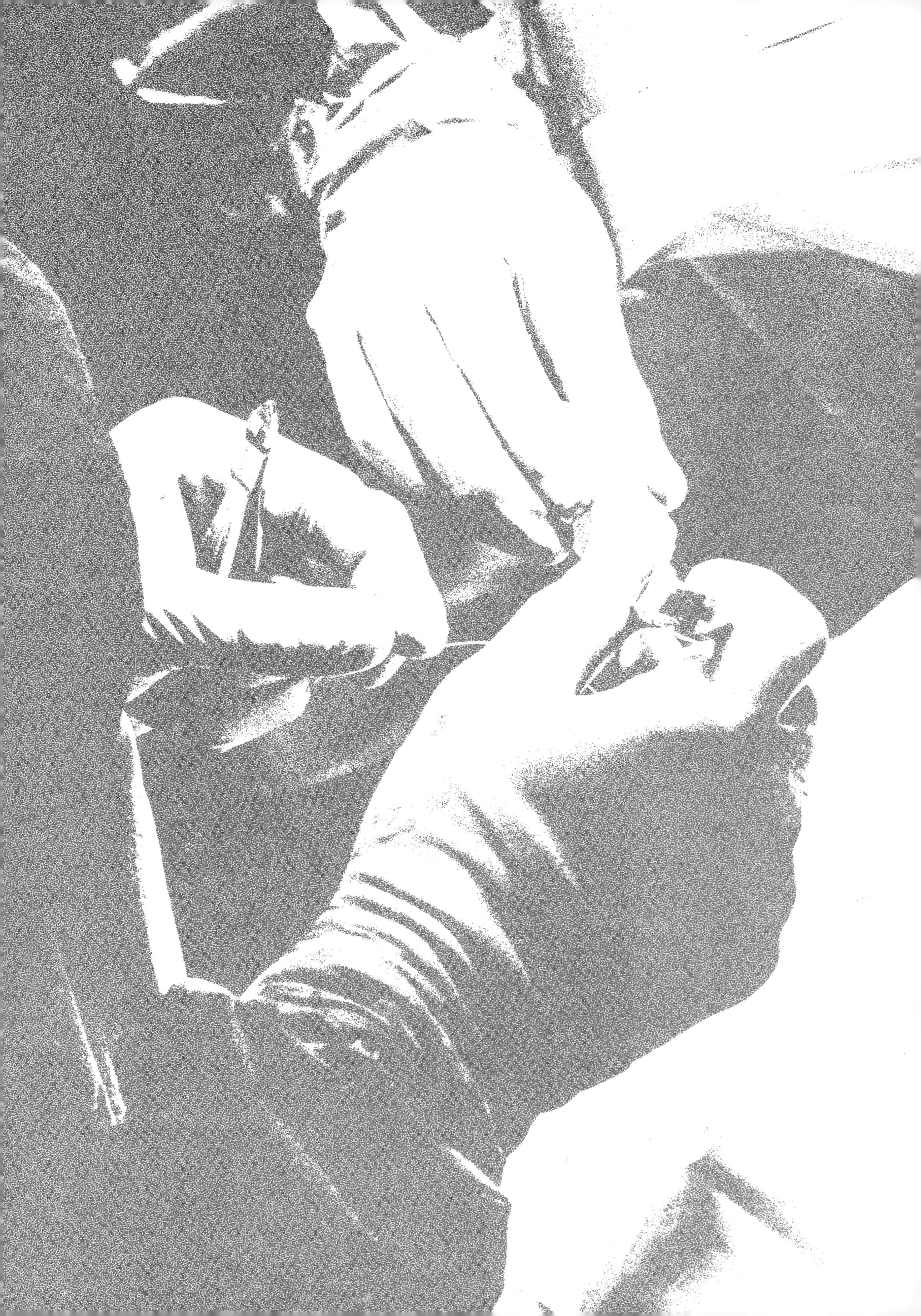

1
CATARACT
SURGERY

ANATOMY OF THE LENS

Frederick H. Davidorf, M.D.

Much has been written about cataract surgery, though the lens itself has received little attention. With greater emphasis on extracapsular procedures and implantation of intraocular lenses, the anatomy of the lens, its anatomic location, and its function as an optical structure are increasingly important.

The lens vesicle develops from an invagination of the surface ectoderm. The primary lens fibers originate from the posterior epithelial cells, which grow anteriorly, obliterating the cavity of the lens vesicle and forming the embryonic nucleus. The crystalline lens is a dynamic structure that grows throughout life. This pattern of growth begins in utero after the first trimester with the development of secondary lens fibers, which surround the embryonic nucleus, EN [1] and begin to form the fetal nucleus, FN [1] [2] .

When secondary lens fibers form the fetal nucleus, they meet to create the Y sutures. The anterior Y suture, AY [1] is erect while the posterior suture is inverted, PY [1] . The location of the Y sutures delineates the extent of the fetal nucleus. After birth, the formation of the new lens fibers creates a more complex sutural arrangement with a stellate configuration [2] . As the lens fibers develop, the more centrally located cortical

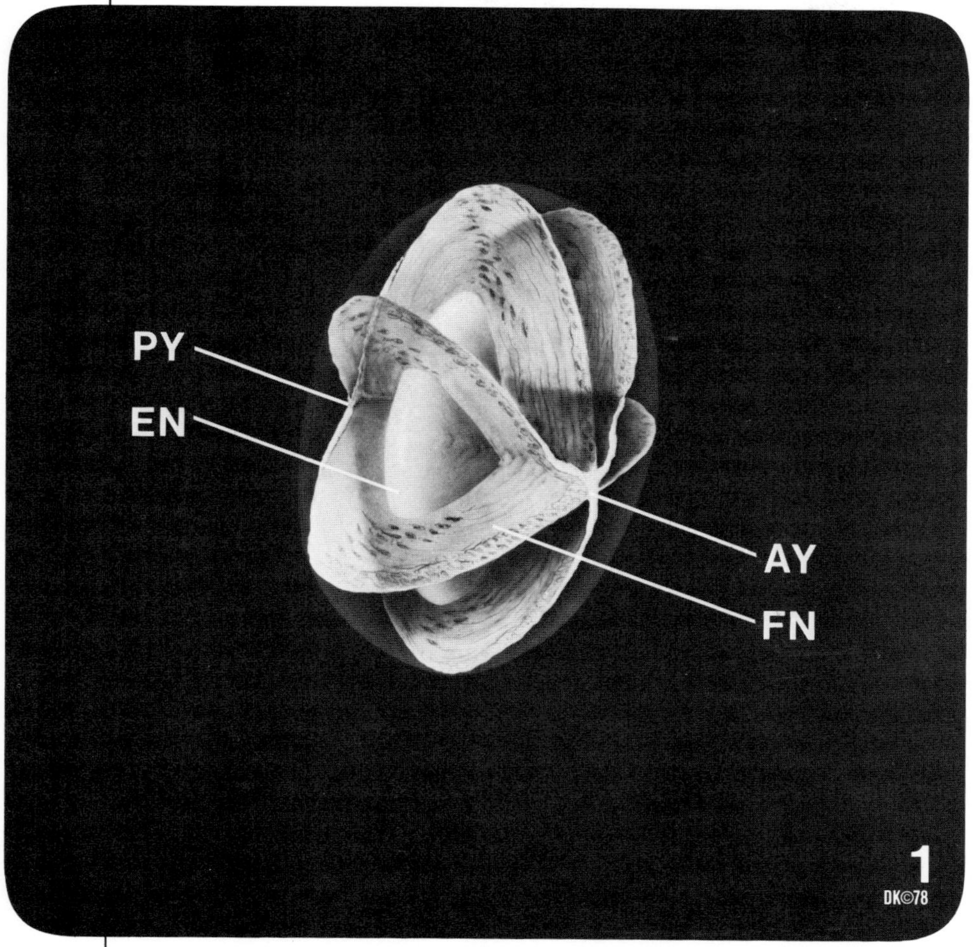

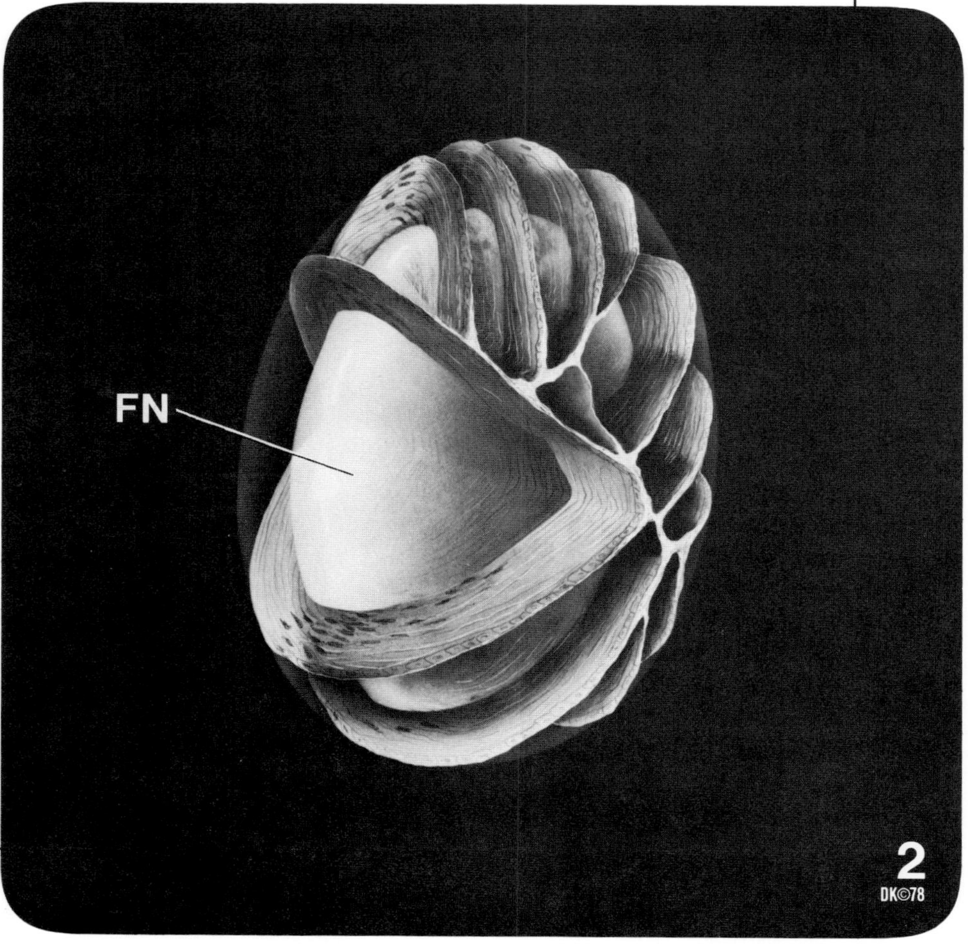

Donald F. Keller

cells lose their nuclei and form the adult nucleus [3]. The newly formed cells peripheral to the adult nucleus, which still contain nuclei, are the lens cortex. Thus, the area of transition between the adult nucleus and cortex is not well defined.

The nuclei of the lens cells are located in the equatorial region, and the anterior and posterior terminations of the lens cells form the lens sutures. The lens capsule, LC [3], the basement membrane of the epithelial cells, thickens until the definitive lens develops. In the young eye, the capsule is elastic and strong; as the lens grows, the capsule becomes thinner and less elastic. Throughout life, the lens enlarges as the secondary lens fibers formed by the anterior epithelium migrate to the equatorial region. The anteroposterior length in newborns is approximately 3.5 mm; it increases to 4.0 mm by age 50 and is nearly 5.0 mm in diameter at age 90.

Zonules, Z [3], the suspensory ligaments of the lens, extend from the ciliary body, CB [4] to the equatorial region of the lens. Their origin is in the nonpigmented epithelium of the ciliary body, in both the pars plicata and pars plana regions. In the pars plicata, the suspensory ligaments are located in valleys between the individual ciliary processes, CP [4]. In the pars plana, the ligaments begin approximately 1.5 mm anterior to the ora serrata and extend toward the equatorial region of the lens. The zonules insert into the lens capsule, forming tent-like configurations at the site of the insertion.

Lens opacities may develop as a result of a variety of mechanisms that alter nutrient transport in the lens fibers. The susceptible areas of the lens are the more metabolically active ones—the epithelium, which lines the anterior aspect of the lens, and the equatorial region, where the lens fibers form continually. Subcapsular opacities appear posteriorly; cortical spoking is a common equatorial finding in early cataract formation. Cortical opacities result from proteolysis and acidification of the lens fibers. As the proteolytic products diffuse from the lens, relative dehydration occurs, and opacification follows.

As changes in the cortex advance and more fibers are involved, the cortex whitens to form a mature cortical cataract. With complete breakdown of the lens fibers, the entire cortex liquefies, with only the nucleus remaining intact. This is a hypermature or morgagnian cataract.

The pathophysiology of nuclear sclerotic cataracts differs from cortical cataracts. The nucleus gradually hardens as the fibers compress, lose their nuclei, and contain less water and protein. This proteolysis causes deposition of urochrome pigment. Initially, the pigmentation is yellow, which may intensify to a dense brown or black, and a brunescent cataract forms.

Although infinite factors may contribute to cataract formation, the two most predominant ones are an individual's general health and genetic make-up.

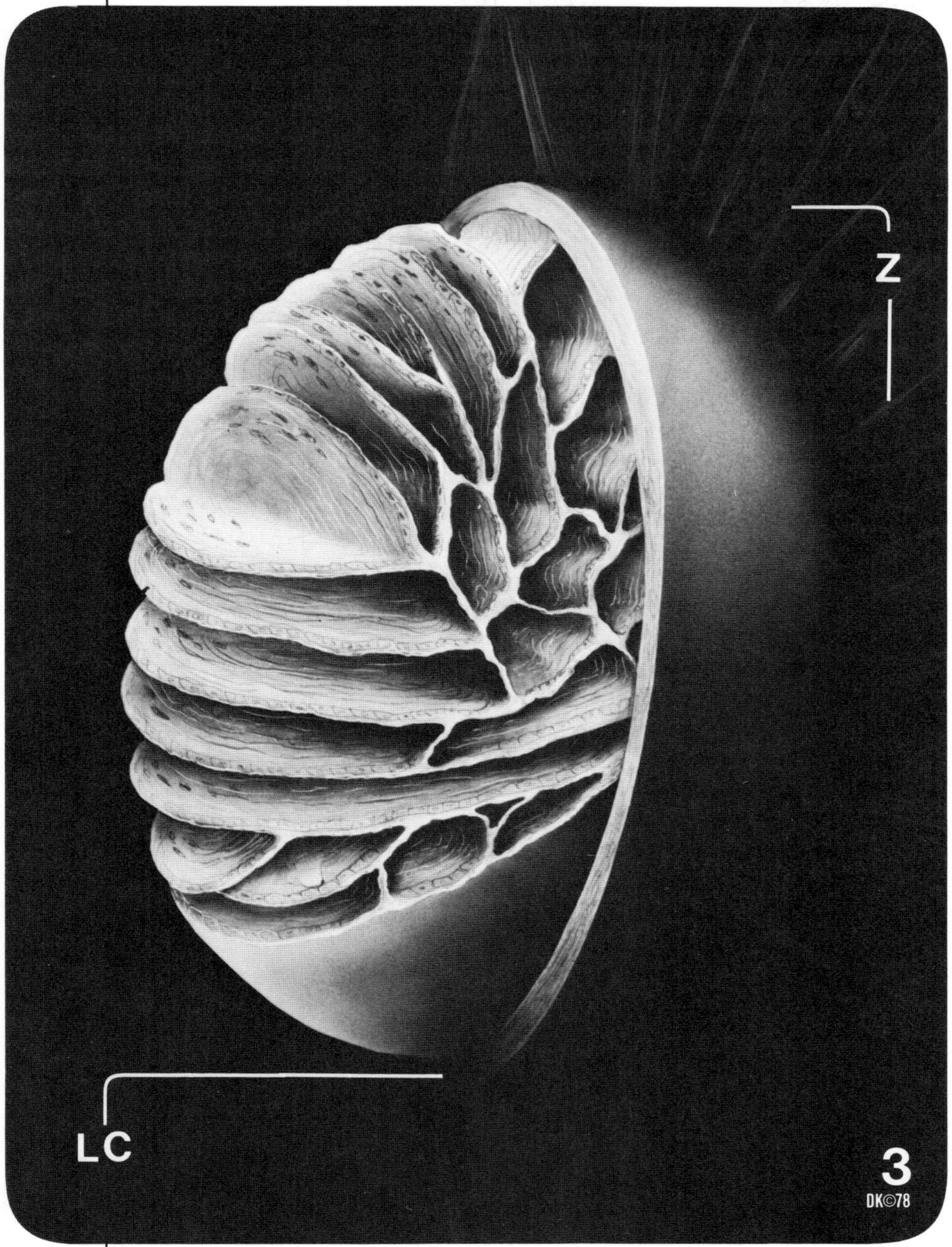

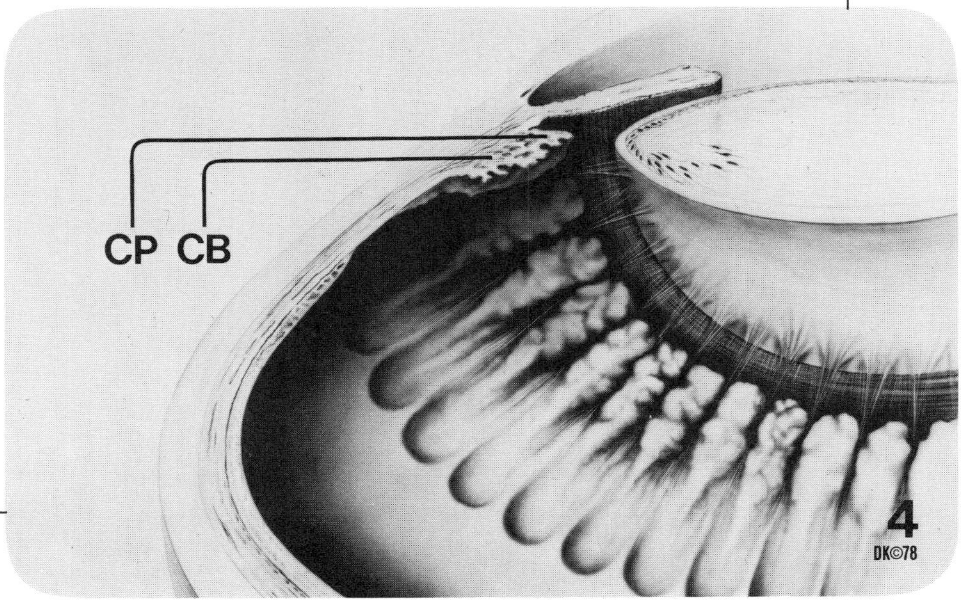

Donald F. Keller

ANATOMY OF THE LIMBUS

Frederick H. Davidorf, M.D.

The corneoscleral limbus is the region of the globe most often encountered by the surgeon's blade. Therefore, sound knowledge of the anatomy of this region is mandatory. The limbus is not a specific structure, but rather an area of transition from the cornea to sclera and includes most of the structures involved in the drainage of aqueous humor. The anterior limit of the limbus is generally defined as a plane passing between the termination of Bowman's line and Descemet's membrane, BL and DM [1] [2]. The posterior limit of the limbus is a plane that passes perpendicularly from the surface of the eye through the scleral spur, SS [1] [2]. The distance between the two planes (the extreme limits of the limbus) on the surface of the globe is approximately 1.5 mm [1].

The most important landmark within the limbus is the blue line, the translucent area between the clear cornea and the white opaque sclera, most readily visible after the conjunctiva is removed. The anterior border of the blue line marks the end of the conjunctiva and the beginning of the corneal epithelium. The blue line varies in width from the vertical to the horizontal meridians. The conjunctival overhang is much greater in the 12- and 6-o'clock meridian than in the 3- and 9-o'clock meridian.

The gradual transition between the cornea and sclera makes it difficult to determine where the cornea ends and the sclera begins. The transparent corneal collagen extends further peripherally than a line drawn between the ends of Bowman's and Descemet's membranes might indicate. In this transition zone, the corneal lamellae mesh with the scleral lamellae, forming a concave junction, dotted line [2].

The conjunctiva covers the limbus externally. The stratified squamous conjunctival epithelium, CE [2], has approximately ten layers and blends into the five-layered epithelium of the cornea.

The trabecular meshwork (TM) lines the internal surface of the limbus. The apex of the corneoscleral meshwork is at Schwalbe's line (SL). The base of the corneoscleral meshwork inserts into the scleral spur and is continuous with the longitudinal portion of the ciliary muscles (LCM). Schlemm's canal

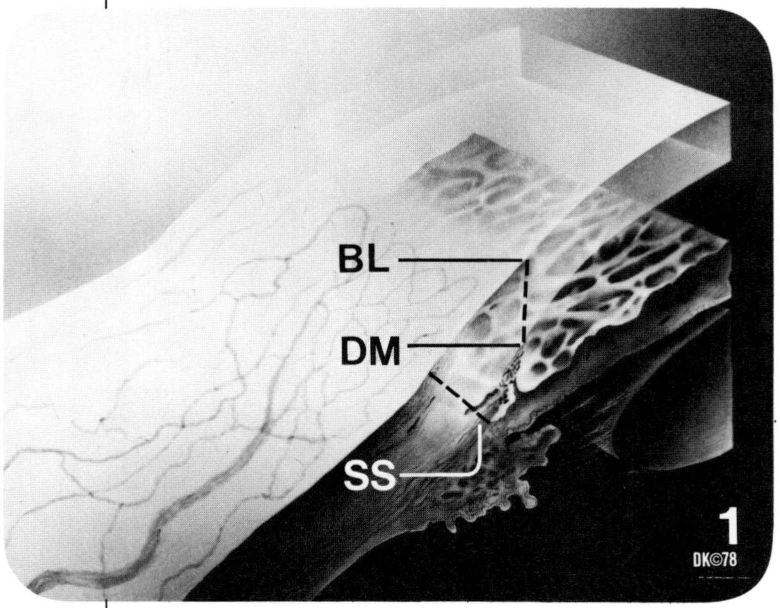

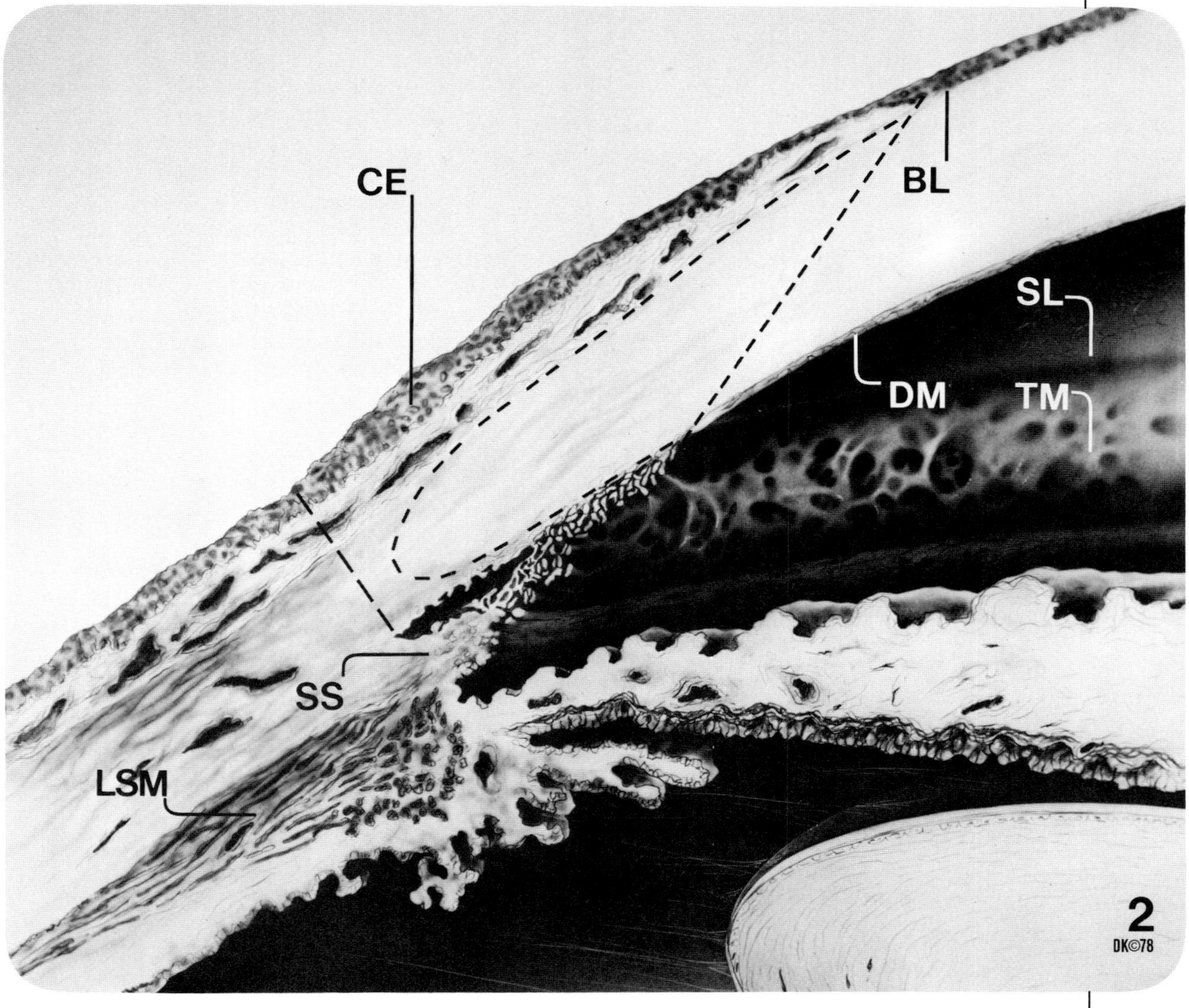

Donald F. Keller

(SC) encircles the globe just adjacent to the base of the corneoscleral meshwork. Aqueous humor passes from Schlemm's canal into either the deep intrascleral plexus or directly to the episcleral veins.

The conjunctiva is firmly attached at the limbus, and rete pegs, RP [3], connect the conjunctiva to the underlying stroma. The pegs form papillae, P [3], that radiate posteriorly from the edge of the cornea and are known as the palisades of Vogt.

Branches of the anterior ciliary arteries comprise the vascular system of the limbus. The anterior ciliary arteries, ACA [3], travel anteriorly in the episclera to a point approximately 4 mm from the corneoscleral junction. This point, called the sulcus sclerae, frequently marked by pigmentation, is the site at which the anterior ciliary arteries divide into two major branches. One branch, the major perforating artery (MPA), traverses the sclera and enters the ciliary muscle where it anastomoses with the long posterior ciliary artery (LPCA) to form the major arterial circle (MAC). The other branch, the episcleral artery (EA), continues to travel anteriorly toward the corneoscleral junction. It gives rise to the conjunctival vessels that form the superficial marginal plexus (SMP). The vessels of this plexus continue their course anteriorly in the papillae of the palisades of Vogt where they further divide and give rise to the recurrent arteries and the terminal branches (PV, RA, and TB). The recurrent arteries travel posteriorly through the palisades of Vogt and supply the perilimbal conjunctiva. The terminal branches comprise the peripheral corneal arcades, an extensive capillary network that then takes the form of venous channels. Atypically, the venous channels of the ciliary system do not correspond to their arterial counterparts in number or in methods of branching, and they do not assimilate the course of their corresponding arteries. Interestingly, they are similar to the veins of the retina, in that neither contains valves.

The drainage vessels from the ciliary body, as well as from the region of the canal of Schlemm, unite to form the deep scleral plexus and the intrascleral plexus. These pass through the sclera and join venous drainage from the conjunctiva and episclera. The veins course posteriorly in the episcleral region and carry blood to the ophthalmic veins. Engorgement of the venous plexus is responsible for ciliary flush, the common sign of anterior segment inflammation.

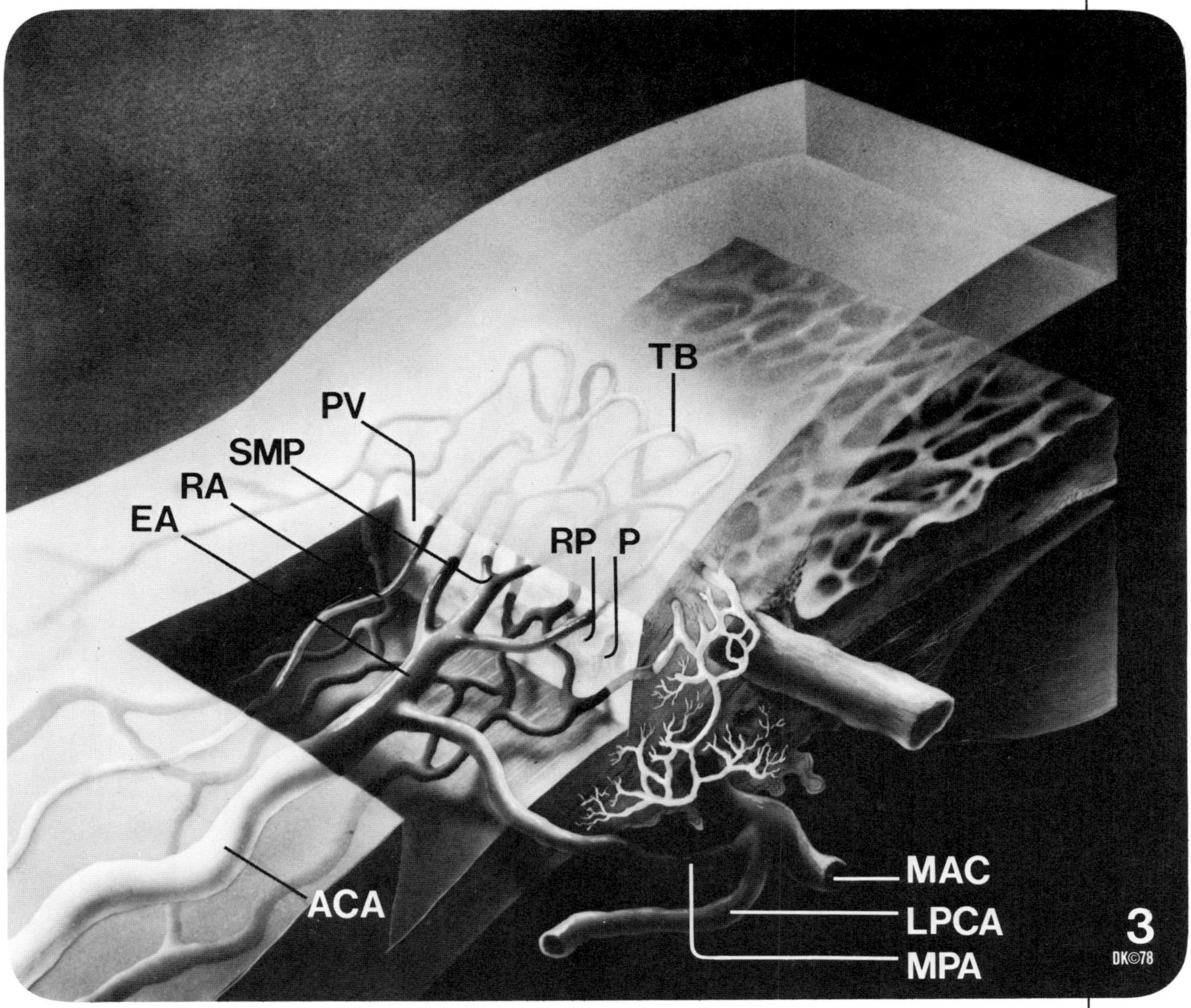

Donald A. Killer

MICROSCOPIC INTRACAPSULAR CATARACT EXTRACTION

Richard H. Keates, M.D.
Frederick H. Davidorf, M.D.

Intracapsular cataract extraction has evolved into a reliable and safe operation. The high success rate of cataract surgery is a result of the development of the operating microscope, modern suture material, finer instruments, and cryosurgery. Refinements in procedure, specifically the methods of handling vitreous loss, have reduced the complication rate. For the aphakic patient, these developments have resulted in more rapid and complete visual rehabilitation.

This chapter describes the techniques for microscopic intracapsular cataract surgery using the 10-0 monofilament suture. Included is a section on the management of vitreous loss.

The obvious advantage of the operating microscope relates to the optimum visualization of the operative procedure. For optimum use of the microscope, the patient is positioned so that the surgical field is in the midzone of the focusing mechanism.

It is essential that the surgeon have maximum exposure during the procedure. We recommend use of either a wire speculum or a Guyton-Parks speculum. If exposure is not adequate, it may be necessary to use superior and inferior lid sutures.

A 4-0 black silk suture is passed through the tendon of the superior rectus muscle. This improves the exposure and allows for repositioning of the globe during the procedure [1]. Starting at the 12-o'clock position, a fornix-based conjunctival flap is dissected with use of a Westcott conjunctival scissors and 0.12-mm Castroviejo forceps. The conjunctiva is cut as close to the cornea as possible [2] [3]. A Colibri forceps stabilizes the conjunctiva as the scissors is advanced. This is done with a walking motion where the scissors, after cutting, lifts the conjunctiva. Residual tissue is almost always present after the conjunctival flap has been reflected. To expose the surgical limbus fully, the surgeon scrapes with a sharp instrument to remove superficial tissue, including epithelium and Tenon's capsule. A No. 64 Tooke knife is ideal for this purpose. The surgeon rotates the blade slightly and cleans the limbus with a wiping motion. This tamponades the superficial vessels and reduces the amount of intraoperative bleeding. Moreover, the view of the blue area of the limbus is clear in preparation for the incision. It is important that hemostasis is obtained prior to incision into the anterior chamber.

It is generally advisable to avoid cauterization at the line of incision since it may weaken the wound. We recommend use of bipolar cautery as it provides maximum cauterization with minimum tissue necrosis [4]. Since bipolar cautery may be used under water, specific bleeding sites may be identified and treated while the assistant irrigates the field. If the surgeon does use one of the older types of cautery, however, it is better to obliterate the vessel away from the line of incision.

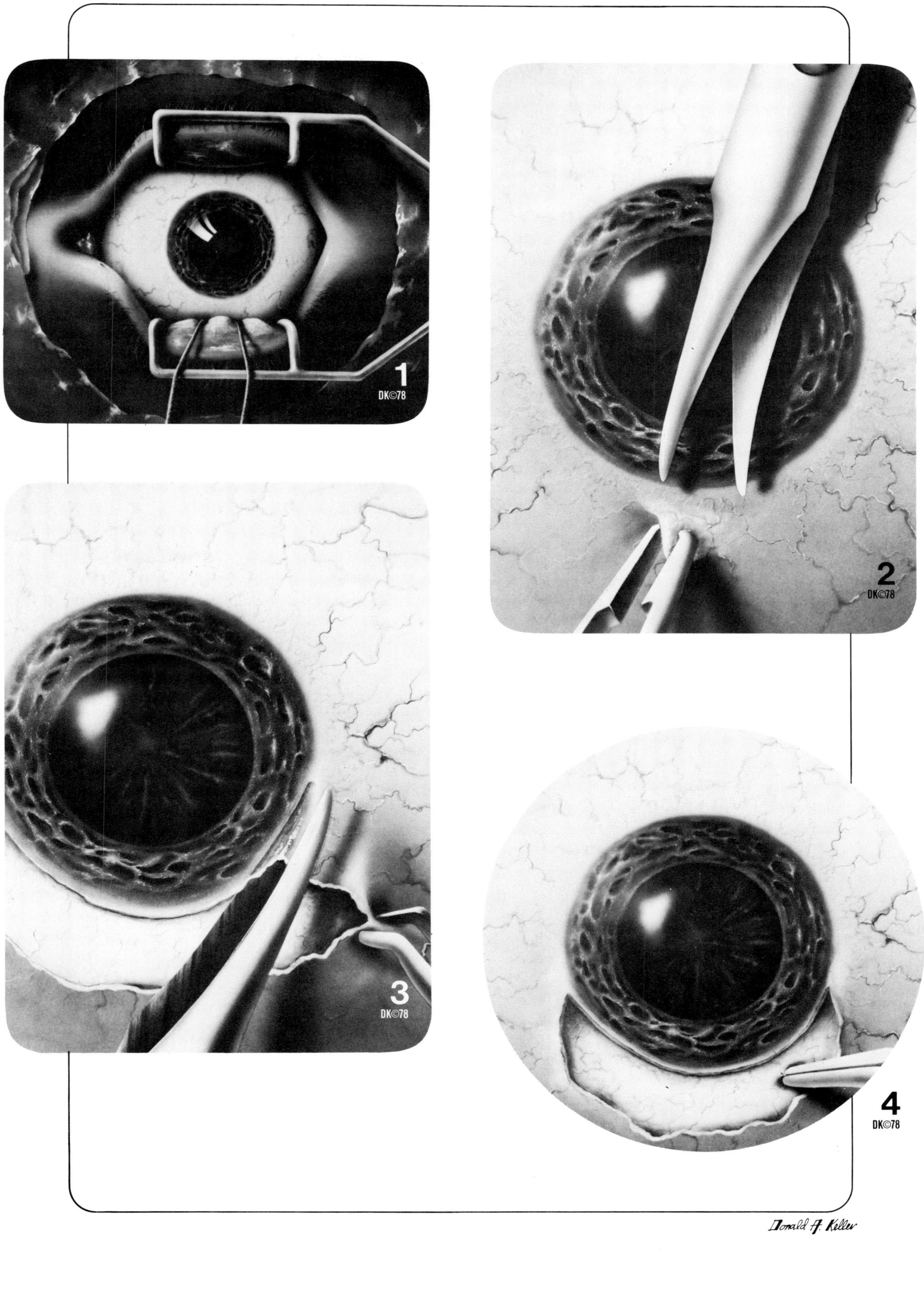

Donald A. Keller

There is considerable controversy concerning the type of incision to be used. Generally, all incisions heal satisfactorily if the edges of the wound are carefully approximated. It is nearly impossible to damage the angle structures if the cataract incision is made through the blue line [5]. This is the area where the radius of curvature of the cornea meets the radius of curvature of the sclera. We prefer a minimally beveled incision at the 12-o'clock position, beginning at the middle of the surgical limbus or blue line.

A sharp instrument, such as a razor blade, can cleanly penetrate corneal tissue with minimal pressure while the surgeon controls the globe with a 0.5-mm Castroviejo fixation forceps [6]. Incisions of this type are more readily made if the blade is used to cut down into the tissue while the forceps stabilizes and lifts close to the area of the incision. The razor blade is inserted until the surgeon sees a drop of aqueous. This depth is maintained while the incision is enlarged. The incision needs to be long enough so that the tips of the scissors can pass easily into the anterior chamber. A 3-mm incision is usually sufficient. The external portion of the incision is usually longer than the internal portion due to the tendency of the surgeon to lift out of the chamber too rapidly, which results in a smaller internal wound. If the interior opening is too small, the surgeon runs the risk of introducing the scissors into the corneal lamella and splitting Descemet's membrane. The tip of the scissors is introduced without resistance, which is facilitated by the surgeon's lifting the wound edge with the forceps. This avoids iris contact that may cause premature contraction of the pupil. If necessary, the razor blade can be used to enlarge the interior wound. Care is taken not to nick the iris or the lens capsule.

Usually, a 120-degree incision from 10 to 2 o'clock provides an adequate opening for an intracapsular cataract extraction. If a marked bevel is used, a slightly larger wound is necessary. Right- and left-handed scissors are used to complete the wound [7]. The wound is enlarged by lifting the cornea with the Colibri forceps and cutting with the tips of the scissors. The scissors are tilted slightly to maintain the beveled incision. Before proceeding, the wound must be enlarged enough to accommodate the lens. The surgeon should avoid cutting into the sclera. This may cause bleeding from the intrascleral plexus of vessels.

With microsurgery, the ability to visualize wound edges and depth of suture placement is so much enhanced that earlier problems of suture placement and wound reapproximation have been largely overcome. Visualization afforded by microsurgery has largely eliminated the need for placing sutures before the wound is completely open.

If the surgeon places preextraction sutures, the wound can be closed rapidly. On the other hand, preplaced 10-0 nylon sutures are quite electrostatic and have a tendency to tangle, which is annoying and may actually interfere with the procedure. We prefer placing the 10-0 sutures after the lens has been removed.

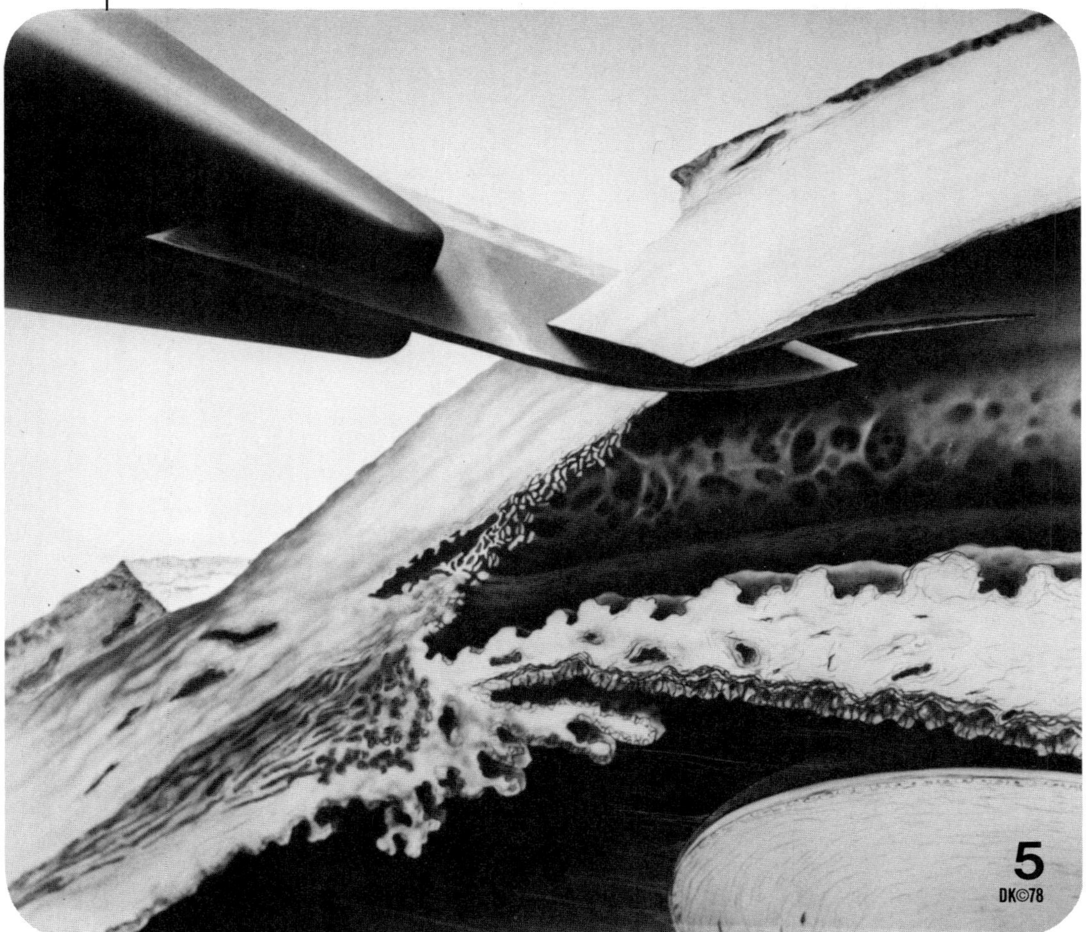

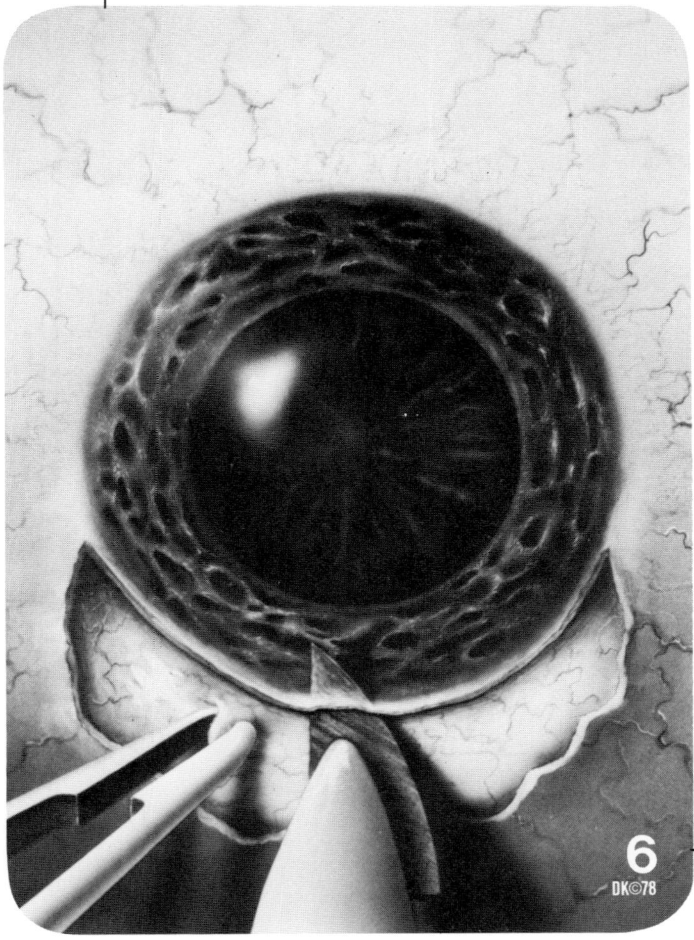

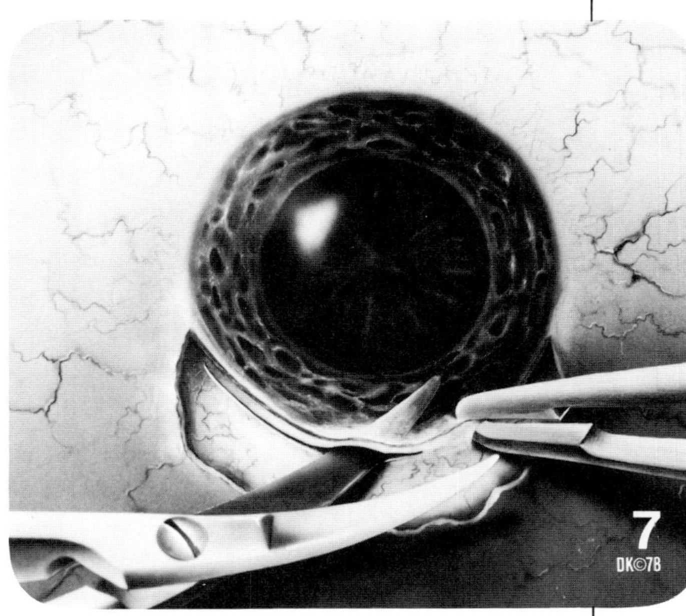

Donald A. Keller

Wound control can be obtained with the use of one 7-0 braided silk safety suture through the corneal and scleral edges of the wound at 12 o'clock [8] . It is placed at one-half the depth of the wound. The suture is looped out of the wound, and when placed on a locking needle holder, it acts as a safety suture which can be rapidly closed if necessary. The advantage of the 7-0 black silk is that it is easier to place on a needle holder, and the cornea is retracted by the assistant without danger of the suture breaking or snapping.

With a routine intracapsular procedure, only one iridectomy is necessary [9] . It is made superiorly at the 12-o'clock position by cutting iris perpendicular to the angle of the limbal wound. The most difficult part of making a small basal iridectomy is grasping the iris. The surgeon's natural inclination may be to grasp and prolapse the iris with the nondominant hand and hold the scissors in the dominant hand. We suggest that it is more reasonable to hold the iris with the dominant hand and cut with the nondominant hand.

The surgeon should attempt to grasp a sufficient knuckle of peripheral iris to include both the iris mesoderm and pigment layers with a Colibri forceps. After the iridectomy is performed, a dull, double-armed spatula is used to check the patency of the iridectomy, with care taken not to damage the lens capsule.

The use of alpha-chymotrypsin has become a routine part of cataract extraction. The action of alpha-chymotrypsin is to weaken the zonules; therefore, it is essential that the enzyme be placed in the posterior chamber [10] . As the lens is removed, the superior zonules are broken first, and the others shear away. Therefore, the critical contact of the enzyme is with the zonules superiorly. The surgeon injects up to 0.2 ml of 1:10,000 solution through the iridectomy or under the edge of the superior iris. The enzyme is injected under the superior edge of the iris while cornea is retracted. Maximum zonulysis occurs after 90 seconds.

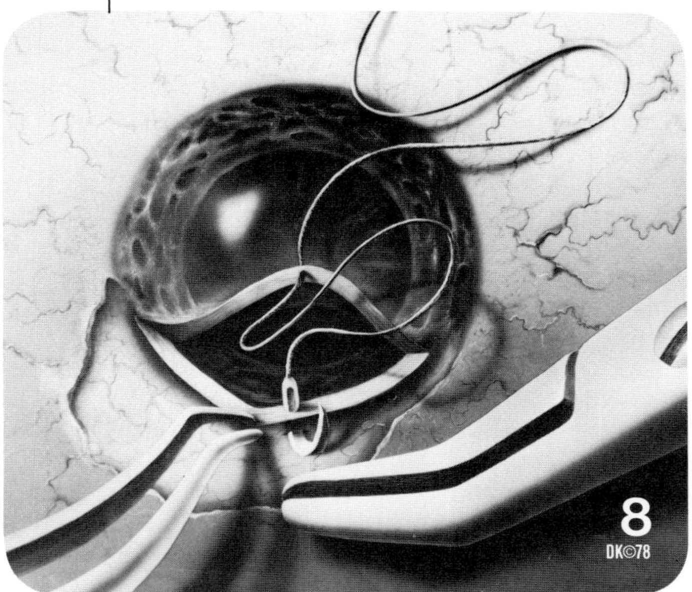
8
DK©78

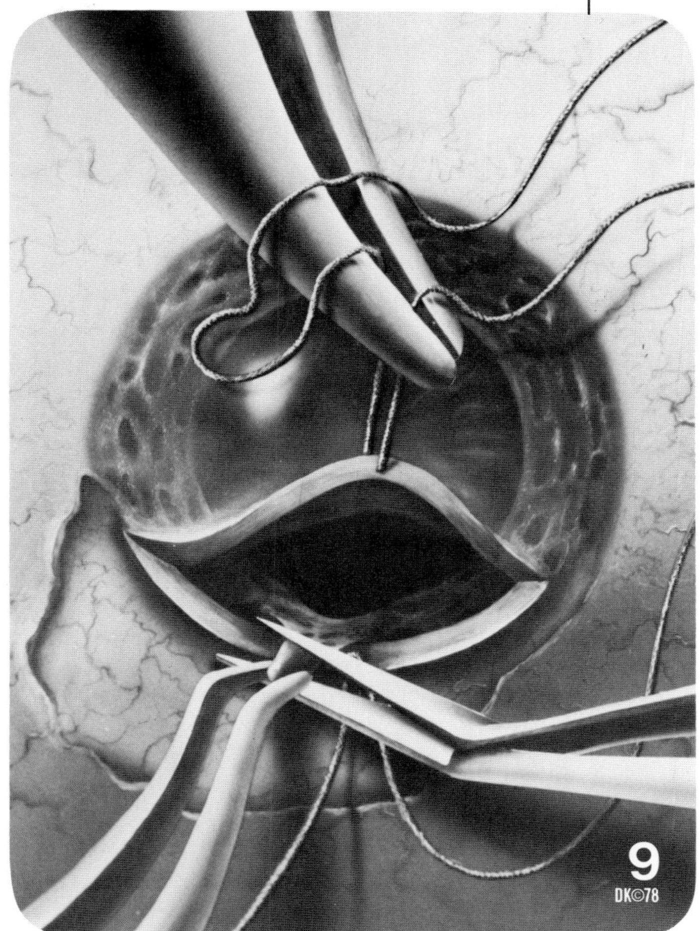
9
DK©78

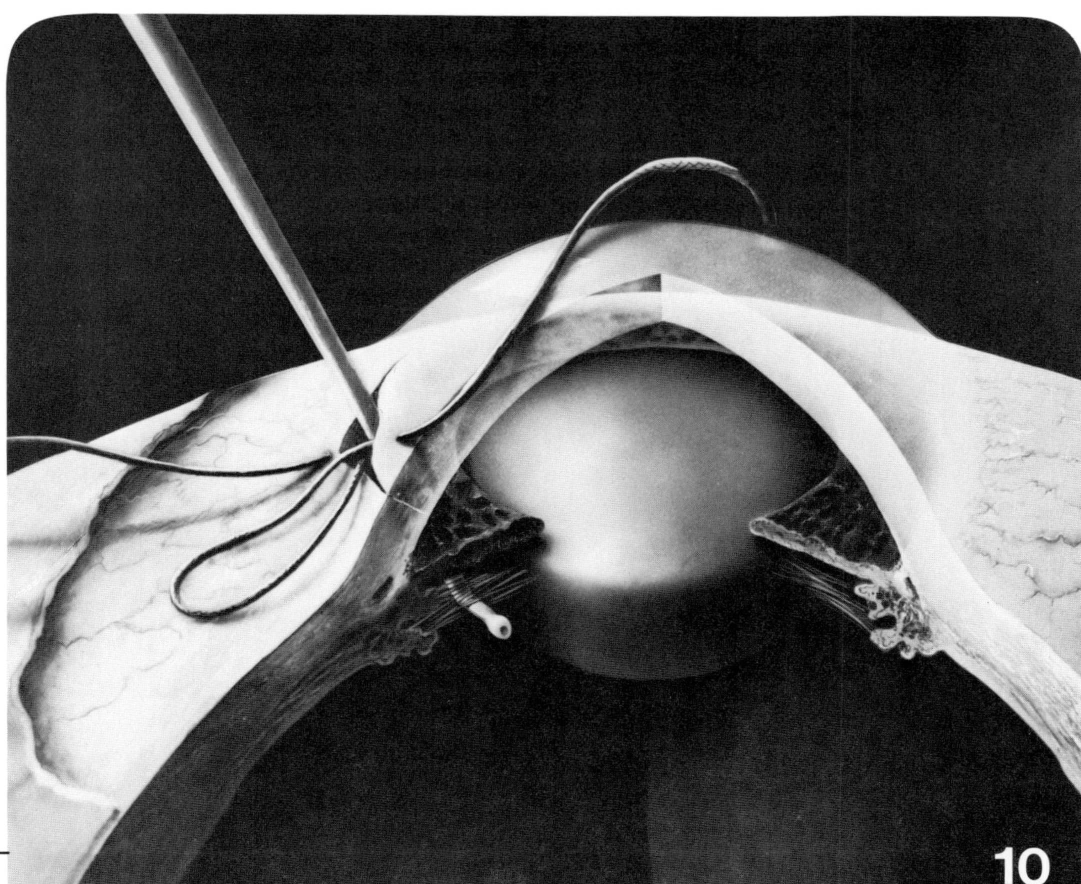
10
DK©78

Prior to removing the cataract, the surgeon again inspects the wound to make sure it is of adequate size to accommodate passage of the lens. The assistant retracts the cornea with the 7-0 braided silk suture. It is important that the sutures are carefully positioned outside the immediate area so that they do not adhere to the ice ball during extraction. Prior to placing the cryoprobe on the lens, the surgeon checks the instrument to make sure that both freezing and thawing are functioning properly. Excessive fluid during cryoextraction may result in inadvertent freezing of the iris. Therefore, a sponge is used to absorb the aqueous fluid before application of the cryoprobe. If the iris is widely dilated, little retraction is required. The Colibri forceps has been found to be the most useful instrument to retract the iris to insure that it does not contact the ice ball. It is used in a closed position and may be used to strip the zonules if necessary.

With the cornea and iris retracted, a microcryoprobe is touched to the superior lens capsule, and the surgeon pauses to allow an adequate ice ball to form [11]. Once this has been achieved, the tip of the microcryoprobe is raised slightly so that the ice ball clears the iris [12]. At first, the surgeon attempts to create tension on the superior zonules, which usually separate spontaneously. If they do not, the surgeon rocks the lens from side to side, which may cause the zonules to shear. If this does not release them, the closed forceps tips may be used to strip the superior zonules manually by applying pressure through the superior iris [13]. Once the zonules release, the iris tends to fall behind the lens, and subsequent zonular separation is achieved rather easily by gentle side-to-side sliding motion of the lens while it is withdrawn from the eye [14].

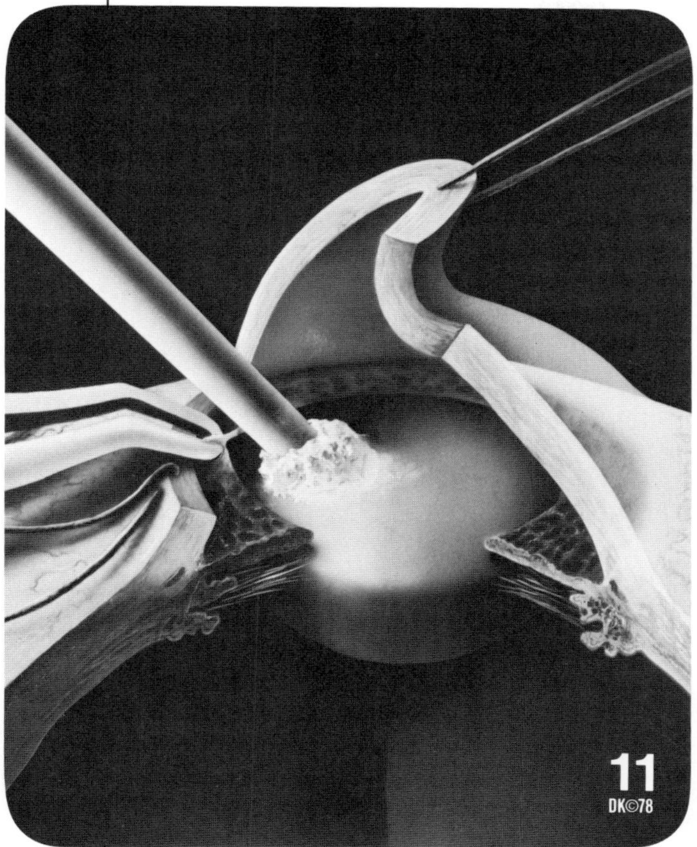

11
DK©78

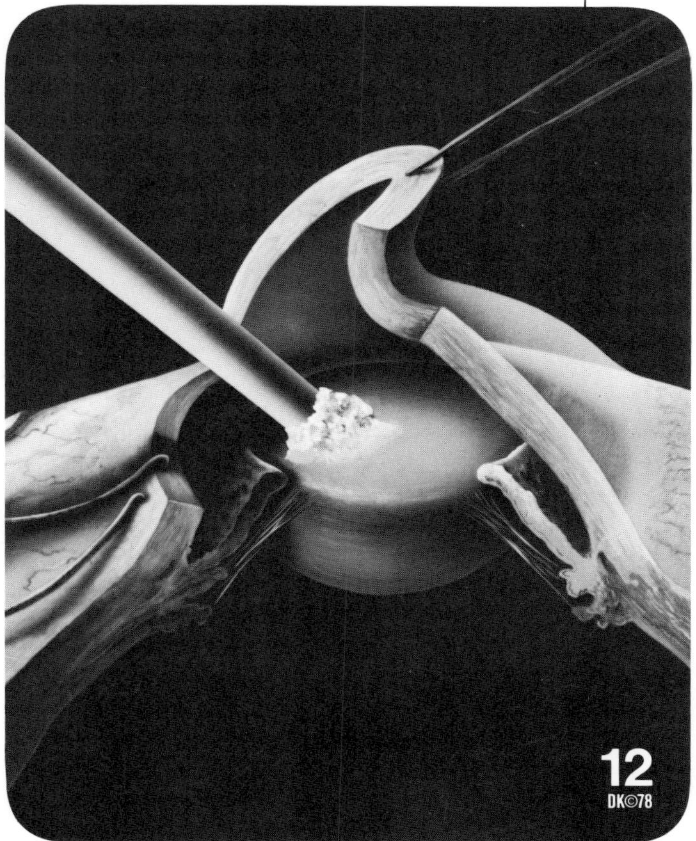

12
DK©78

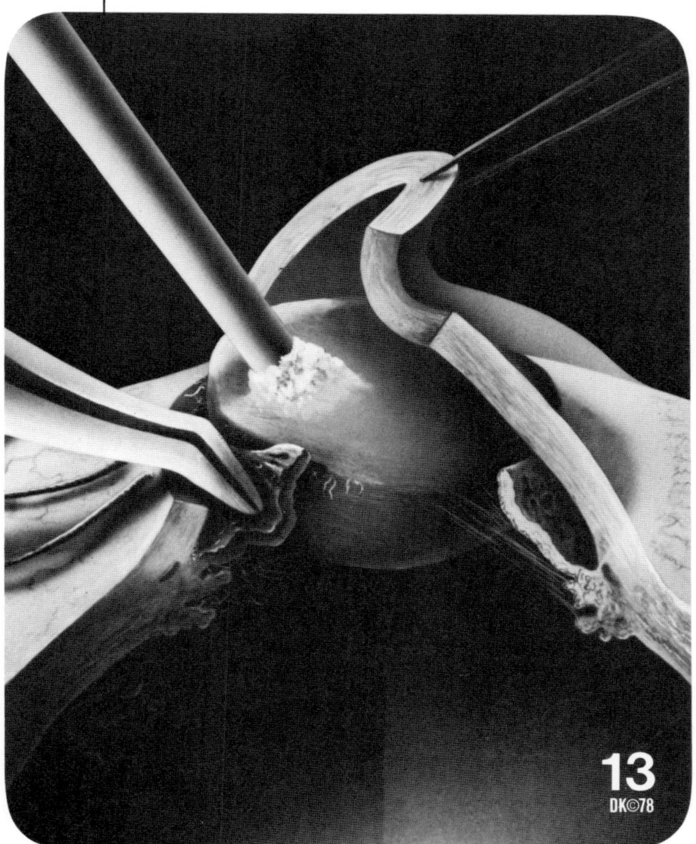

13
DK©78

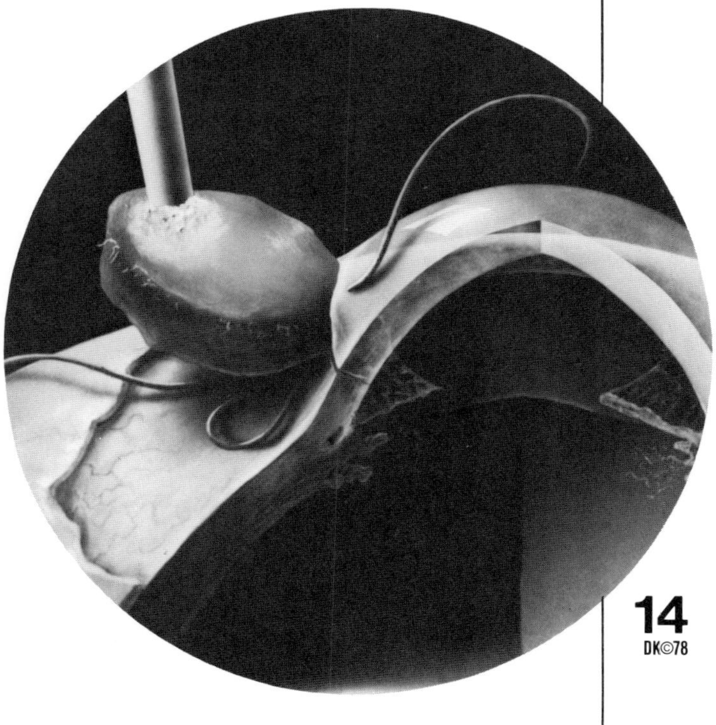

14
DK©78

Donald A. Keller

When the ice ball is outside the eye, the assistant begins to release the corneal traction to minimize pressure on the eye as the lens is removed. This reduces the likelihood of vitreous loss. When the cryoprobe and the lens are removed completely from the eye, the assistant releases the safety suture and the wound usually closes without tying. It is extremely important not to cause any pressure or to jerk on the suture. The assistant releases the locked needle holder but does not pull away. The surgeon removes the 7-0 suture from the needle holder so as to avoid the assistant's inadvertently pulling away and snapping the suture. Any undue pressure may cause the iris to prolapse. If this occurs, the safety suture should be tied, and the iris reposited by irrigation or with a cyclodialysis spatula. A small amount of acetylcholine chloride is extremely helpful at this time. If there is any question in the surgeon's mind that there is posterior pressure, the use of a large air bubble at this point frequently helps the surgeon estimate the location of the vitreous face and also keeps the vitreous back until the wound is further closed. Immediate loss of the air is a strong warning sign to the surgeon of impending vitreous loss.

Thanks to the evolution of modern techniques, vitreous loss during cataract surgery does not have the disastrous consequences it once did. Vitreous loss takes two forms: subtle vitreous loss, which is inferred from persistent tenting of the pupil during wound closure, and overt vitreous loss, in which vitreous presents at the wound and is unmistakable in appearance.

Goals in the management of vitreous loss are to eliminate vitreous from the wound and to decompress the vitreous body so that vitreous falls posterior to the iris plane. In the case of minimal or impending vitreous loss, the vitreous body can be decompressed by aspiration of liquid vitreous. Nearly all eyes requiring cataract surgery show marked vitreous syneresis. Aspiration of fluid vitreous reduces the volume of the vitreous cavity, and the formed vitreous recedes from the anterior chamber. To remove liquid vitreous, a blunt 18-gauge needle on a 2-mm syringe is directed through the iridectomy toward the center of the eye for approximately 10 mm. When the needle is inserted into the pocket of liquid vitreous, aspiration meets little resistance. Usually removal of 1 ml of liquid vitreous allows the vitreous to fall away from the incision 15 16 .

The needle is withdrawn, and air is instilled in the anterior chamber. By watching the air bubble and the shape of the pupil, the surgeon can tell whether the vitreous is sufficiently decompressed.

Even if the vitreous appears sufficiently decompressed, the surgeon should lift the corneal edge of the wound and use a cellulose sponge to check along the length of the incision to find any remaining vitreous strands. If any are found, adequate excision must be carried out, as it is the failure to remove the vitreous sufficiently that leads to most complications.

When extensive vitreous loss occurs, an anterior vitrectomy is necessary. Cellulose sponges are used to identify and engage the formed vitreous which is cut with a Westcott scissors 17 . The cornea is elevated to expose the iris and pupil. As the vitreous is engaged, the surgeon raises the sponge and excises the vitreous 18 . This process is repeated with fresh cellulose sponges until solid vitreous falls well behind the pupil. It is important at this point to refill the eye with saline and recheck the wound for subtle vitreous strands.

Decompression of vitreous in this manner is effective. Similar results can be accomplished with use of any one of a number of vitrectomy instruments.

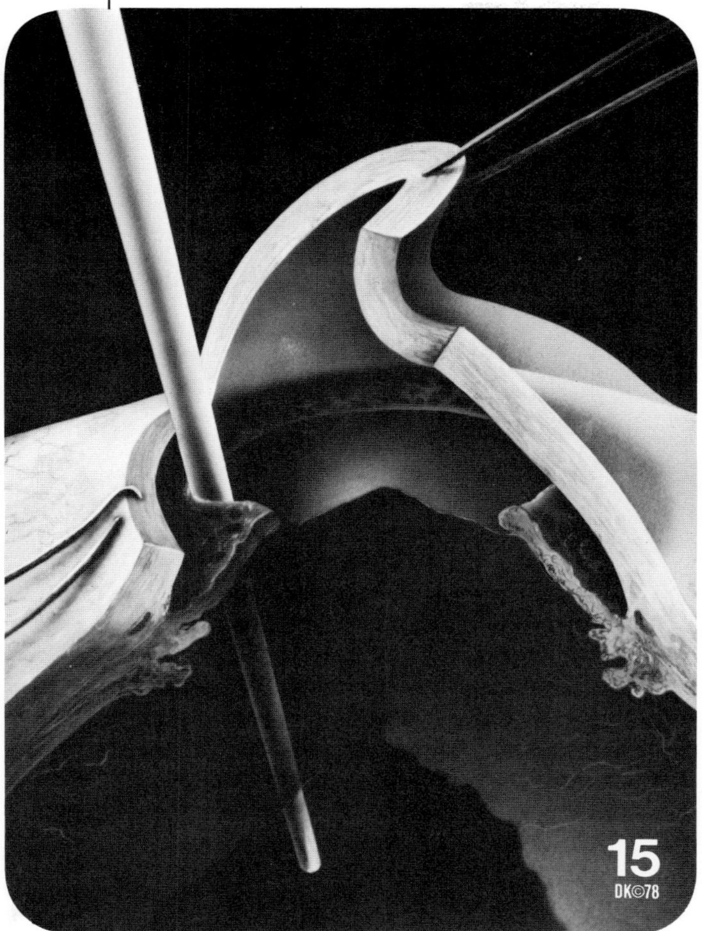

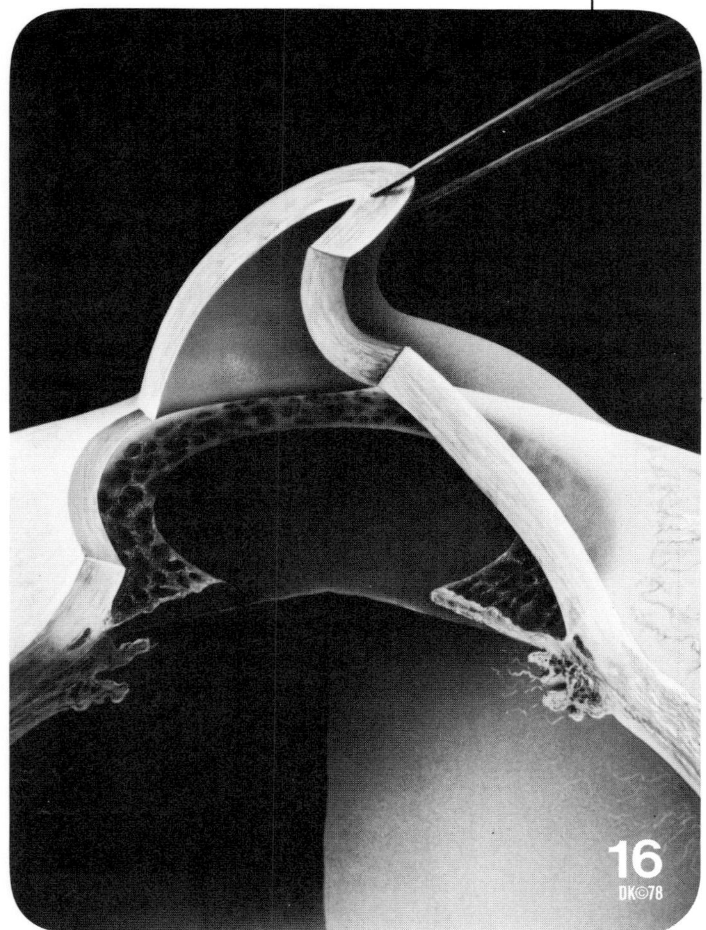

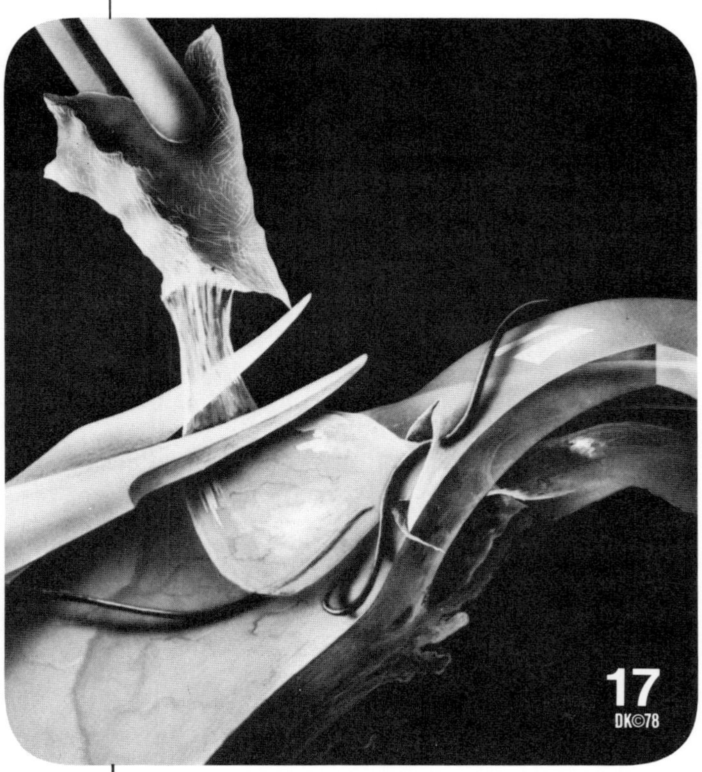

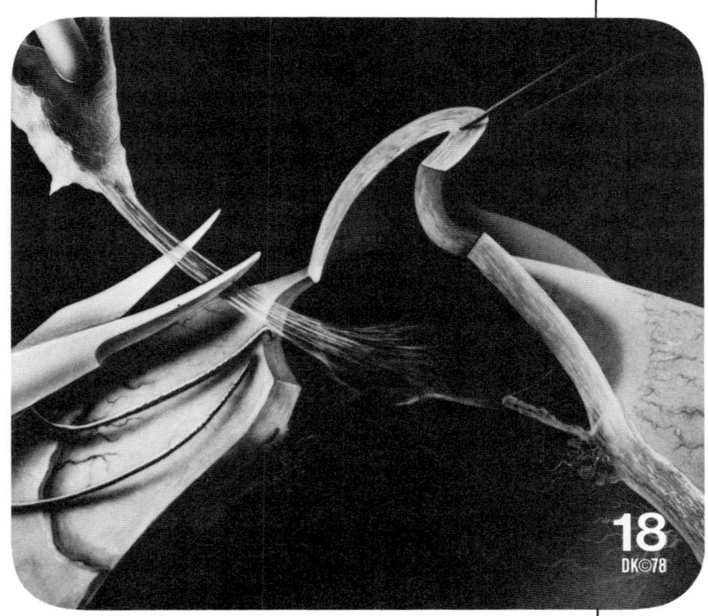

Donald A. Keller

The incidence of unplanned extracapsular cataract extraction has fallen markedly since the advent of cryoextraction. Nevertheless, rupture of the lens capsule may occur, especially in eyes where the lens is swollen and the capsule is fragile. When the capsule ruptures, the most important concern is that the nucleus is removed. It is usually frozen to the cryoprobe, leaving behind cortex and capsule. The surgeon removes as much of the anterior capsule as possible, using two capsule forceps with a hand-over-hand motion to maintain a grip on the broken capsule. Frequently, cortex is hidden beneath the iris and this can usually be removed by simple irrigation as described in the extracapsular cataract extraction section. The surgeon should attempt to assess the integrity of the posterior capsule, because excessive irrigation at this point, if the posterior capsule is not intact, causes mixing of the vitreous and cortex. It is probably better to leave some cortex to absorb than to cause vitreous loss. If opacities persist on the posterior capsule, discission is performed with a needle knife after the wound is closed. Should the posterior capsule be opacified, incision with a needle knife is recommended.

After the lens is removed and the anterior chamber is free of vitreous, the eye is closed. We recommend using seven interrupted 10-0 nylon sutures. A half-circle spatula needle is the most suitable for microsurgery. It is exquisitely sharp and can be placed deeply into the tissue without taking a large bite. A fine Colibri forceps grasps the corneal edge of the incision, and the surgeon places the needle as close to the forceps as possible for maximum control. After the needle has passed through the corneal side of the wound, the needle tip is used to engage the scleral side. The Colibri forceps stabilizes the sclera as the surgeon completes the suture tract. The needle penetrates one-half to three-quarters the thickness of the cornea, equally on both sides of the wound **19** . We prefer to make small, deep bites rather than more superficial, large bites that cause buckling. Inadvertent placement into the anterior chamber may not be as harmful as once thought. The suture is tied to reapproximate the wound edges without creating tension. If there is disparity in placement of the suture on the apposing edges, a lateral displacement or overriding of the wound may interfere with normal healing.

Tying a 10-0 nylon suture requires more skill than does larger suture material and is best accomplished with one straight and one curved MacPherson forceps. A three-layered square knot is necessary for security. The first tie, a three-looped surgeon's knot, holds the wound in position during tying of a second single-looped knot **20** . The tying of a 10-0 suture is illustrated in the section on Wound Healing and the Control of Postoperative Astigmatism. Care must be taken not to tie the second loop too tightly since the second tie locks the knot. Too much tension causes stress on the cornea that cannot be released. Should corneal tension lines be present, the suture is removed and a new one positioned. The third and final tie is a single loop that completes the square knot. The suture ends are cut as close to the knot as possible. The seventh, and last, suture replaces the 7-0 silk safety suture.

One mistake made by surgeons unfamiliar with 10-0 suture material is to leave the ends too long. The surgeon should use a sharp razor blade knife to cut ends as close as possible to the knot without actually cutting the knot **21** . Long ends may protrude through conjunctiva and cause persistent irritation to the patient. Before the surgeon covers the sutures with the conjunctiva, the suture is grasped near its entrance into the cornea and is pulled toward sclera. It is extremely important for the surgeon to check each knot mechanically by pulling on it at the same time that the knot is swung toward the scleral side and into the suture tract. It is much better to replace the sutures in the operating room rather than the next day.

The conjunctival flap is pulled over the incision and secured with either interrupted 10-0 nylon sutures cut extremely short or with use of the wet field bipolar cautery **22** .

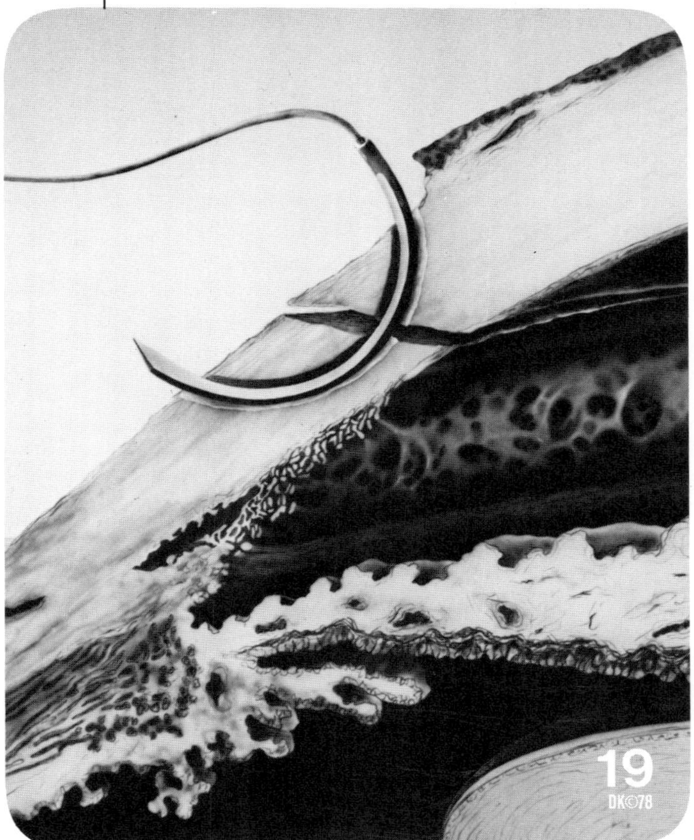

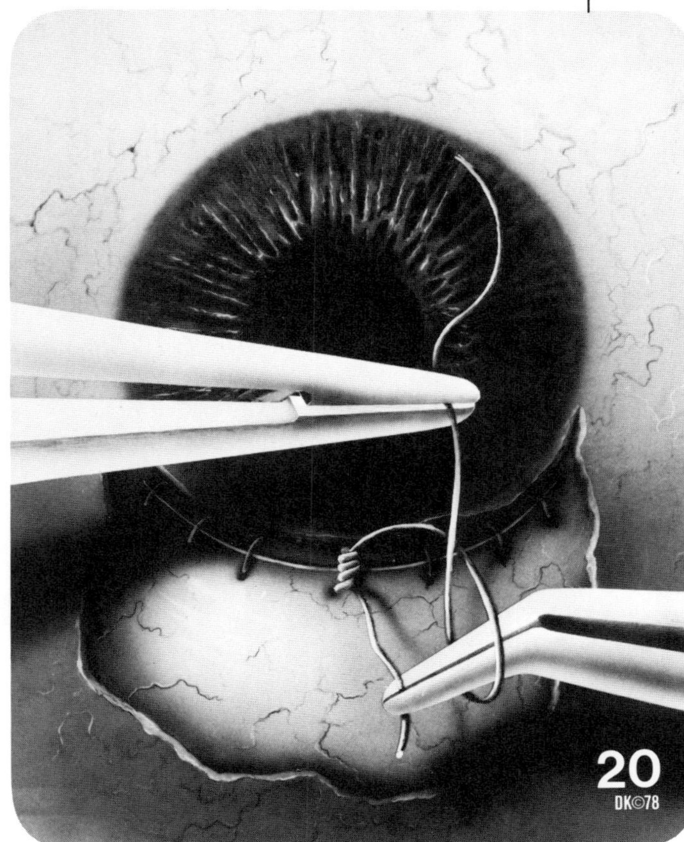

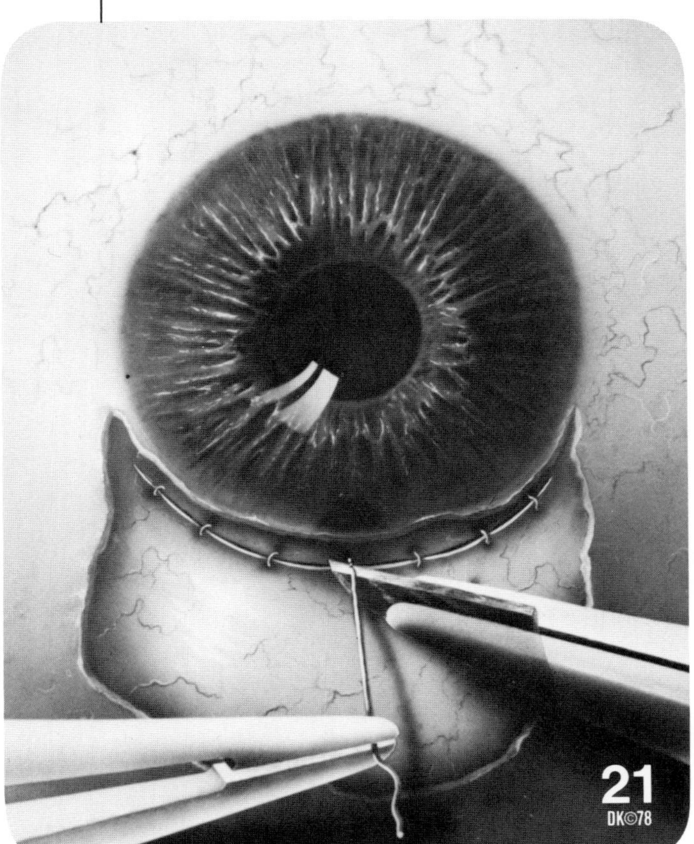

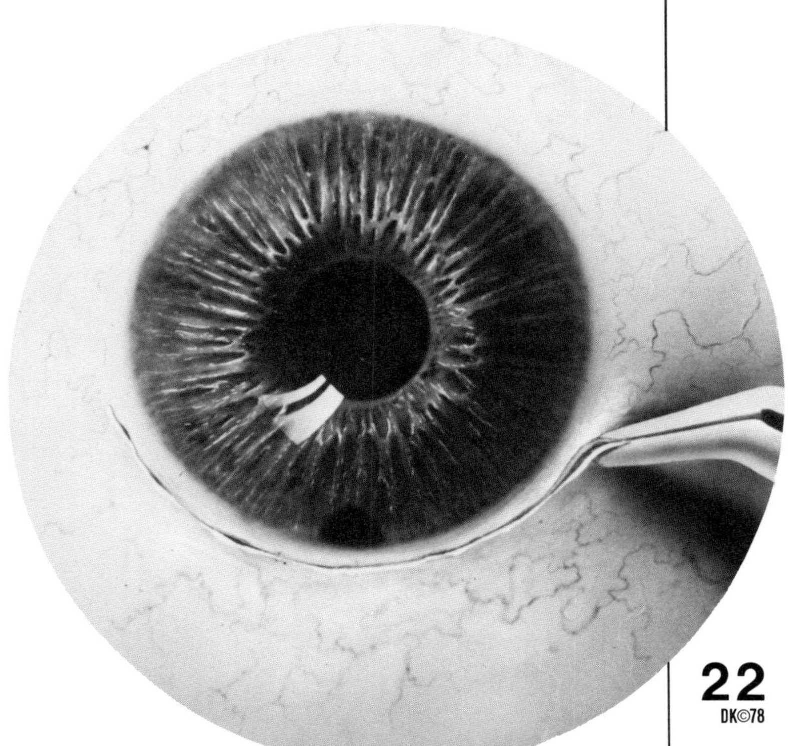

Donald A. Keller

PLANNED EXTRACAPSULAR CATARACT EXTRACTION

Extracapsular cataract extraction procedures are most suited for young patients in whom intracapsular extraction might be complicated by vitreous loss. The vitreolenticular connections, which persist to about age 30, are strong in patients under the age of 20, particularly in those with congenital cataracts. As the vitreous liquefies during the third decade, the vitreolenticular connections loosen. Extracapsular cataract extraction allows for the removal of opacified lens material without disturbance of the vitreous.

Many surgeons believe that an extracapsular extraction offers the most suitable fixation within the capsular bag for placement of intraocular lens. Some believe that the incidence of aphakic retinal detachments and cystoid macular edema is reduced in patients who have an intact posterior capsule.

This chapter will describe an extracapsular cataract extraction with the use of phacoemulsification. In addition, a discussion on the technique for the manual expression of a hard nucleus is included.

PHACOEMULSIFICATION

Richard H. Keates, M.D.
Richard G. Lembach, M.D.

We recognize that many excellent mechanical devices exist for the performance of extracapsular cataract extractions. Our discussion will be limited to the use of the Kelman Cavitron unit. This was the first of these units to be introduced and has remained one of the best designed, most reliable, and consequently most popular units available.

Maximal dilation should be achieved prior to surgery. The surgeon should be sure that the pupil is at least 7 mm wide before proceeding. A wire speculum usually provides adequate exposure and is small enough not to limit the movement of the handpieces during surgery. The use of lid sutures may improve access to the globe, especially in children. An Elschnig forceps grasps the tendon of the superior rectus muscle, and the surgeon passes the 4-0 black silk bridle suture through the muscle tendon and secures it to the drape. The inferior rectus muscle is secured with a bridle suture in a similar manner.

A small, triangular, limbus-based conjunctival flap is fashioned [1] [2] . The flap is used to retract the cornea for access into the anterior chamber. It also serves as a valve to seal the wound in order to maintain the depth of the anterior chamber during surgery.

Prior to the incision, a Tooke knife is used to remove the redundant tissue at the limbus [3] . This tamponades the superficial limbal vessels and causes a reduction in the amount of bleeding at the time of the incision. Vessels that continue to bleed are cauterized. With a 1-mm needle knife, a beveled incision is made into the anterior chamber temporally at the limbus through clear cornea [4] . This creates a watertight, self-sealing wound and

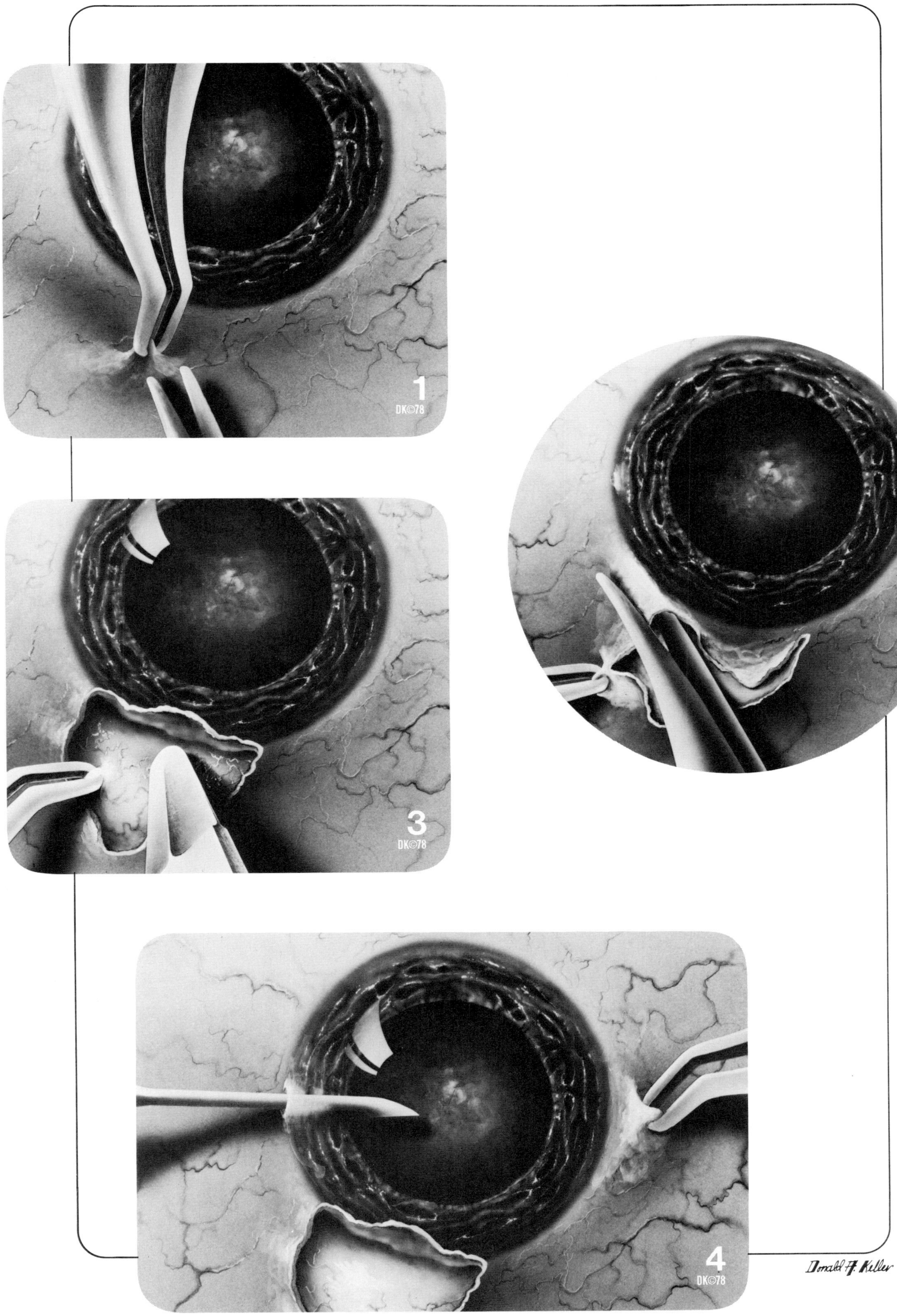
1
DK©78
2
DK©78
3
DK©78
4
DK©78

provides separate access into the anterior chamber. Before entering the anterior chamber, a distance of 2 mm is marked at the incision site [5] . A razor blade incision, measuring 2 mm both internally and externally, should be made in the middle of the blue line [6] .

An irrigating cystitome is ideally suited to create a large opening in the anterior capsule to expose the cortex. The cystitome is introduced into the anterior chamber through the superior incision [7] , and the tip of the cystitome is rotated at the 6-o'clock position to engage the anterior capsule [8] . Drawing the instrument from 6 to 12 o'clock tears the capsule in a Christmas-tree shape [9] . As the cystitome is removed, if the anterior lens capsule comes out with it, it is cut with a scissors. If the capsule does not come out, it is grasped with extra long, angled, toothed, McPherson forceps and cut with a scissors. In an alternative method, the surgeon makes multiple dog-eared incisions in the peripheral region of the capsule to create an opening [10]. If the capsule does not adhere to the cystitome as the cystitome is withdrawn, the McPherson forceps is used to remove it [11].

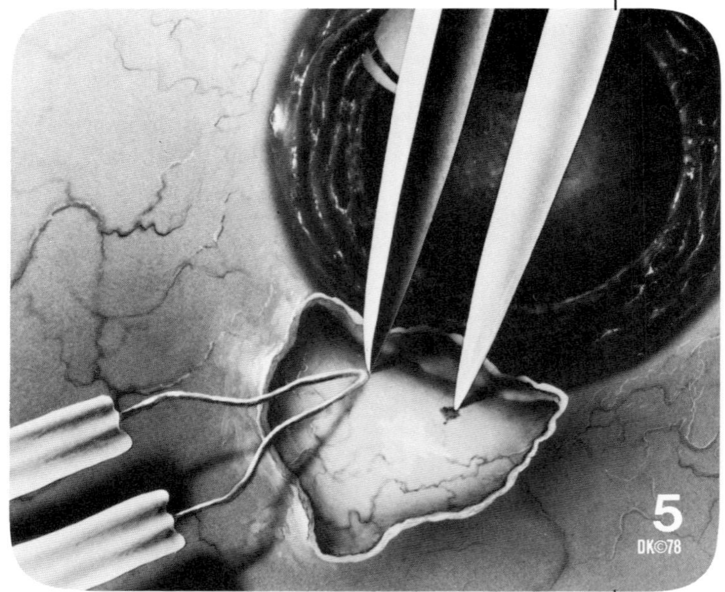

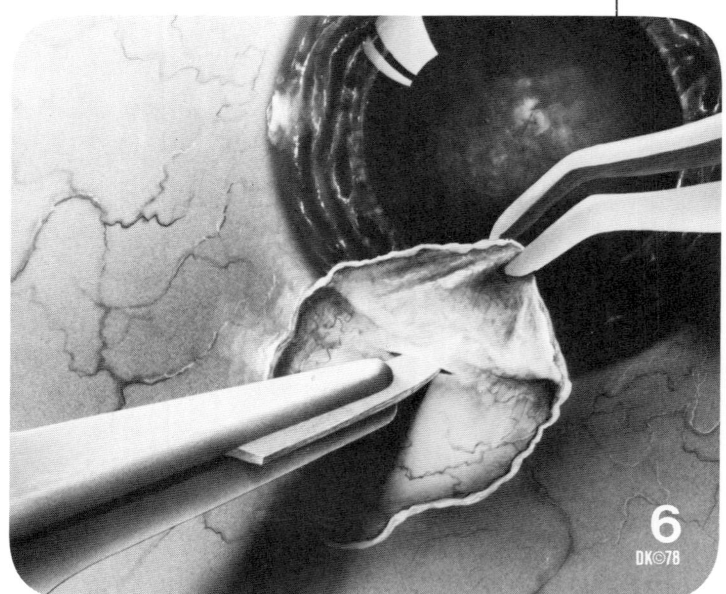

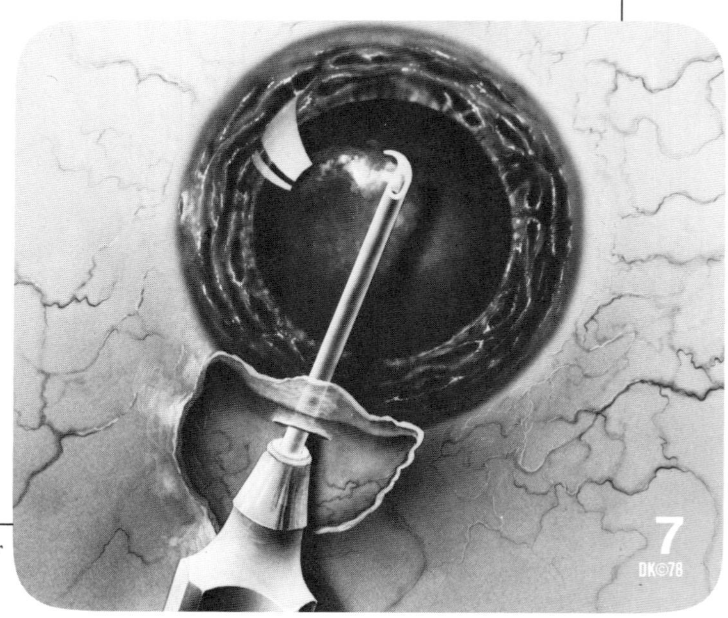

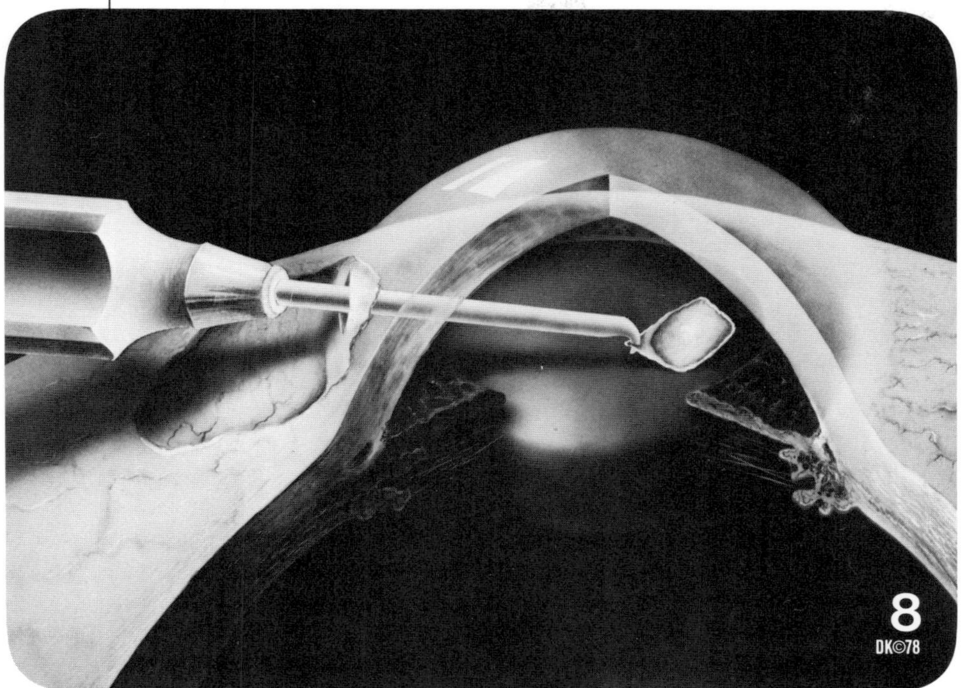

8
DK©78

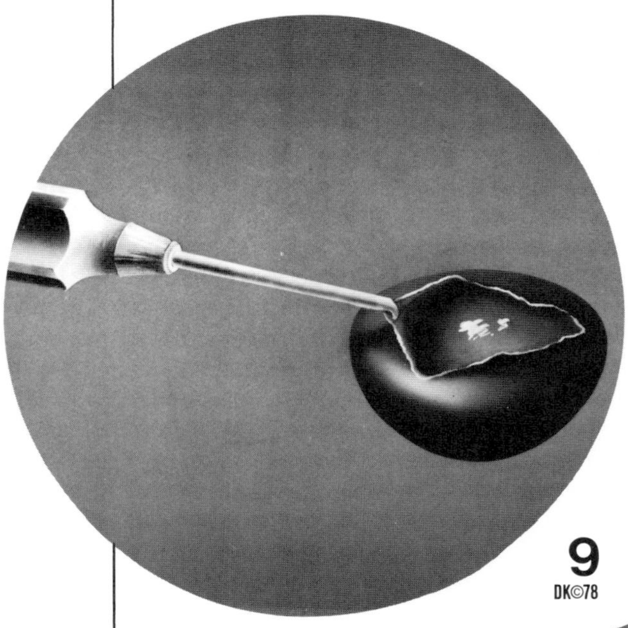

9
DK©78

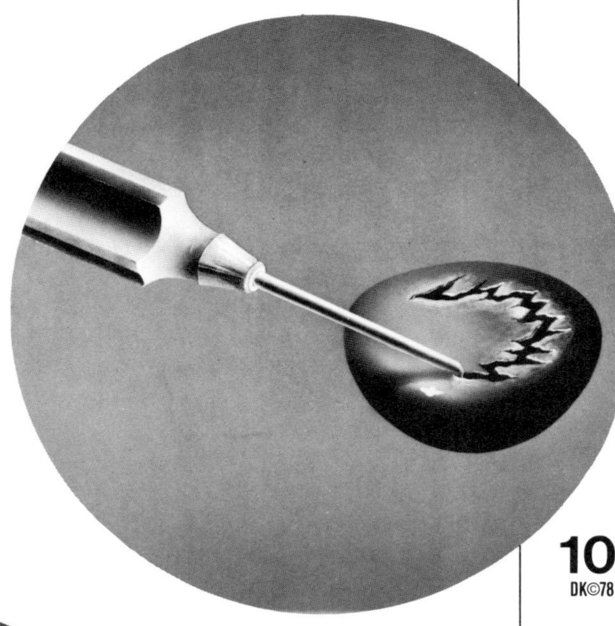

10
DK©78

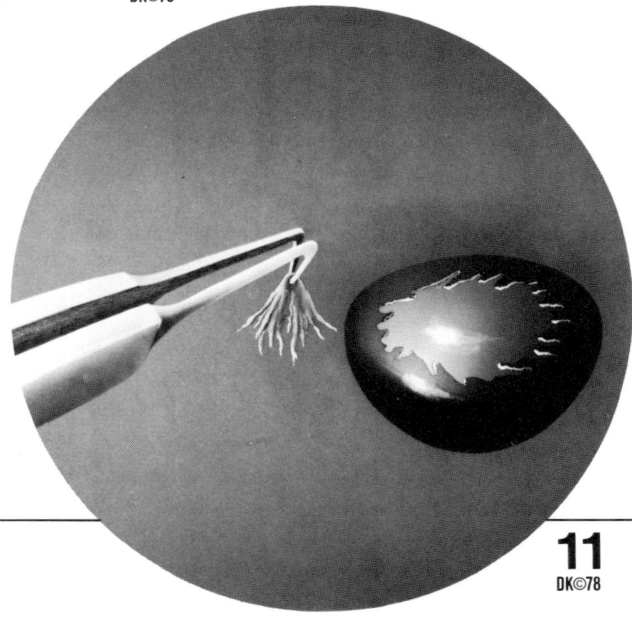

11
DK©78

Donald A. Keller

Because of its consistency, the nucleus is the most difficult portion of the lens to remove. If it is prolapsed into the anterior chamber, the nucleus is more easily emulsified and aspirated, thus minimizing trauma to the iris. The surgeon engages the nucleus with the tip of the cystitome at the 6-o'clock position [12] . The cystitome is elevated to lift the inferior pole of the nucleus, which allows the inferior iris to drop behind it [13] . Next, the nucleus is rotated temporally, and the nasal edge of the nucleus slides in front of the iris. Once the nasal iris is behind the nucleus, it is slid nasally and inferiorly. This allows the temporal and superior iris to fall into position and completes the prolapse [14]. The cystitome is then removed. If the nucleus will not prolapse and the pupil begins to constrict, the surgeon should enlarge the incision and remove the lens manually with either a cryoprobe or lens spoon.

After the nucleus is in the anterior chamber, the wound is enlarged to 3 mm to accommodate the ultrasonic tip [15] [16] . If the incision is too small, the silicone sleeve of the handpiece may catch on the wound edges and impede its flow. If the wound is too large, too much fluid may leak during the procedure which might allow the anterior chamber to collapse. Should this leakage occur, the surgeon can place a 10-0 nylon suture at one edge of the wound. The ultrasonic tip measures 2 mm in diameter and consists of a 1-mm titanium needle that vibrates 40,000 times per second and is covered with a soft silicone sleeve. The vibration of the tip fragments the lens material. The tip also is equipped with an infusion-aspiration mechanism. The infusion pressure is automatically regulated not to exceed 25 mm Hg. This allows the anterior chamber to be maintained as the lens material is suctioned. Before the ultrasound tip is introduced, the surgeon uses the power settings to insure that the machine is tuned properly. The suction and irrigation mechanisms also are checked. The harder portions of the nucleus are removed

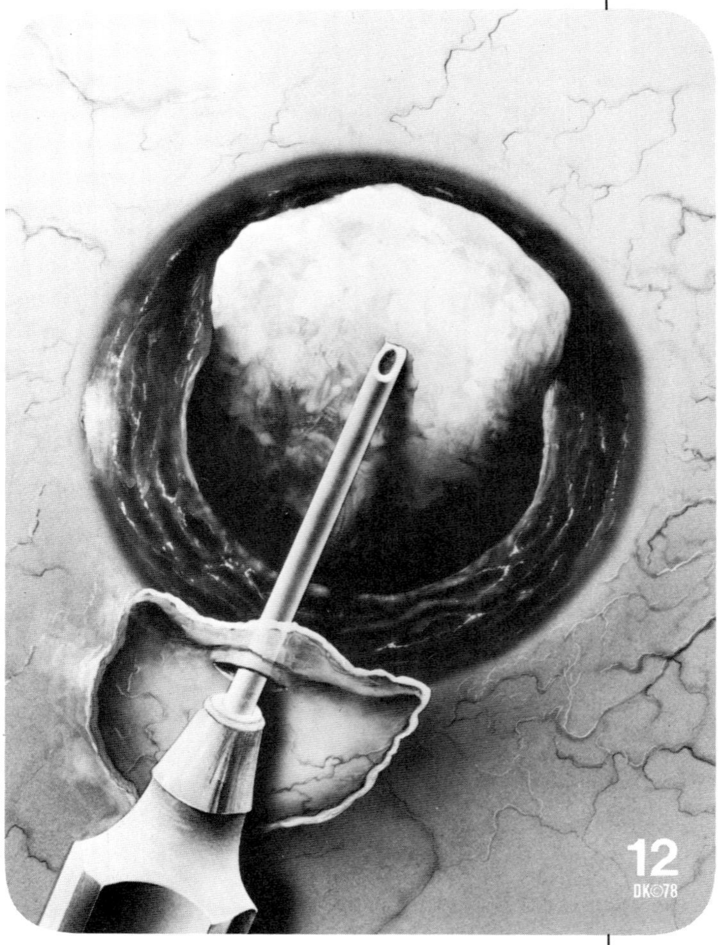

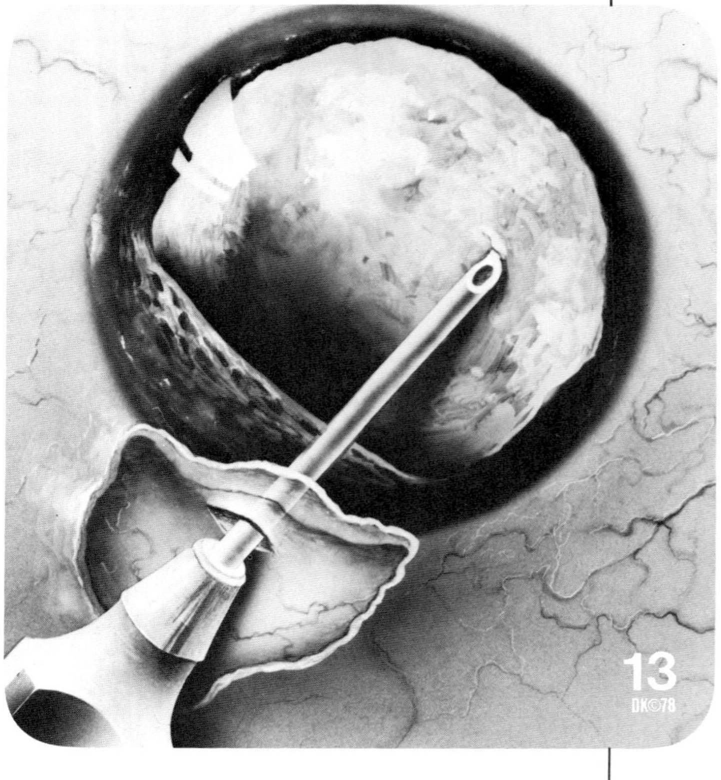

Donald A. Killer

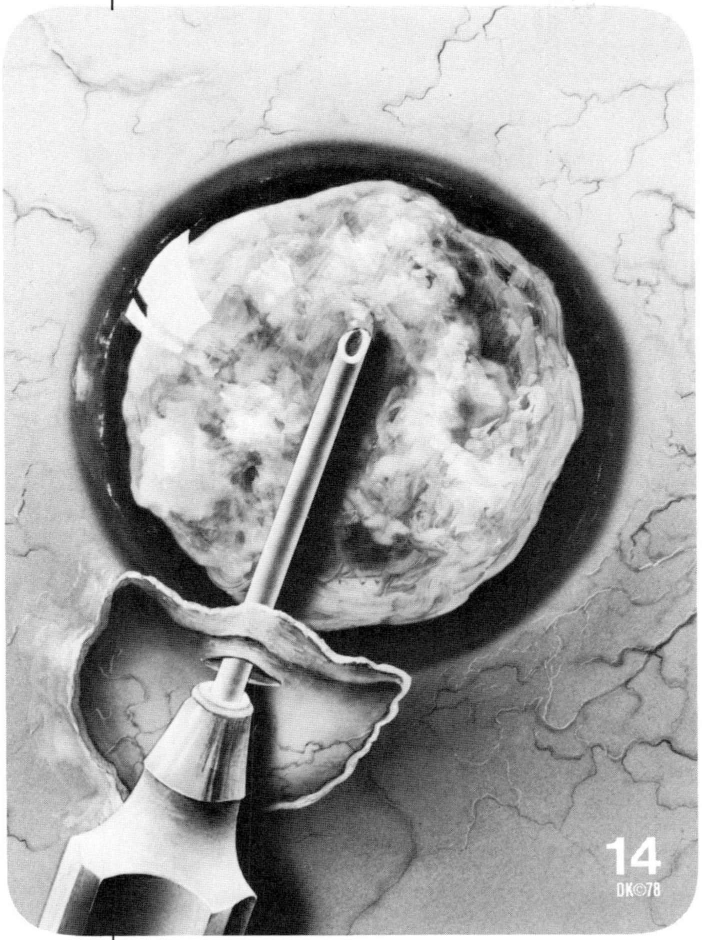

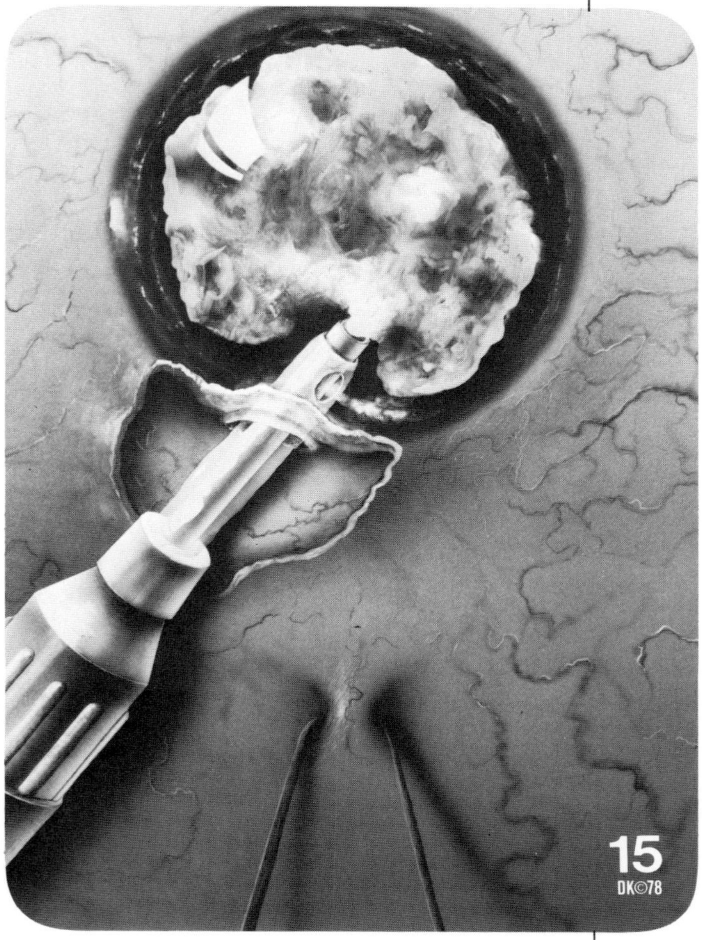

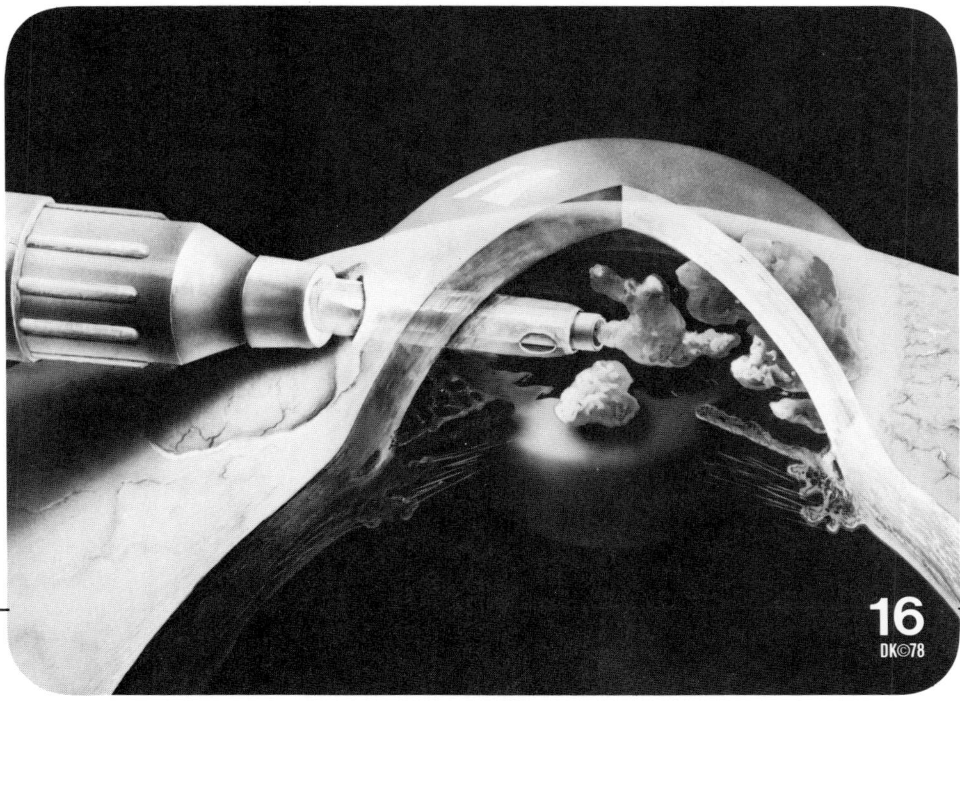

Donald F. Keller

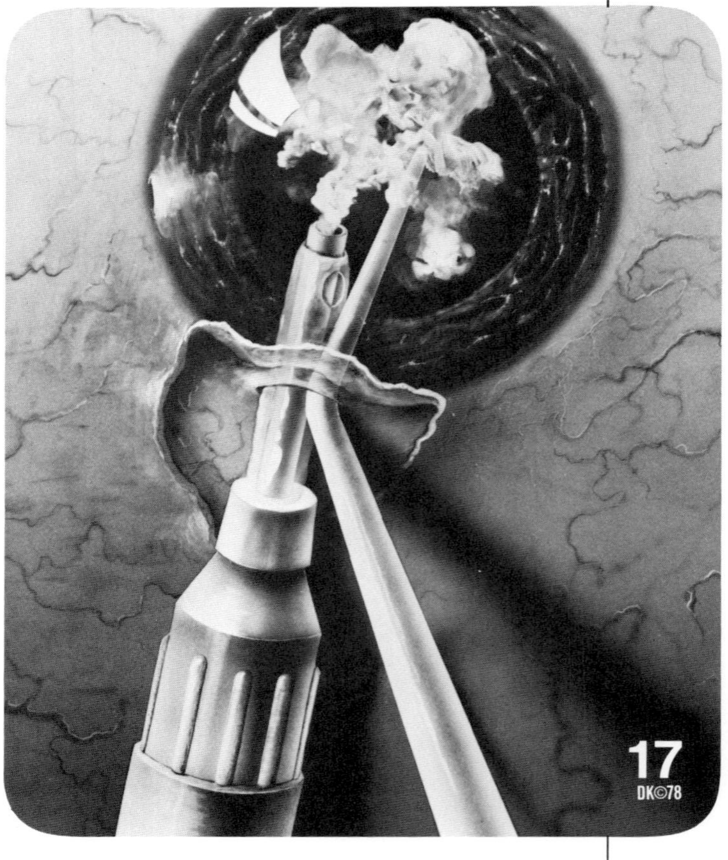
17
DK©78

first with short bursts of ultrasonic power. Occasionally, the lens nucleus begins to tumble. If this occurs, a Castroviejo spatula, placed through the incision, steadies the nucleus [17]. After the nucleus has been emulsified and aspirated, the surgeon withdraws the ultrasonic tip and introduces the infusion-aspiration handpiece, which is smaller in diameter than the ultrasonic tip [18] . This nonultrasonic tip removes the remaining cortical material and cleans the posterior capsule. During this last maneuver, the power is reduced by half to prevent inadvertent rupture of the posterior capsule. Residual cortical material may be swept from under the iris with a cyclodialysis spatula through either the needle knife incision or the 12-o'clock incision. When the surgeon is satisfied that all cortical material is removed, the handpiece is withdrawn. A peripheral iridectomy is made superiorly [19] .

One or two 10-0 nylon sutures close the corneoscleral wound [20] . The wound edges are approximated with no tension on the adjacent cornea and sclera. The knots are brought to the scleral side and cut. This provides a small, watertight wound.

In a considerable number of patients under age 60, opacification of the posterior capsule occurs. For these individuals, we recommend a discission of the capsule at the end of the procedure. If a discission is performed, it is preferable for the anterior chamber to be slightly less than aphakic depth. The Haab needle knife is passed through the needle knife tract to create a vertical opening in the posterior capsule [21] . This produces an oval tear approximately 3 mm in its longest diameter. If the tear is too small, it can be enlarged with the back of the blade, but care must be taken not to disrupt the vitreous face. Alternatively, the fine Castroviejo spatula can be inserted through the needle knife tract and used to enlarge the opening in the posterior capsule. Acetylcholine chloride solution is then injected through the needle tract into the anterior chamber. No sutures are required to close the flap.

Postoperatively, the patient is fully ambulatory. Because of the small incision, surgically induced astigmatism is minimal.

Donald F. Keller

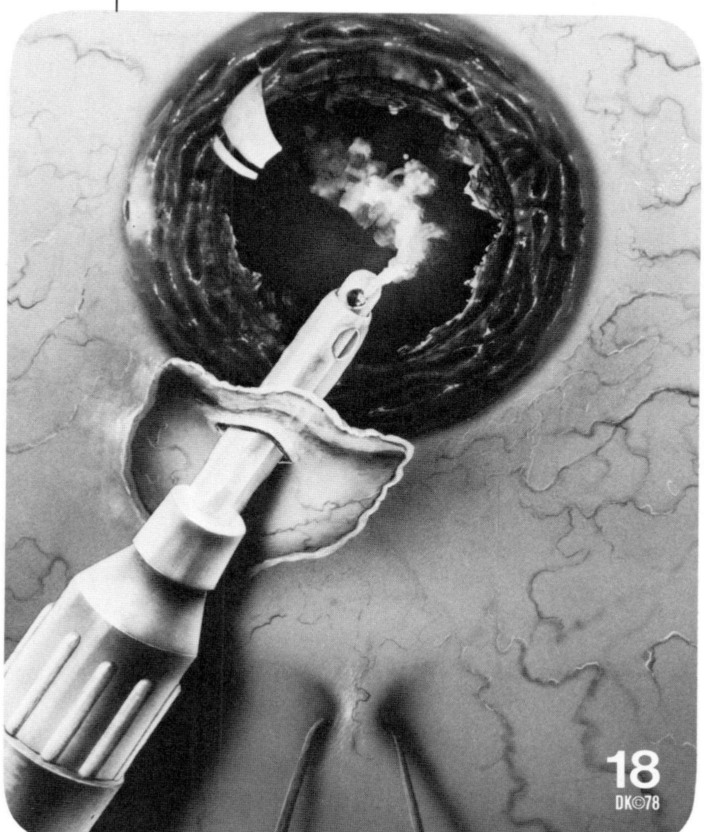

18
DK©78

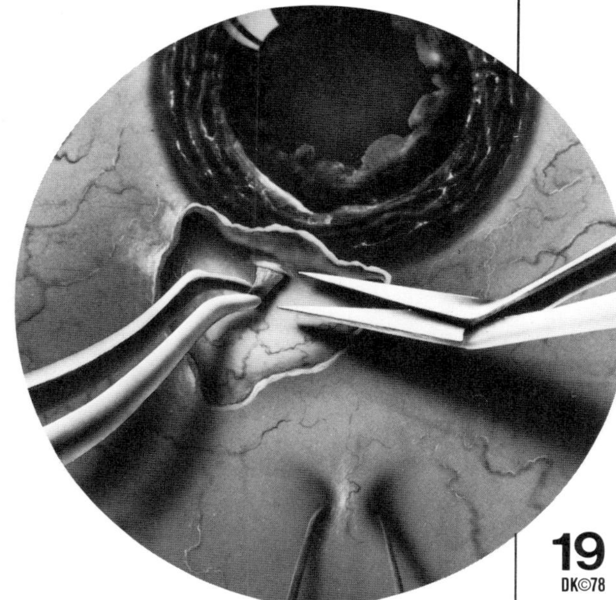

19
DK©78

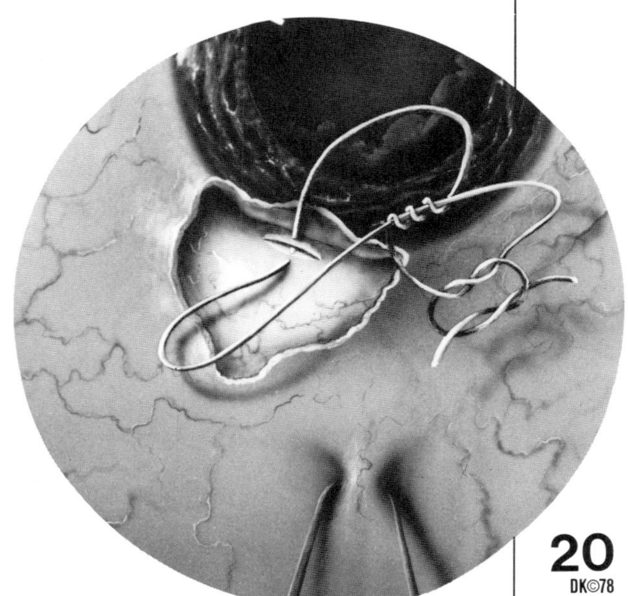

20
DK©78

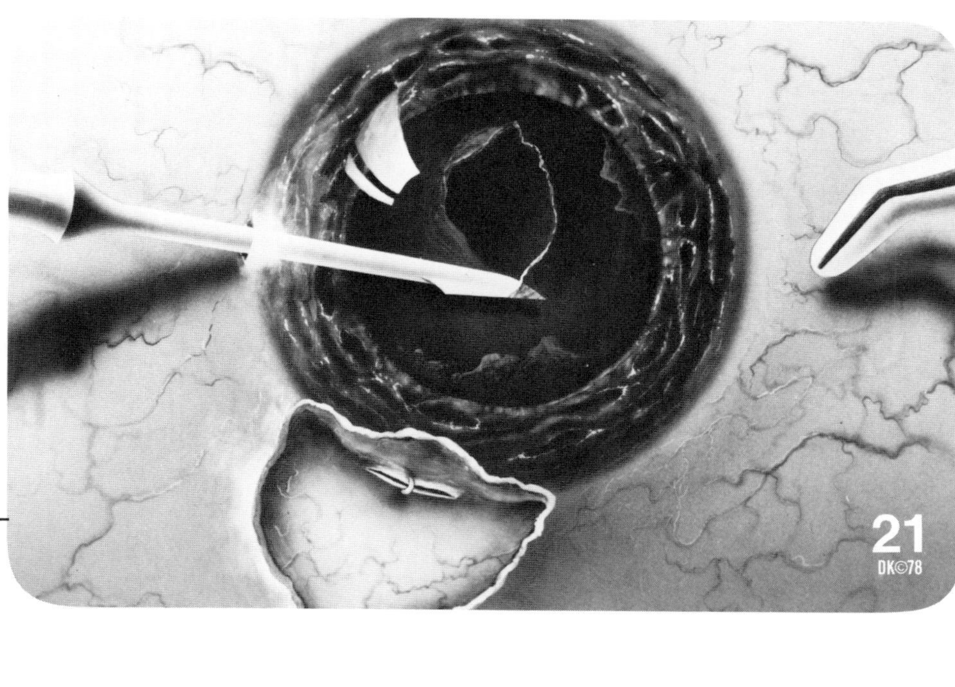

21
DK©78

Donald A. Keller

MANUAL EXPRESSION OF THE LENS

Richard H. Keates, M.D.
Richard G. Lembach, M.D.

The surgeon must be familiar with a technique for the manual expression of a hard nucleus when performing an extracapsular cataract extraction. In certain cases, the surgeon may plan to remove the lens by phacoemulsification but intraoperatively discovers that the nucleus is too hard. In these patients, the surgeon must be able to convert from phacoemulsification to manual expression of the nucleus. In other instances, as with the implantation of an intraocular lens which uses capsular fixation, the surgeon plans preoperatively to use both manual expression and phacoemulsification.

The preliminary steps in the manual expression of the nucleus are identical to those described in phacoemulsification. The major exception is the preparation of a large fornix-based conjunctival flap instead of a smaller limbus-based flap. The dislocation of the nucleus into the anterior chamber is also the same as previously described. After the prolapse of the nucleus into the anterior chamber, the 2-mm incision is enlarged to 120 degrees with fine corneal scissors. A 7-0 silk traction suture is placed at 12 o'clock. The simplest and least traumatic method to remove the nucleus is with the use of the infusion-aspiration handpiece from the phacoemulsification instrument. The tip is inserted into the anterior chamber through the temporal side of the incision [1] . The infusion fluid creates an eddy current that pushes the nucleus through the lips of the wound.

If the nucleus does not prolapse through the wound, the scleral lip of the wound is depressed with a forceps at 12 o'clock. The surgeon then depresses the inferior cornea with a lens loop [2] . This engages the nucleus and forces it through the wound superiorly as the loop is advanced along the corneal surface . When a portion of the nucleus is outside the eye, the surgeon uses a forceps for stabilization and a cyclodialysis spatula to cartwheel the nucleus completely out of the anterior chamber [3] . Once the

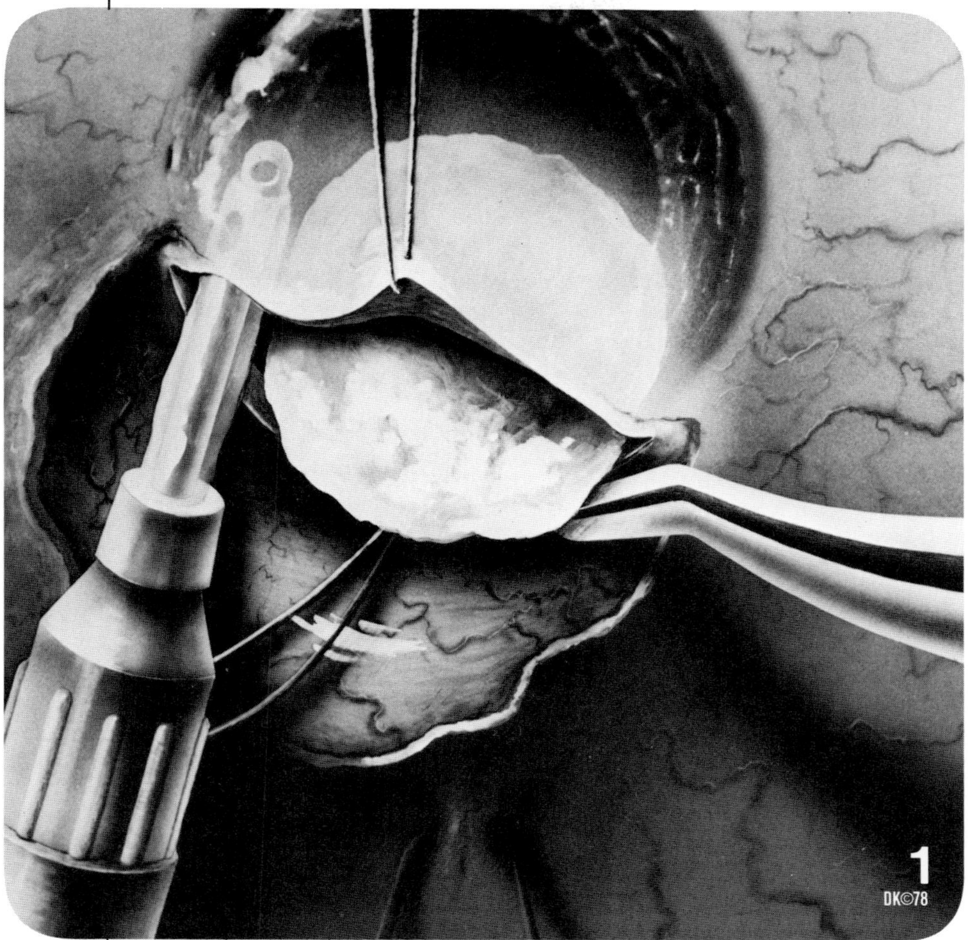

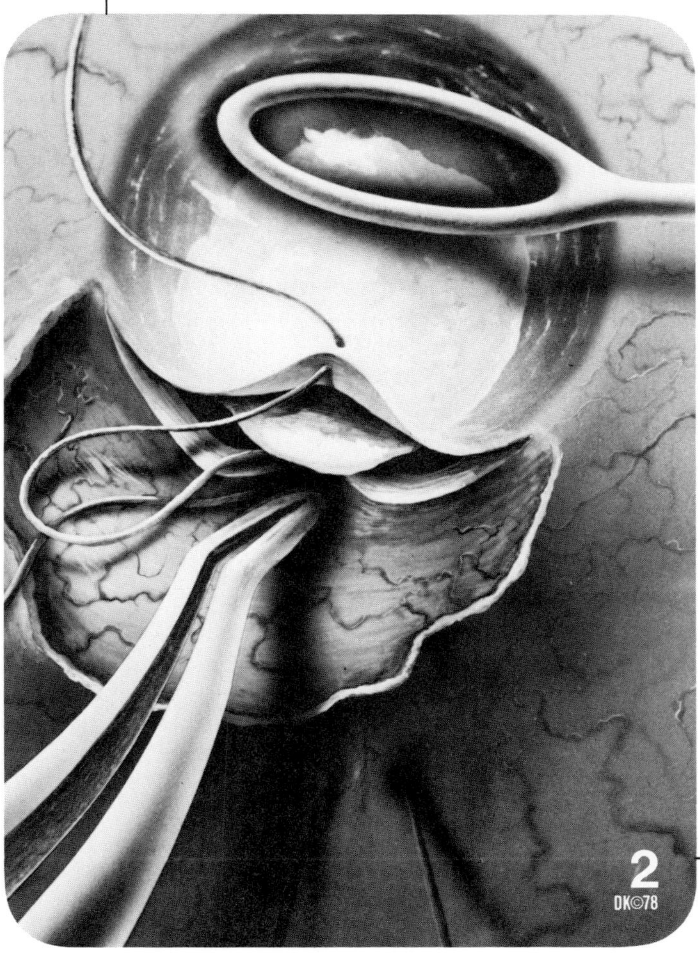

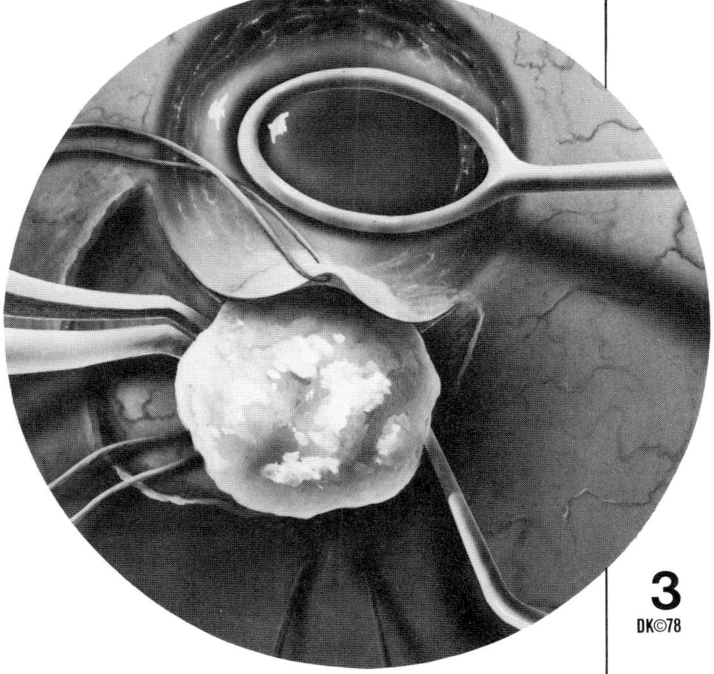

3
DK©78

Donald A. Keller

nucleus has been removed, the incision is closed with 10-0 interrupted nylon sutures, leaving a 3-mm opening in the wound [4]. The remainder of the cortical material is removed with the infusion-aspiration handpiece [5], as described previously in phacoemulsification. One 10-0 nylon suture closes the corneoscleral wound [6].

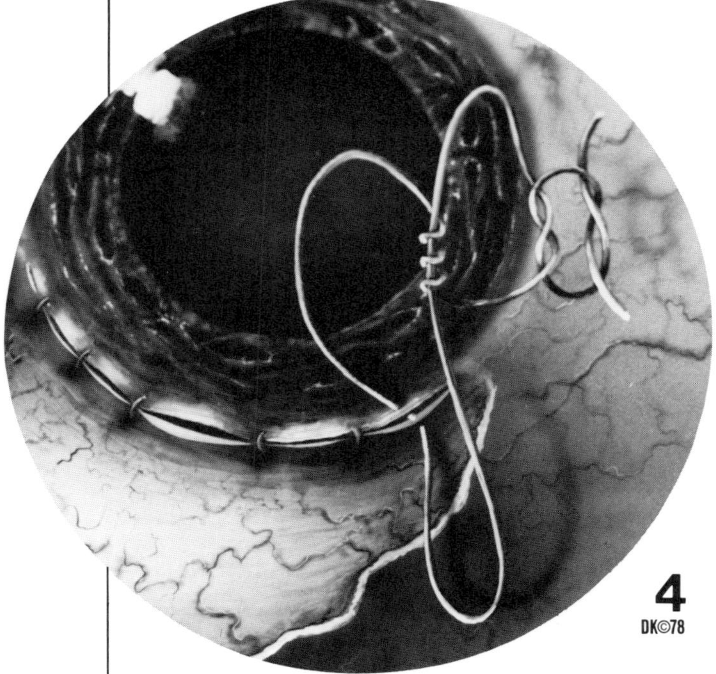

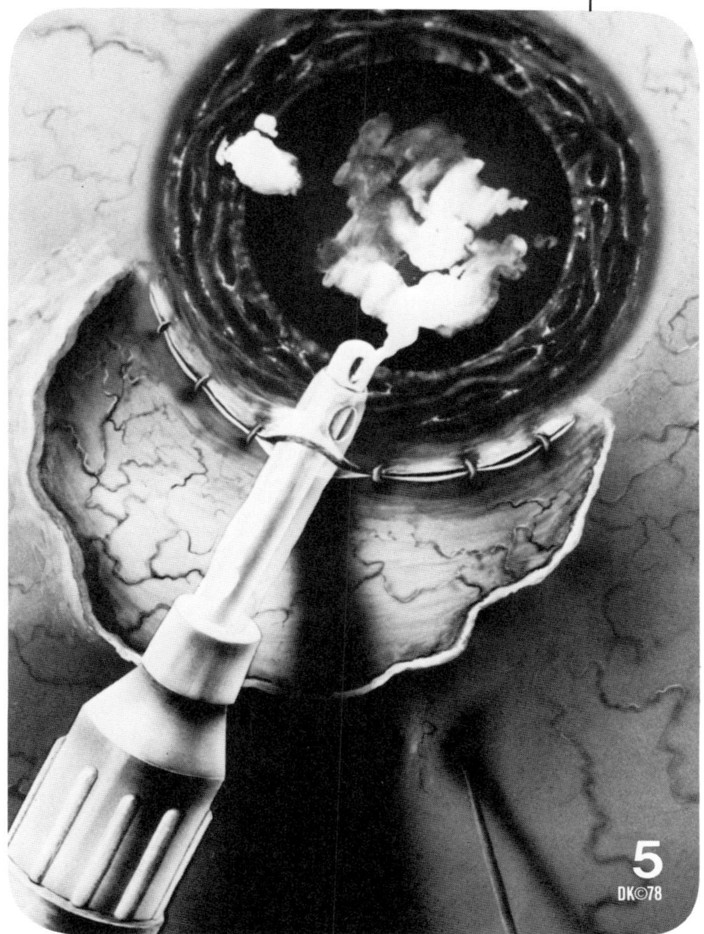

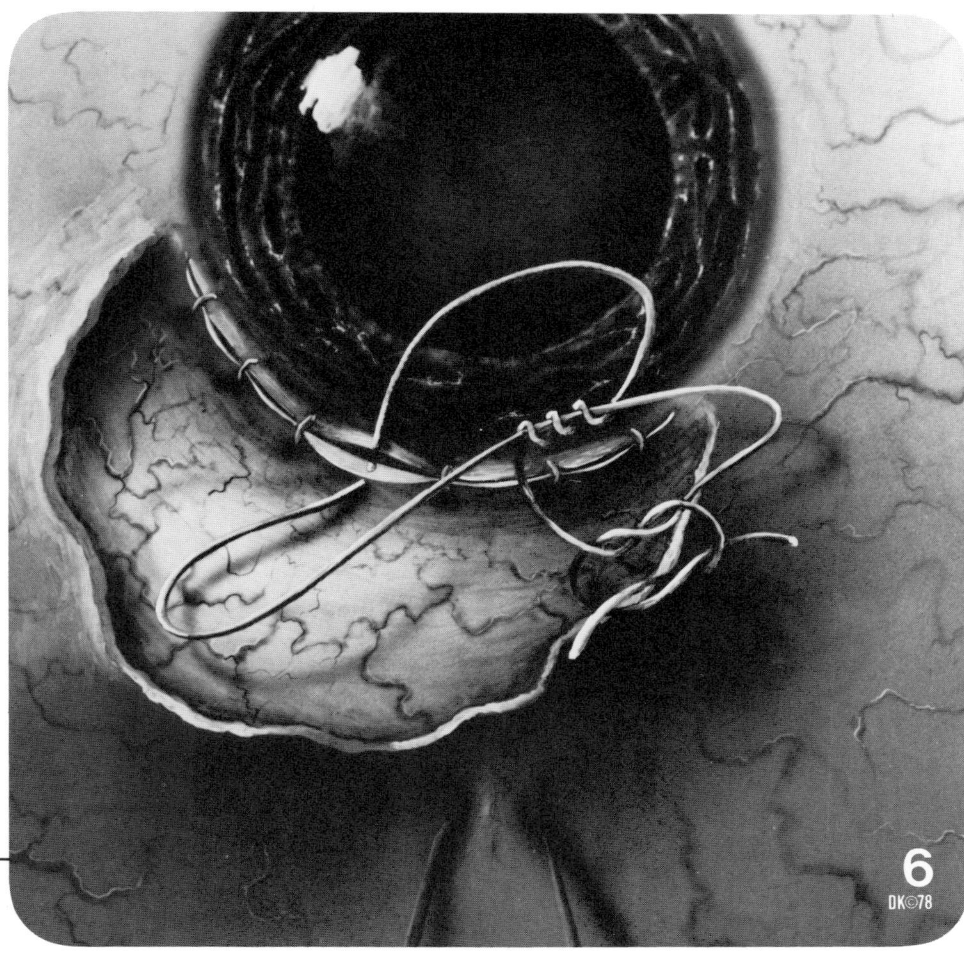

Donald A. Keller

INTRAOCULAR LENS IMPLANTATION

Indications for the use of intraocular lenses vary greatly, depending on the philosophy of the individual surgeon. Most advocates agree that the elderly patient, who has an intolerance to spectacle correction and who physically would be unable to manipulate and wear a contact lens, is the ideal candidate for intraocular lens placement.

In order to diagnose and treat ocular disorders after surgery, the examiner must be able to dilate the pupil fully without dislocating the lens. The anterior chamber lens, which rests on the sclera, and the two-loop lens, which is fixed to the capsule, are the most stable intraocular lenses. These lenses permit free iris dilation without fear of dislocation.

The decision to use an anterior chamber lens or a two-loop lens depends on the type of cataract extraction to be performed. In patients requiring an intracapsular extraction, we use an anterior chamber lens. In younger patients, from whom the cataract can be removed most efficiently by means of an extracapsular procedure, we recommend the use of a two-loop capsular fixation lens.

The power of the intraocular lens is quite important since a variable amount of aniseikonia is induced, depending on postoperative refractive error. If an eye is made emmetropic after the implantation of an intraocular lens, the magnification is approximately 3 percent. If the myopia in an implanted eye measures 1.5 diopters, aniseikonia is minimal.

Ultrasound is definitely indicated prior to the implantation of an intraocular lens. The power of the cornea (or corneal curvature), the axial length of the globe, and the depth of the anterior chamber are used to calculate the lens power. Nomograms have been developed to aid in this determination. In spite of this information, inaccuracies are common, and an error of ± 1 diopter occurs in nearly all intraocular lens implantations. The clinician can avoid significant refractive errors after surgery with the use of preoperative axial length measurements. The exact power of the lens to be implanted is calculated before the patient is admitted for surgery.

ANTERIOR CHAMBER LENS

Richard H. Keates, M.D.
Richard G. Lembach, M.D.

The two most commonly used anterior chamber lenses are the Choyce Mark VIII lens and the Tennant lens. These lenses can be inserted immediately after routine intracapsular cataract procedures or can be implanted secondarily. They are the most stable intraocular lenses because they rest on the sclera.

The selection of the lens also depends on the size of the eye. The external appearance of the limbus is oval, primarily due to the conjunctival overhang of the limbus at the 12- and 6-o'clock positions. The internal limits of the limbus are truly circular; therefore, the corneal diameter is measured in the horizontal plane from the white sclera of one side to the same position 180 degrees away [1]. A lens 1 mm larger than this measurement usually is the correct choice. The lens should fit snugly in the scleral recess, free of the chamber angle.

When the lens has been selected, the surgeon performs a routine intracapsular cataract extraction. We believe that use of the operating microscope optimizes the intraoperative and postoperative results of cataract extraction and lens implantation.

Creation of a tract into the anterior chamber permits instillation of air or fluids during lens implantation [2]. Prior to the limbal incision, the surgeon places a needle knife tract temporally, using a 1-mm needle knife. To stablilize the eye as the anterior chamber is entered, countertraction is placed at the limbus 180 degrees away. As the knife is removed, the incision is slightly enlarged for insertion of a 30-gauge cannula. Instead of one iridectomy at the 12-o'clock position, we recommend two basal iridectomies [3]. Since the intraocular lens is 6 mm wide, the iridectomies should be 8 mm apart [4]. The

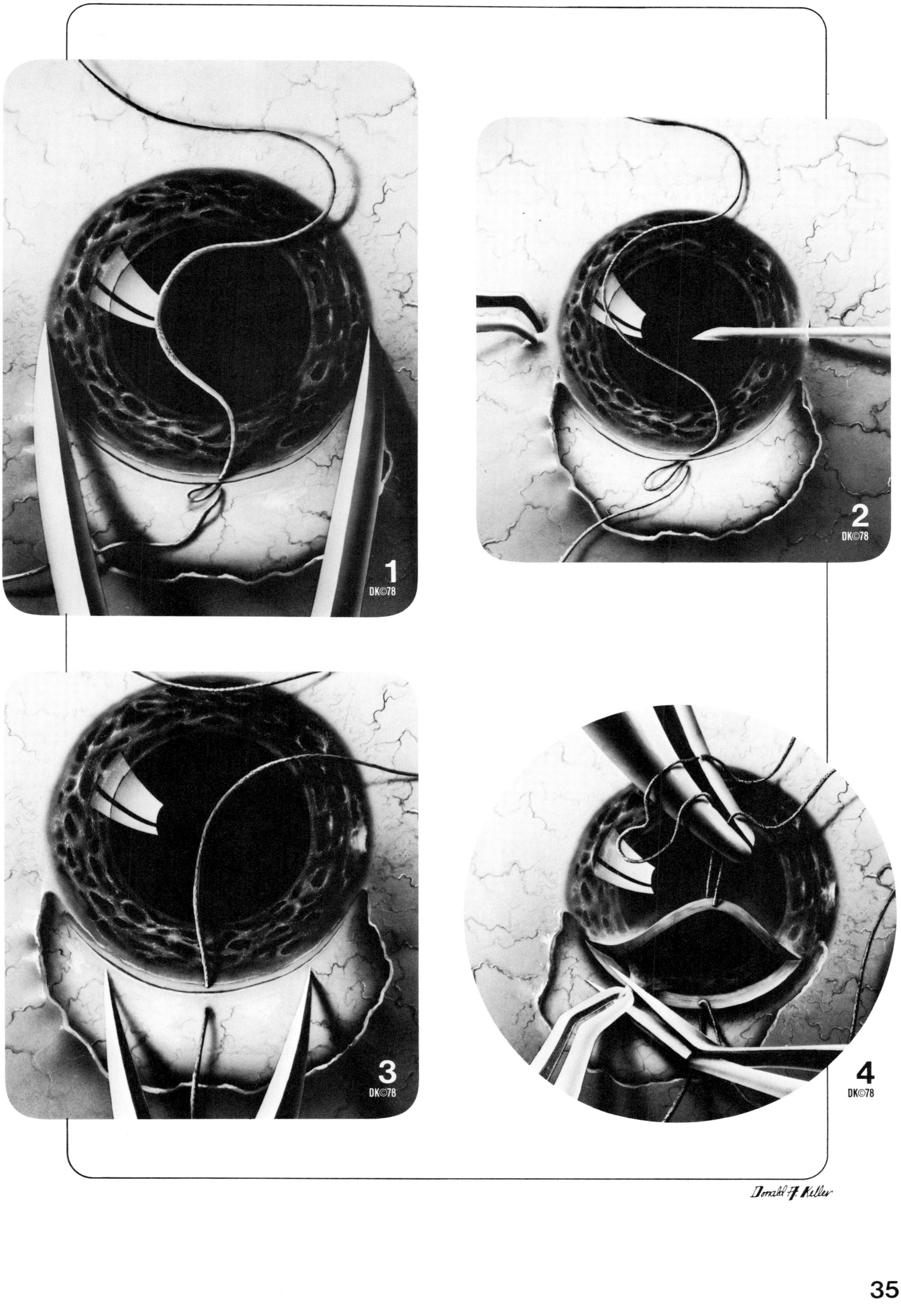
1
DK©78
2
DK©78
3
DK©78
4
DK©78

patency of the iridectomy is checked with a cyclodialysis spatula [5]

After the cataract is removed (see microscopic intracapsular extraction), the pupil is constricted with acetylcholine chloride. Air is injected into the anterior chamber with a 30-gauge cannula to re-form the anterior chamber. If the lens is inserted over a dilated pupil, it may engage the peripheral iris roll and incarcerate it between the feet of the implant and the scleral recess. Insertion of the lens over a dilated pupil may also disrupt the anterior hyaloid. The instillation of air should be sufficient to re-form the anterior chamber and flatten the iris plane [6]. Too much air in the anterior chamber may cause the feet of the implant to engage the body of the iris rather than the base.

Prior to the insertion of the lens, the surgeon grasps the superior foot with a curved needle holder and inspects it under the operating microscope for warping and chipping [7]. Intraocular lenses are quite electrostatic, and occasionally foreign material adheres to the surface. The surgeon can easily remove any foreign material with irrigation or a cellulose sponge.

The actual insertion of the lens is the most difficult part of the intraocular lens procedure. Throughout the procedure, care must be taken to avoid trauma to the cornea and iris. Three basic maneuvers are utilized when placing the lens into the anterior chamber [8]. In the first maneuver, the surgeon inserts

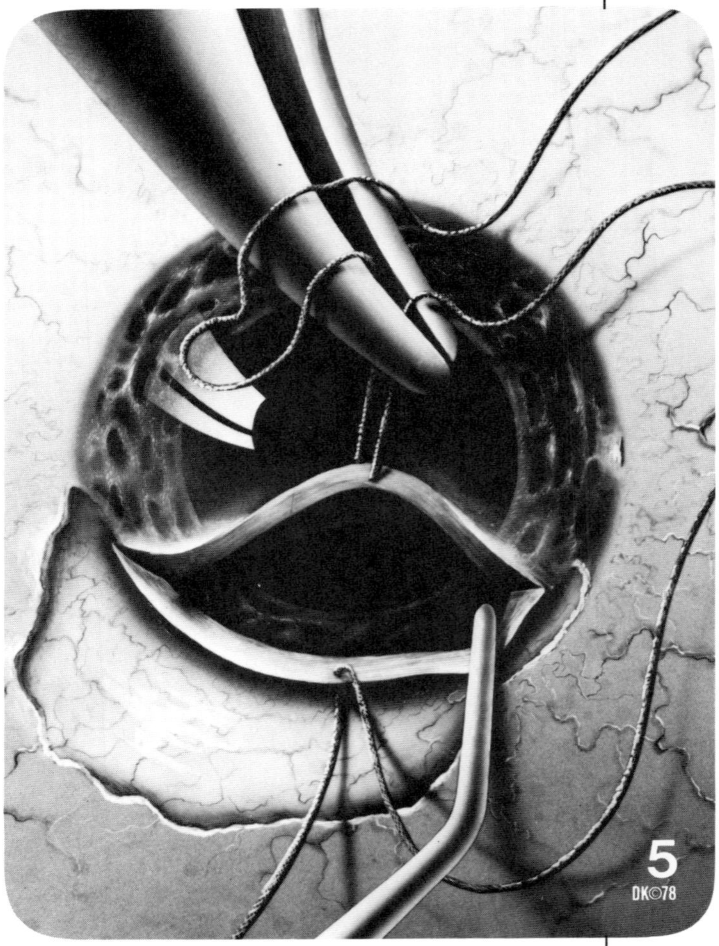

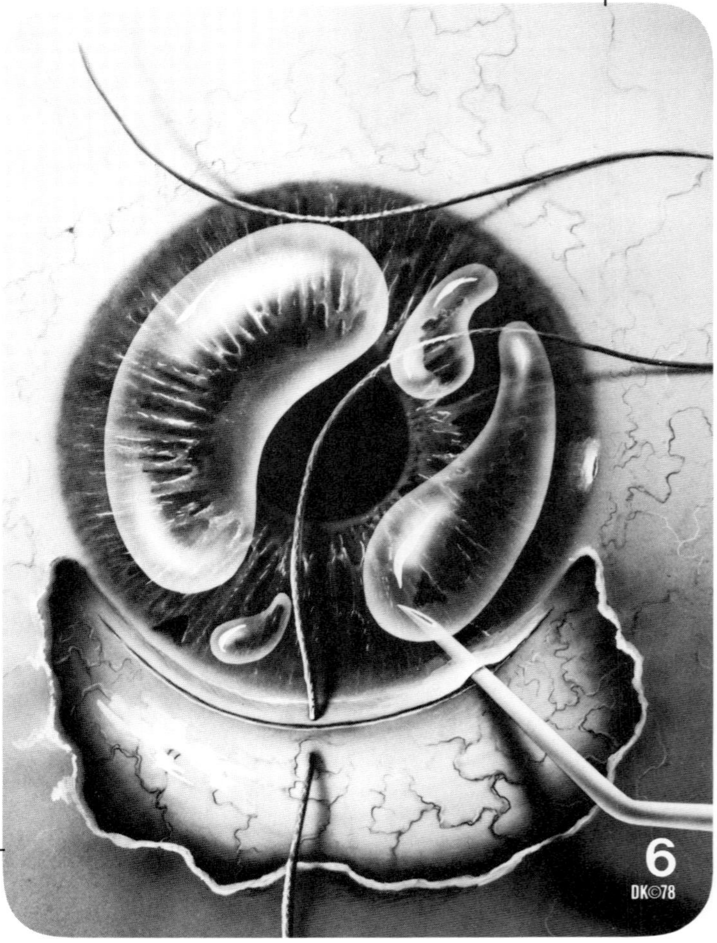

Donald F. Keller

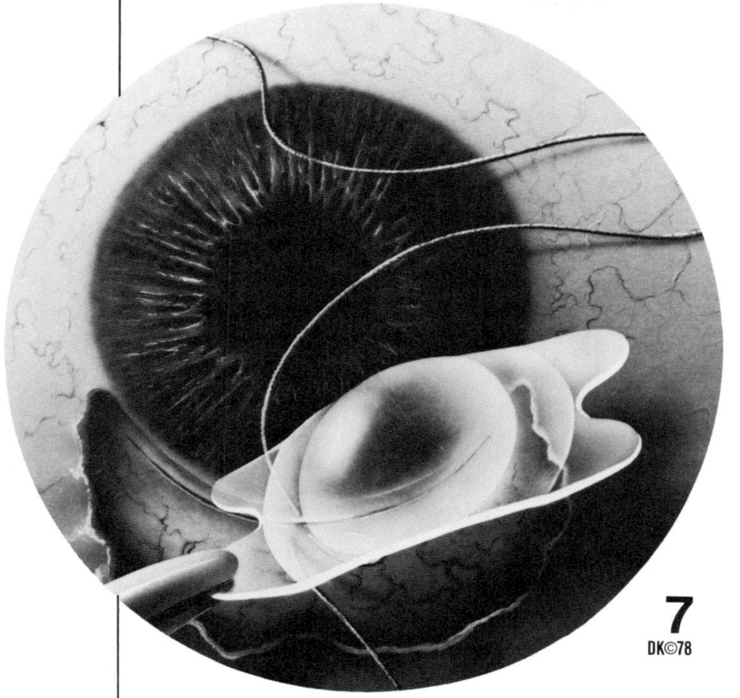

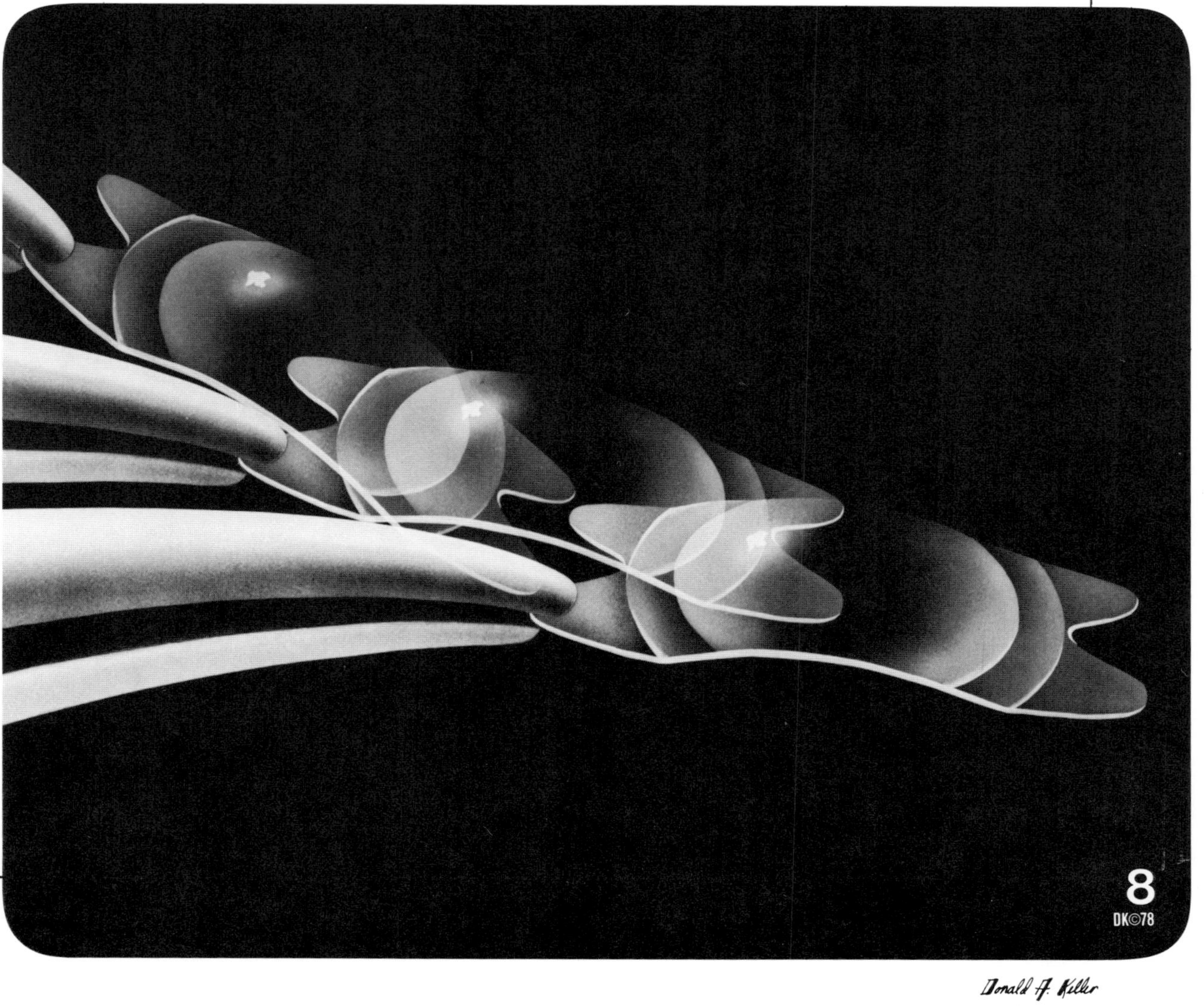

Donald A. Kilb

the lens through the wound at an oblique angle [9] [10]. The lens is passed under the air bubble, while care is taken not to engage the peripheral iridectomies. During this procedure, it may be necessary to elevate the lip of the cornea slightly if the surgeon encounters some resistance.

In the second maneuver, the surgeon flattens the plane of the lens as he advances it [11] [12]. This avoids engaging the pupillary margin.

Finally, once the distal feet pass the pupillary margin, the plane is flattened further to clear the remainder of the iris [13] [14]. If the feet of the lens engage the iris, the pupil becomes oval. When the distal feet are snugly in the angle recess, the proximal feet extend 1 mm beyond the edge of the wound.

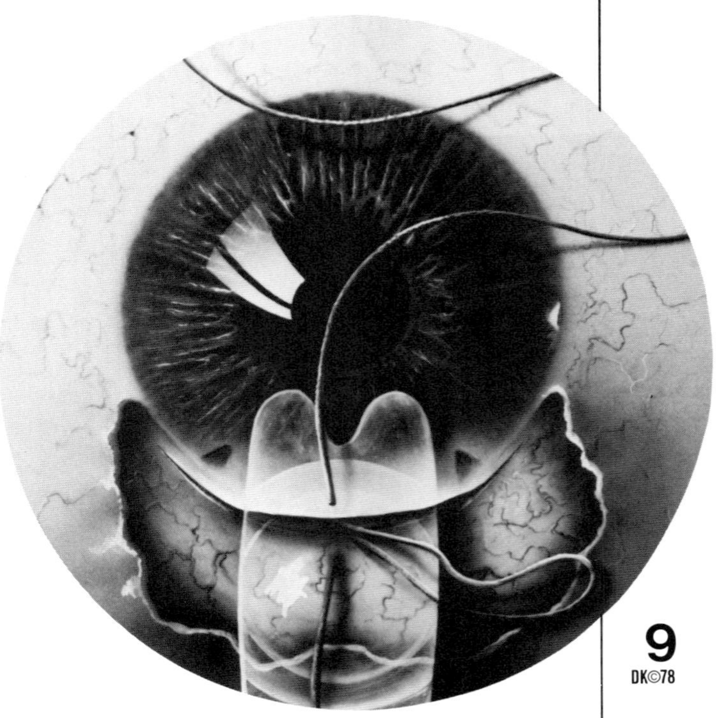

9
DK©78

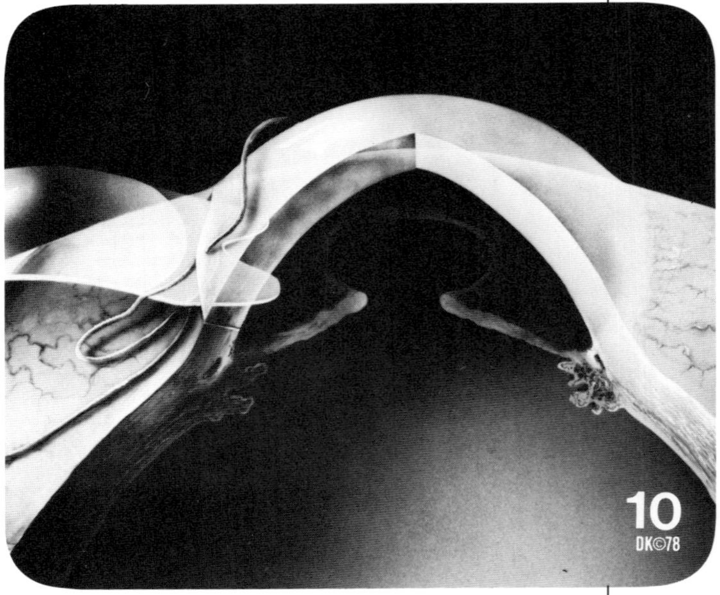

10
DK©78

Donald F. Keller

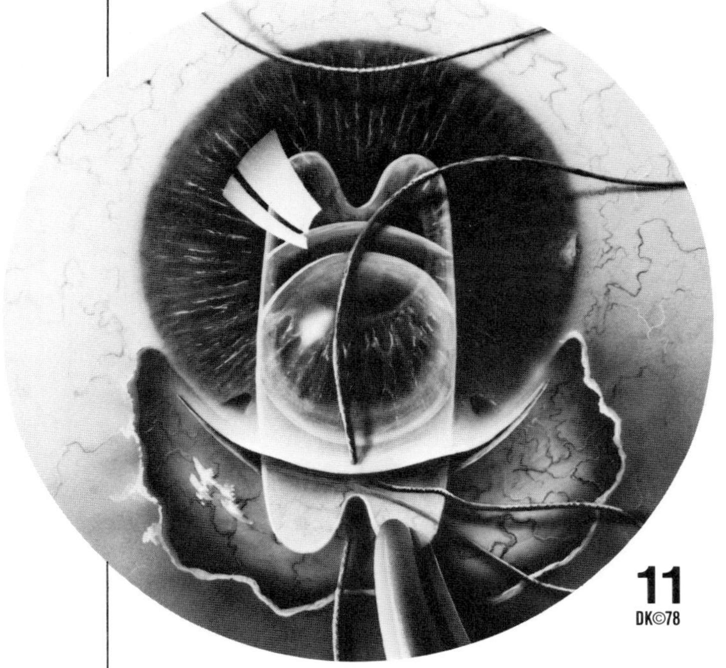

11
DK©78

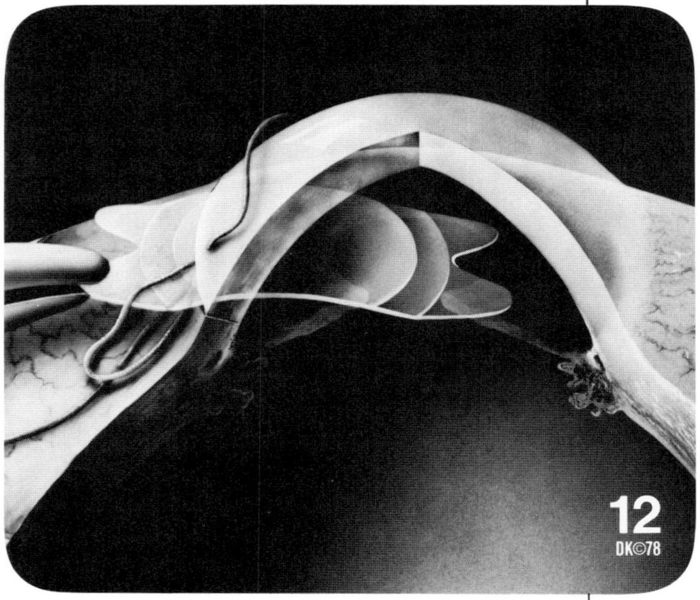

12
DK©78

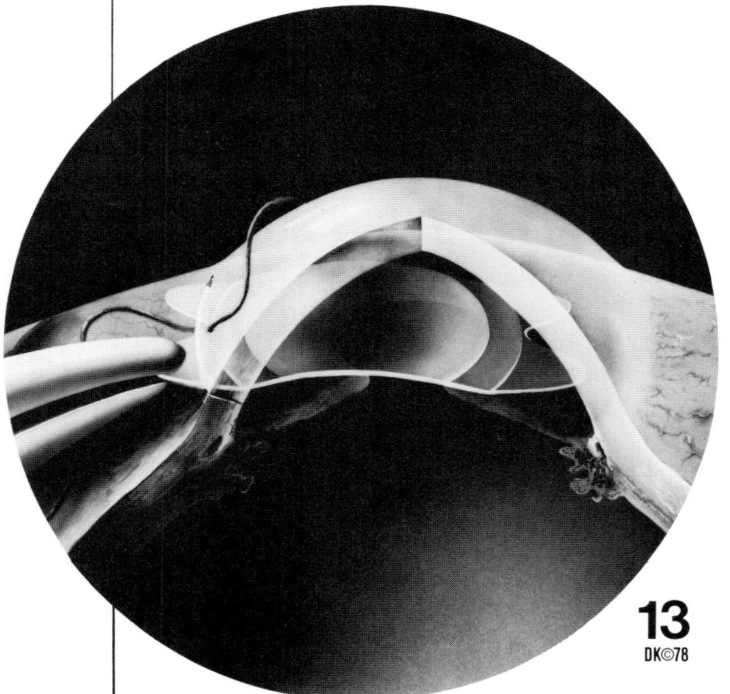

13
DK©78

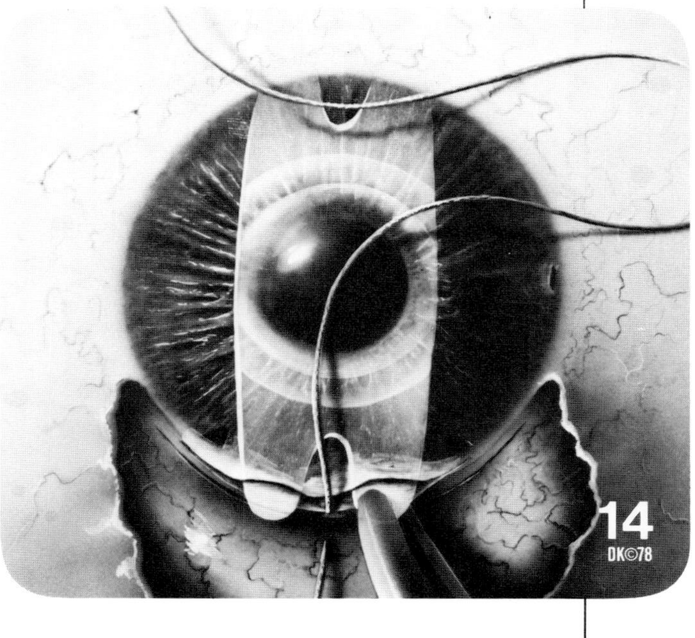

14
DK©78

Donald F. Killer

When these three maneuvers are completed, the proximal feet are inserted [15] [16]. The surgeon stabilizes the lens with a cyclodialysis spatula and retracts the sclera. With minimal downward pressure, the surgeon inserts the feet into the angle recess. If the lens is too long, it is impossible to pull the sclera firmly enough to insert the lens. It is important not to exert force toward the 6-o'clock position; this may cause undue pressure on the inferior angle, traumatize the iris and ciliary body, and cause hemorrhage. If the feet do not move into position easily, the lens may be too large, and the surgeon must use a smaller lens.

If the lens is too small and not properly seated in the angle recess, it may rotate or tilt forward causing chronic irritation. To avoid this, the lens is checked both after placement and before suturing.

After placement of the lens into the anterior chamber, the surgeon places a cyclodialysis spatula between the superior feet of the lens and gently nudges it [17]. The lens will recoil to its original position if it is situated properly and is the correct length. If the lens is too short, however, the nudge will dislocate the lens and bring the proximal feet into view from beneath the edge of the wound.

After the surgeon re-forms the anterior chamber with saline and ties the safety suture, he again checks the position and size of the lens with a tap test [18]. The sclera is tapped with a needle holder near the temporal limbus. The iris should move beneath the lens while the lens remains stable. If there is movement, the lens is too small.

If the lens is properly positioned, the feet are securely situated, posterior to the scleral spur in the angle recess [19].

At the close of the procedure [20], the pupil is vigorously dilated, for any contact between the iris and the lens may cause the formation of peripheral anterior synechiae. Normally, the use of a cycloplegic agent is necessary for approximately one month. Considerable anterior chamber reaction requires the use of topical steroids. In the immediate postoperative period, the surgeon must reaffirm that the lens is in place. Virtually no movement of the lens should occur with ocular movement.

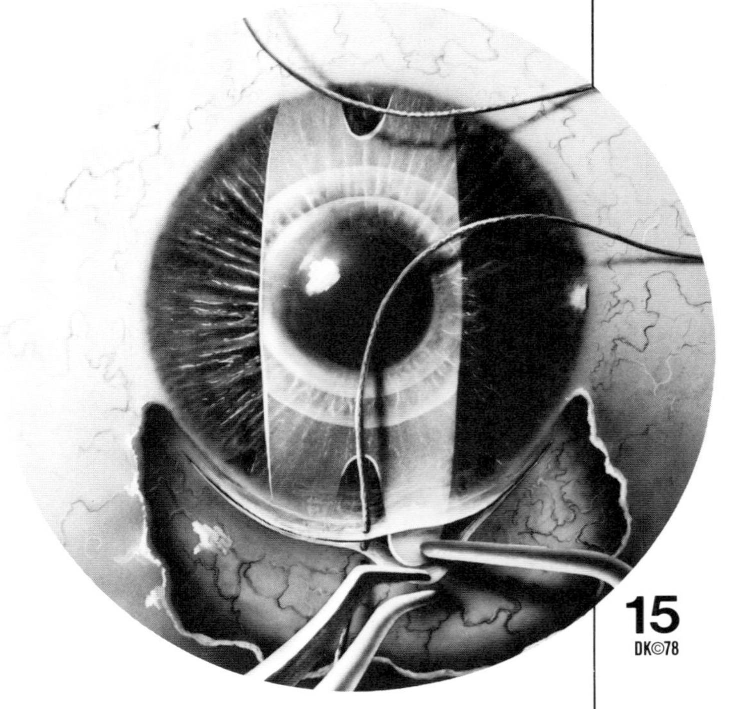

15
DK©78

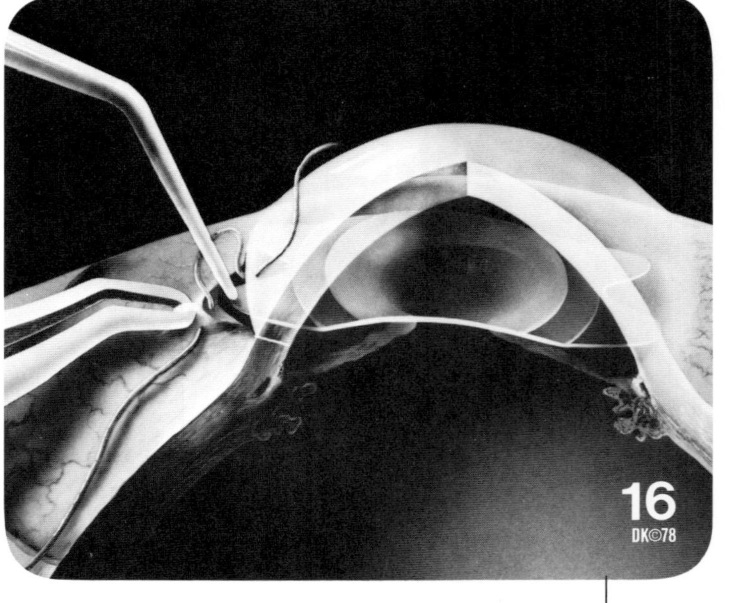

16
DK©78

Donald F. Killer

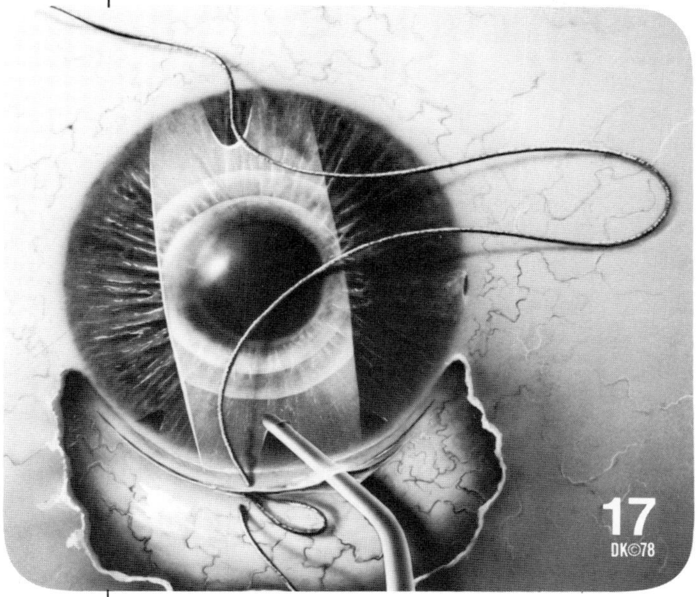
17
DK©78

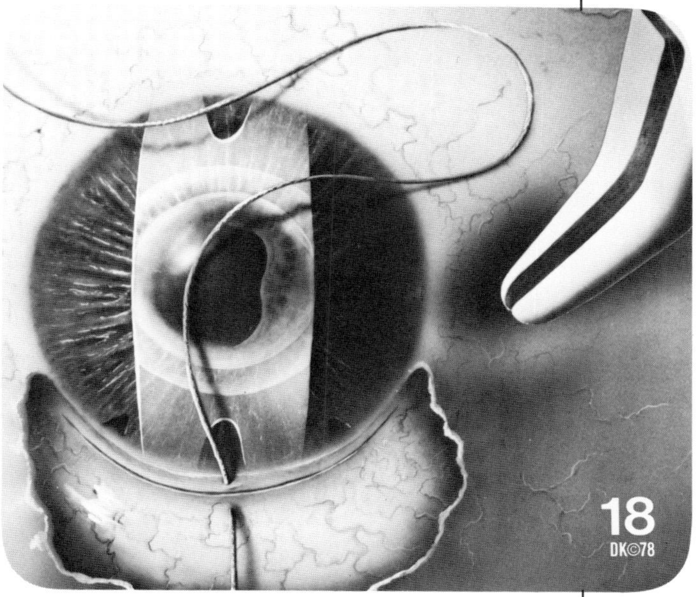
18
DK©78

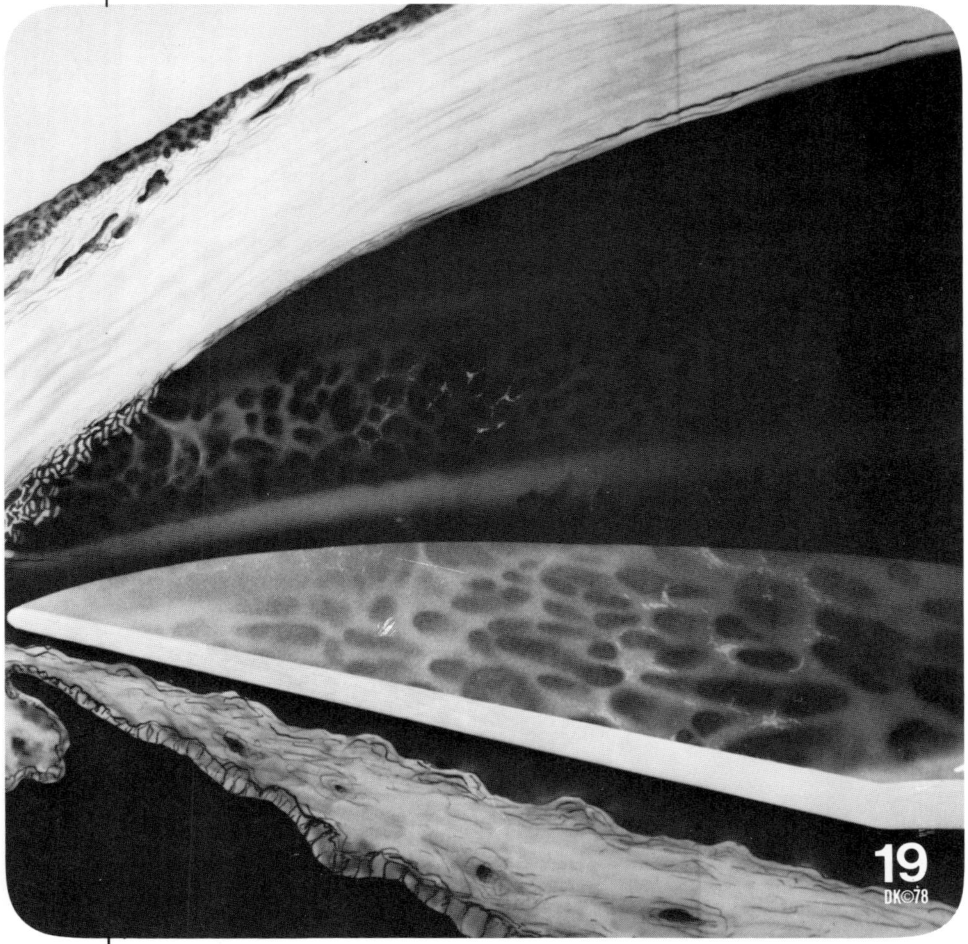
19
DK©78

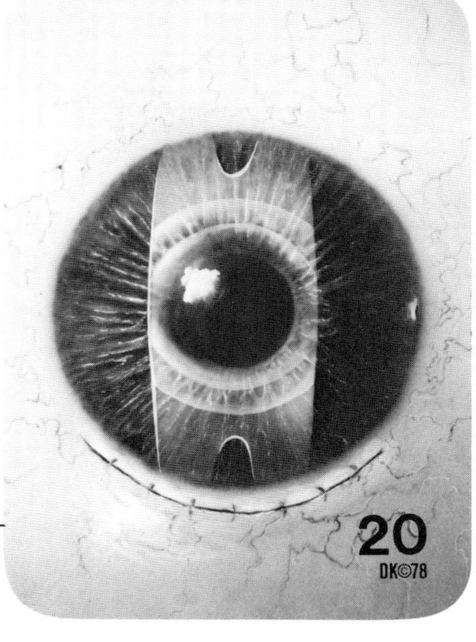
20
DK©78

TWO-LOOP CAPSULAR FIXATION LENS

Richard H. Keates, M.D.
Richard H. Lembach, M.D.

If the surgeon decides to insert an intraocular lens in a younger patient in whom an extracapsular cataract extraction is indicated, we recommend the use of a two-loop capsular fixation lens. Using a 30-gauge cannula, the surgeon introduces air into the anterior chamber until it is completely filled, yet not overfilled. If the air shows any tendency to escape when the posterior lip of the wound is gently depressed, placement of additional wing sutures provides an airtight seal for later lens insertion. The 7-0 black silk safety sutures are reposited to the sides of the incision, and the lens is grasped with a McPherson forceps by either the temporal or nasal feet. Prior to insertion, the lens is inspected and irrigated. The anterior chamber is maintained with air throughout the insertion to prevent lens contact with the endothelium. With the loops oriented vertically, the cornea is elevated slightly, and the lens is introduced into the anterior chamber beneath the air bubble. The surgeon must avoid touching the endothelium or stripping Descemet's membrane. If air escapes at this time, the lens is removed, and the speculum and bridle suture are checked for any signs of pressure. If air continues to leak from the anterior chamber, the incision is too large, and additional corneoscleral sutures are placed until the chamber does hold air.

As the lens is introduced into the anterior chamber, the inferior loop is directed beneath the inferior iris and anterior capsule, while the optical portion of the lens is positioned anterior to the iris [1] [2] . If the pupil is dilated moderately, the surgeon can position the superior loop under the iris by gently advancing the lens inferiorly [3] [4] . If this cannot be accomplished easily, the surgeon can use a cyclodialysis spatula to stabilize and depress

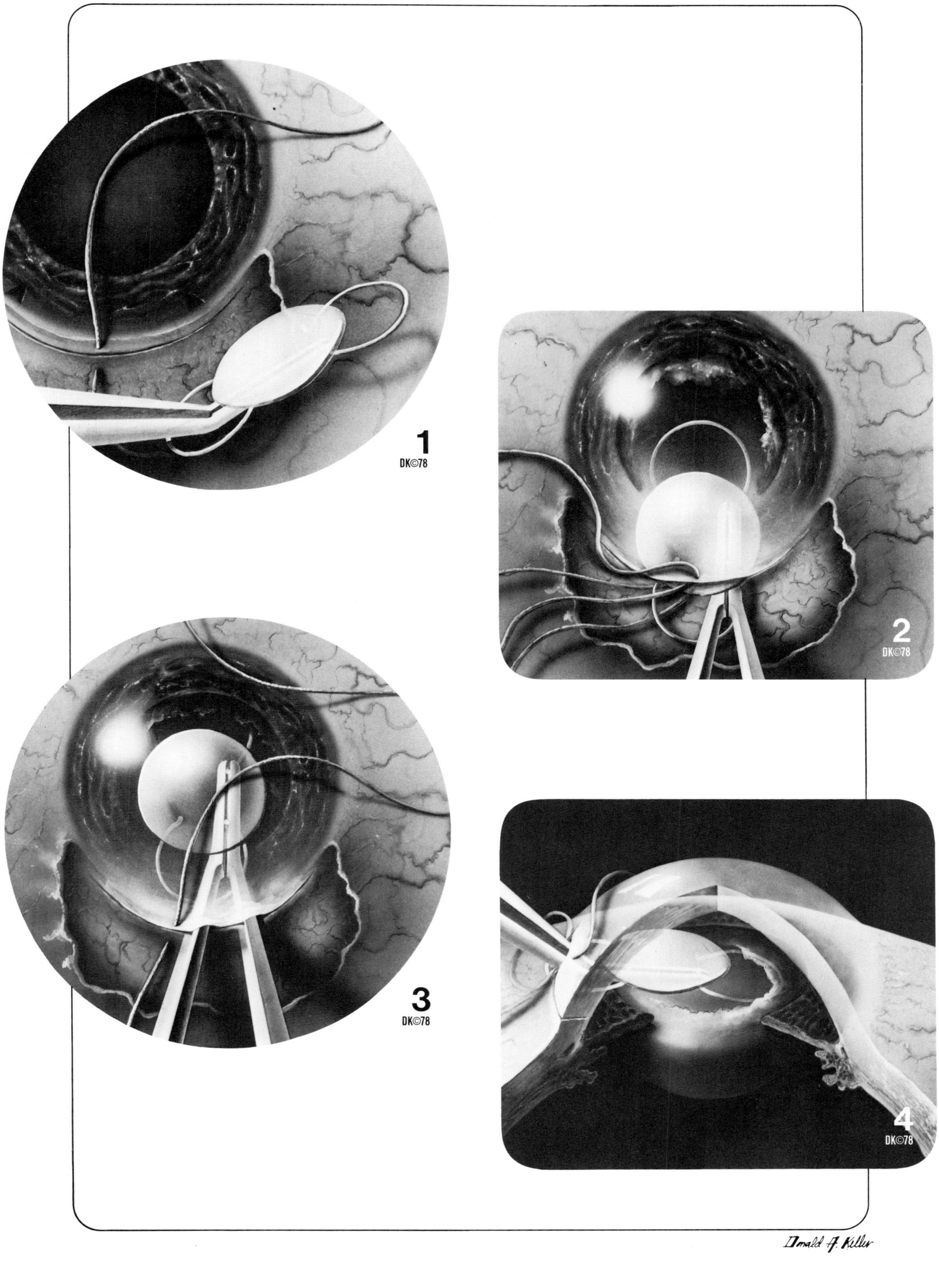

Donald A. Keller

the lens while an iris hook elevates the iris and capsule over the superior loop of the lens [5] [6] . The two loops now should rest in the lens capsule, and the optical portion should lie anterior to the iris plane. To check the position of the lens, the surgeon inserts a spatula through the needle knife incision [7] . As the lens is gently pushed, the surgeon looks for wrinkling of the remnants of the anterior capsule inferiorly. This confirms capsular fixation. Acetylcholine chloride is injected through the temporal incision with a 30-gauge cannula to help center the lens. The surgeon then closes the wound with 10-0 nylon interrupted sutures [8] . Subconjunctival gentamicin sulfate and aqueous dexamethasone are given. One drop of 1 percent pilocarpine hydrochloride may be applied to the cornea before a patch and shield are applied. The patient should be observed several hours after surgery to insure that the lens is in position.

Ideally, adhesions will form between the loops of the lens and the capsule and usually are complete at one week. It is important to avoid synechiae between the lens and iris; therefore, we prescribe short-acting cycloplegics and antibiotic-steroid drops postoperatively.

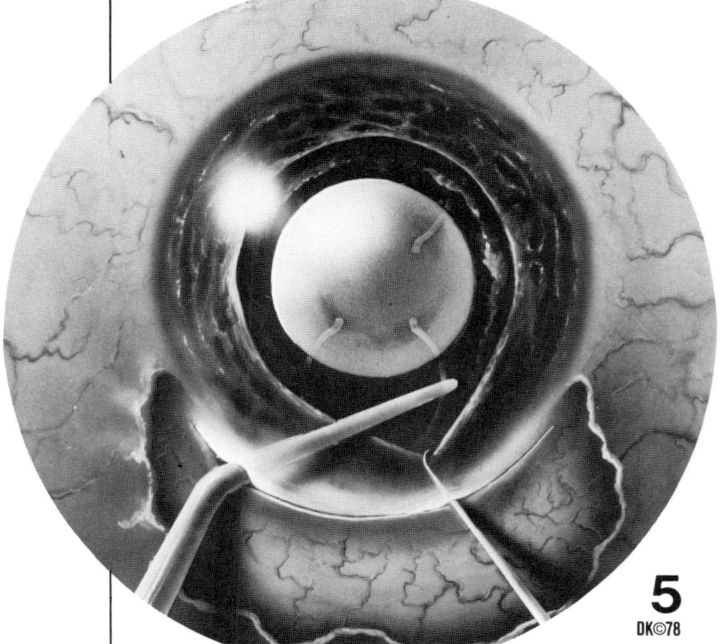

5
DK©78

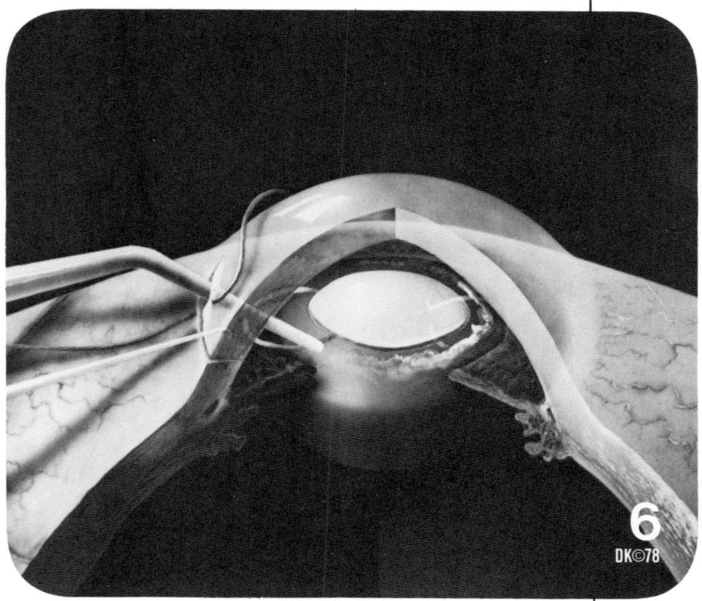

6
DK©78

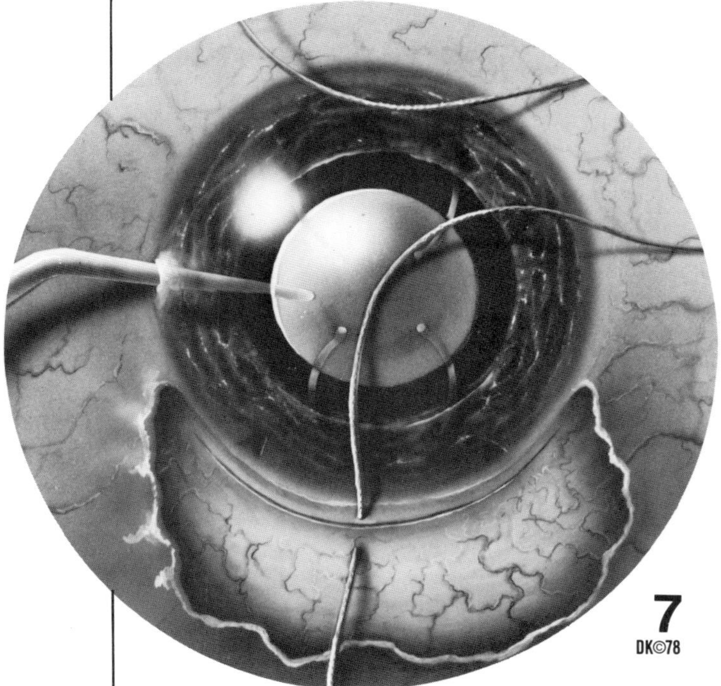

7
DK©78

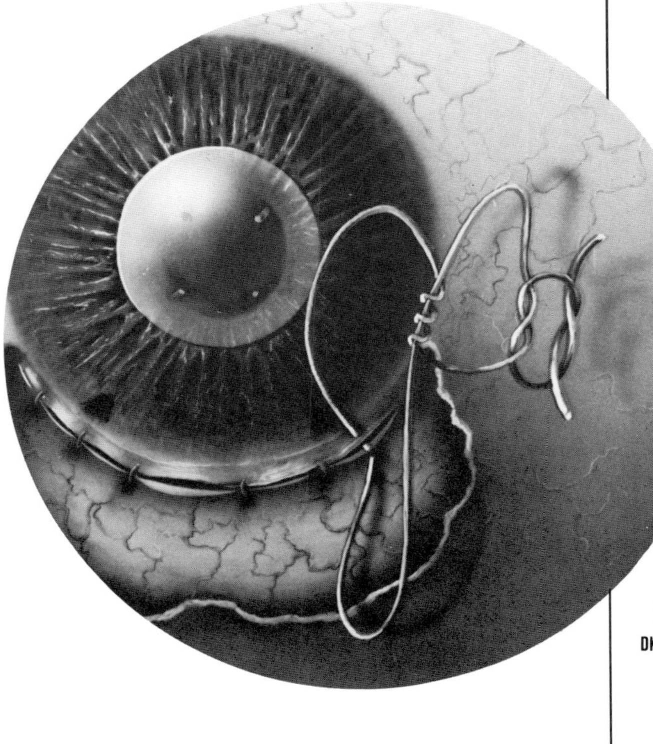

8
DK©78

WOUND HEALING AND THE CONTROL OF POSTOPERATIVE ASTIGMATISM

Frederick H. Davidorf, M.D.

Over the years, modern technology has enabled manufacturers to produce progressively smaller caliber suture materials, yet maintain tensile strength. The immediate benefit of the fine-caliber sutures has been the dramatic reduction in postoperative discomfort. While the increasing popularity of 10-0 monofilament nylon has reduced postoperative ocular morbidity, it has created new problems that relate primarily to wound healing and its effect on postoperative corneal astigmatism.

With an increasing interest in soft and continuous-wear contact lenses for aphakic patients, controlling surgically induced astigmatism is vital to the cataract surgeon. Generally, no more than 1 to 1½ diopters of with-the-rule astigmatism can be tolerated if a soft contact lens or extended-wear contact lens is to be used.

We will review several factors that affect the postoperative astigmatic error and discuss ways to control it intraoperatively and postoperatively. Before discussion of the management of surgically induced astigmatism, however, it is important to describe the stages of wound healing.

The healing of a cataract wound is a dynamic process. The ultimate tensile strength of the wound depends on the integrity of the stroma. The initial healing of the stroma is completed by approximately six weeks; therefore, if the surgeon is to alter the wound, it should be done by this time. Wound remodeling may occur as late as several years after surgery.

In the immediate postoperative period, five to seven days [1] , the strength of the wound depends on the sutures. If the incision is made through the blue line, the strength of the wound comes from the conjunctival flap and underlying connective tissue. The external portion of the wound is bridged by the conjunctival flap, which is edematous in the immediate postoperative period. There is fibrovascular proliferation in the episcleral and subconjunctival connective tissue in this area. The subconjunctival connective tissue contains a mixed population of cells; it is from here that fibroblasts, which gradually migrate into the stroma and participate in stromal healing, originate. There is stromal edema at the edges of the wound, but no stromal healing takes place during this period. Fibroblasts and collagen fibers are oriented parallel to the edges of the incision. This represents a relatively weak union. The edges of Descemet's membrane retract somewhat and are very slowly regenerated by endothelium. Between 24 and 48 hours after surgery, the endothelium slides over the internal defect of the wound.

The conjunctival flap is firmly adherent to the underlying stroma by dense connective tissue. By two weeks, the fibroblasts have extended through the entire thickness of the wound [2] . As remodeling of the stroma occurs, the wound gains strength.

By six weeks [3] the stroma is firmly healed but incompletely remodeled. Initially, the remodeling occurs in the central stroma and consists of a reorientation of the collagen fibers so that they run parallel to the scleral and corneal lamellae. This remodeling of the wound occurs slowly over an extended period of time, perhaps two years or longer, before the entire cornea is involved. The corneal curvatures change only slightly during the remodeling process.

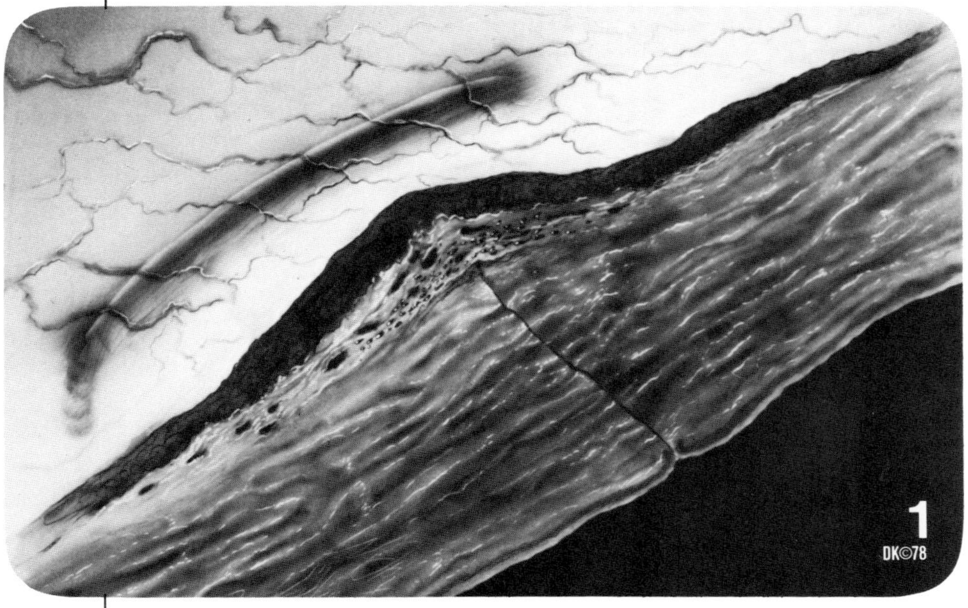
1
DK©78

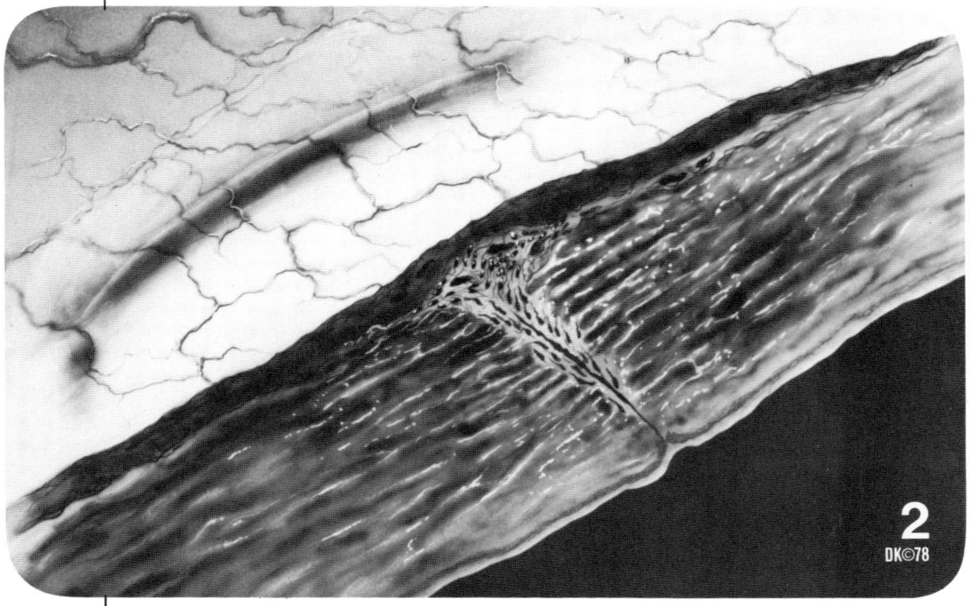
2
DK©78

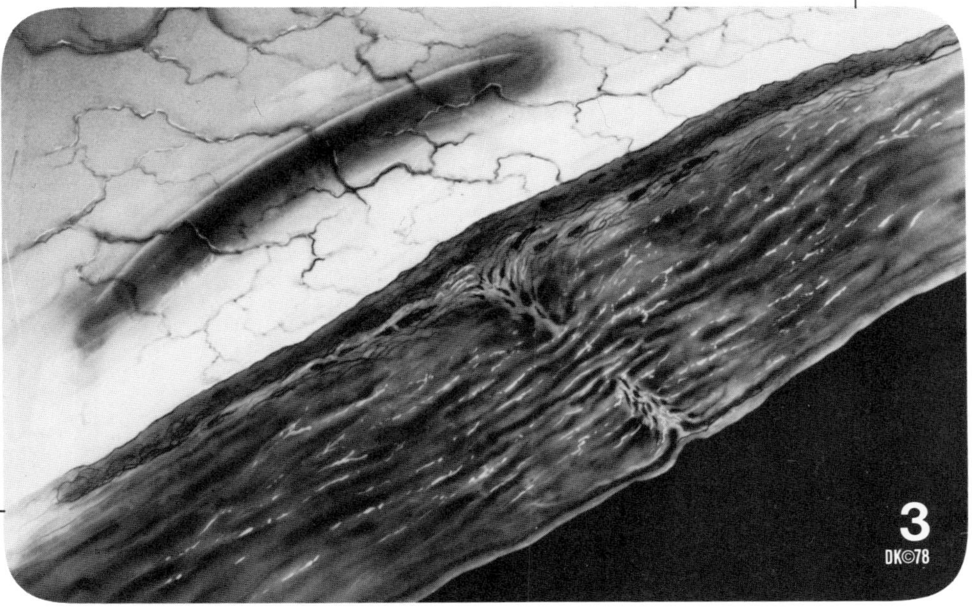
3
DK©78

With an understanding of wound healing, we can now turn our attention to surgically induced astigmatism. The closure of a cataract wound is the single most important factor in its control. The primary goal of wound closure is to maintain alignment of the edges of the incision as the wound heals. Therefore, in the ideal wound closure, the sutures should serve to hold the edges together without causing distortion. Any technique that distorts the edges of the wound may induce astigmatism. Absorbable suture material is much more forgiving than the 10-0 monofilament material now recommended. With use of absorbable suture, the amount of astigmatism diminishes gradually over a period of time. The wound tends to assume the preoperative shape as the sutures lose their tensile strength. However, 10-0 monofilament suture does not weaken during the immediate postoperative period. Therefore, any wound distortion resulting from this type of suture must be dealt with by the time stromal healing is completed at six weeks.

When using 10-0 monofilament suture, we recommend deep, short bites that should be placed from three-quarters to full thickness of the cornea with equal depth on both sides of the wound [4] . Ideally, the suture will lie just superficial to Descemet's membrane to insure adequate apposition of the wound edges. This type of suture technique is facilitated with the use of the half-circle spatula needle. The 10-0 monofilament suture can be placed at this depth since the size and composition of the suture material cause little tissue reaction.

In addition to using deep sutures, we recommend short bites as they encompass less tissue and consequently produce less wound distortion. If a suture is placed too superficially (less than half the depth of the tissue) or if there is a considerable difference in suture depths on either side of the wound, a gaping or misalignment of the internal portion of the wound may result [5] [6] . Any misalignment of the endothelium interferes with wound healing, which may result in chronic corneal edema.

The most common cause of postoperative corneal astigmatism with 10-0 monofilament sutures results from tying the suture too tightly [7] . The tying of a 10-0 monofilament

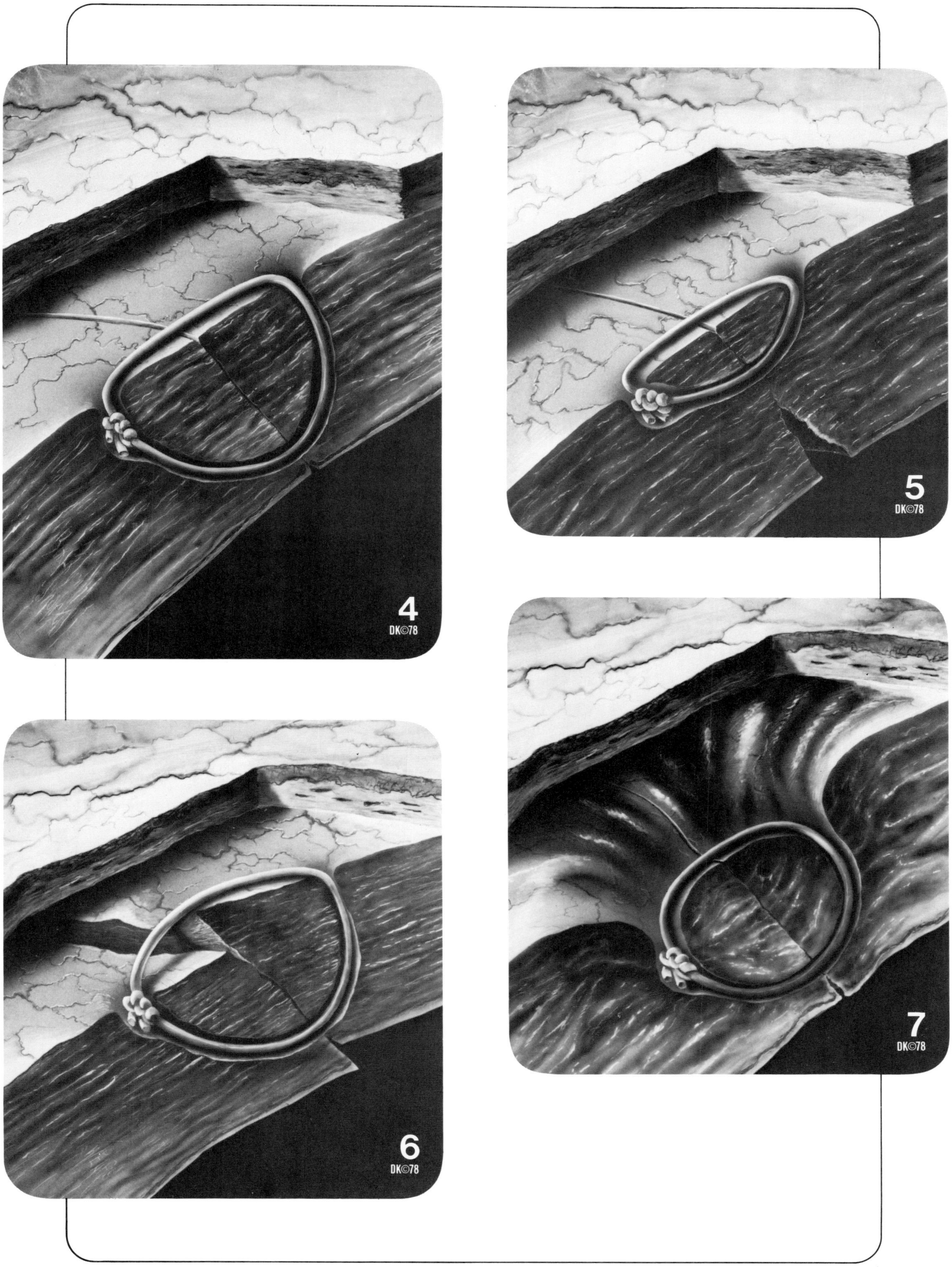

Donald A. Keller

suture is an art that requires practice to master. Because the suture is quite electrostatic, it has a tendency to adhere to the drape, tissue, and instruments, and can be quite difficult to manipulate. The process is facilitated with the use of two fine tying forceps [8] [9]. The first portion of the knot utilizes a triple-throw surgeon's knot [10]. This is self-locking and approximates the wound edges while the operator ties the second and third loops of the knot [11] [12]. When the wound closure is completed, the corneal side of the wound should be inspected for excessive tension adjacent to a suture. Should this be present, the suture should be cut and replaced.

In spite of careful suturing techniques, it is not uncommon to find a suture that is too tight postoperatively. Therefore, we recommend preoperative recording of keratometry readings on all patients undergoing cataract surgery. This is important in determining whether the postoperative astigmatism is surgically induced. A tight suture creates a steep meridian parallel to the orientation of the suture.

If an astigmatic error of greater than 1½ diopters is present during the first postoperative visit, keratometry should be done to confirm the axis of the steepest corneal meridian. Marked edema of the wound in this area may indicate that the astigmatism is a result of poor apposition of the wound edges and is not caused by a tight suture. If wound apposition is good, however, and the cornea is not edematous in the area of the suspected tightness, the examiner sees indentation of the epithelium and/or tension lines within the corneal stroma. The identification of a tight suture may be enhanced with the use of fluorescein. There will be a small triangular area of pooling on the corneal side of a tight suture.

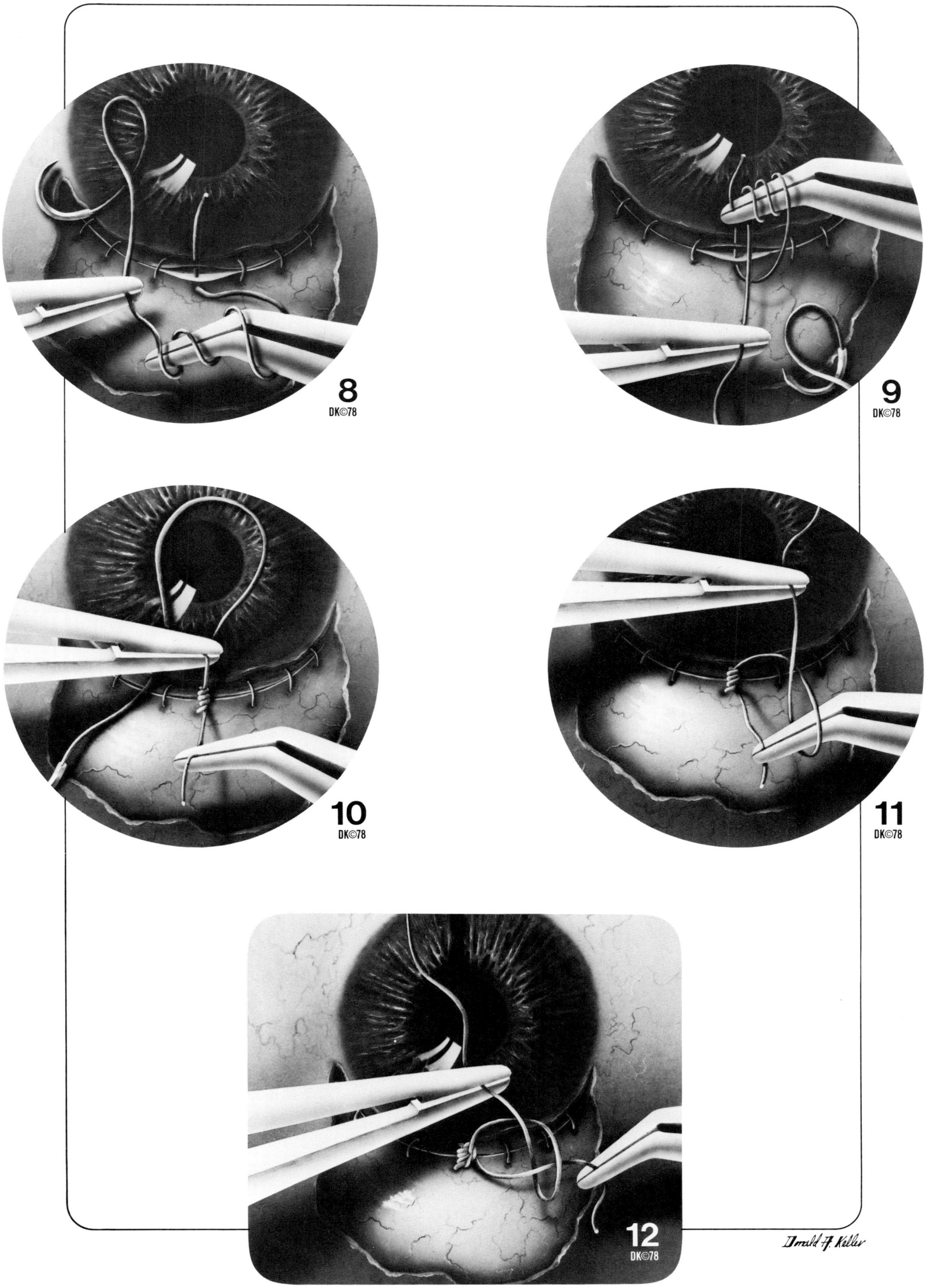
8
DK©78
9
DK©78
10
DK©78
11
DK©78
12
DK©78

If the astigmatic error persists after two to three weeks, stromal healing has been sufficient, in most instances, to safely cut a suture to release its tightening effect. If a patient has been receiving corticosteroid therapy, it is better to wait at least three weeks before removing a suture. At times, it is possible to remove a suture as late as two months after cataract surgery and still effect a relaxation in the induced astigmatism. The longer the time since surgery, however, the less chance there is of relaxing an incision.

The technique of cutting a tight suture to relieve induced postoperative astigmatism is quite simple and safe and can be done in the office with the help of a slit lamp, topical anesthesia, and an assistant to hold the lid. Before removing a suture, the surgeon must reassure the patient that the wound is healing satisfactorily but that cutting or relaxing a particular suture will improve the ultimate surgical outcome. While the patient looks down, the assistant elevates the upper lid using the index finger to exert pressure on the orbit so that the patient cannot close the lids during the procedure. The fixation light is positioned so that good exposure of the surgical limbus is obtained. We recommend use of a No. 11 disposable scalpel to cut the suture **13** . With the hand resting on the patient's cheek to avoid damage to the eye due to sudden movements of the patient's head, the surgeon inserts the blade through the conjunctiva under the suture. The suture is cut by gently rotating and lifting the tip of the blade **14** . If the cut end of the suture is exposed, the surgeon removes it with a fine toothless forceps. It is advisable to remove the suture from the scleral side so that the knot does not pass through the corneal tissue. If both ends of the cut suture retract and are covered by tissue, it does not need to be removed. After approximately 10 to 15 minutes, repeated keratometry is suggested to determine if any relaxation has been effected by cutting the one suture. In some situations, it is necessary to remove more than one. The patient should be instructed to use topical antibiotics for two days after the suture is cut to decrease the chance of infection. Patching of the eye is not required in most instances.

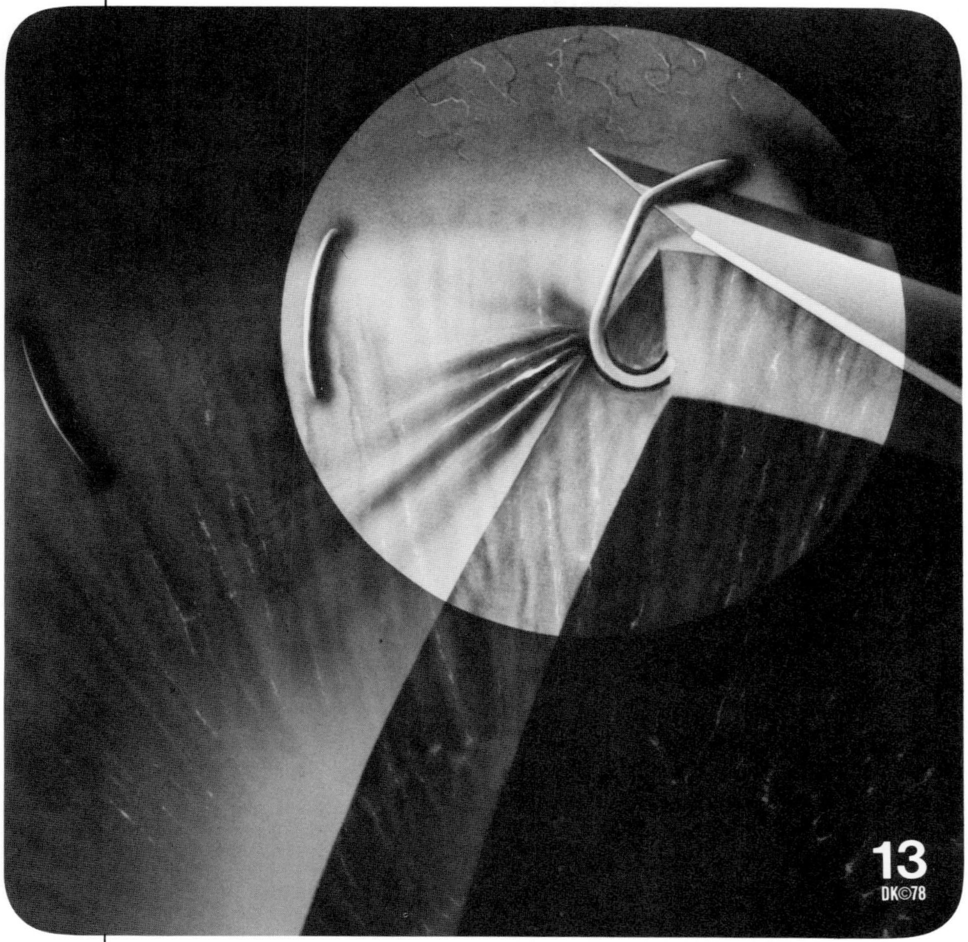
13
DK©78

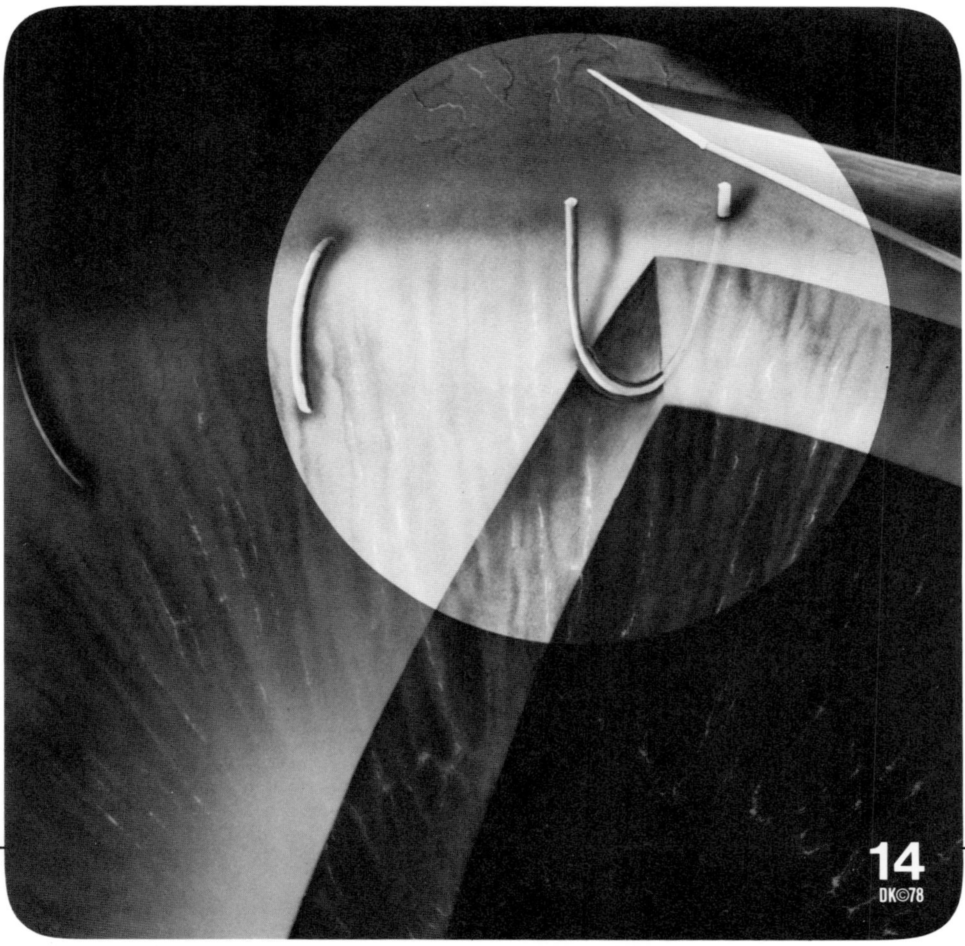
14
DK©78
Donald F. Keller

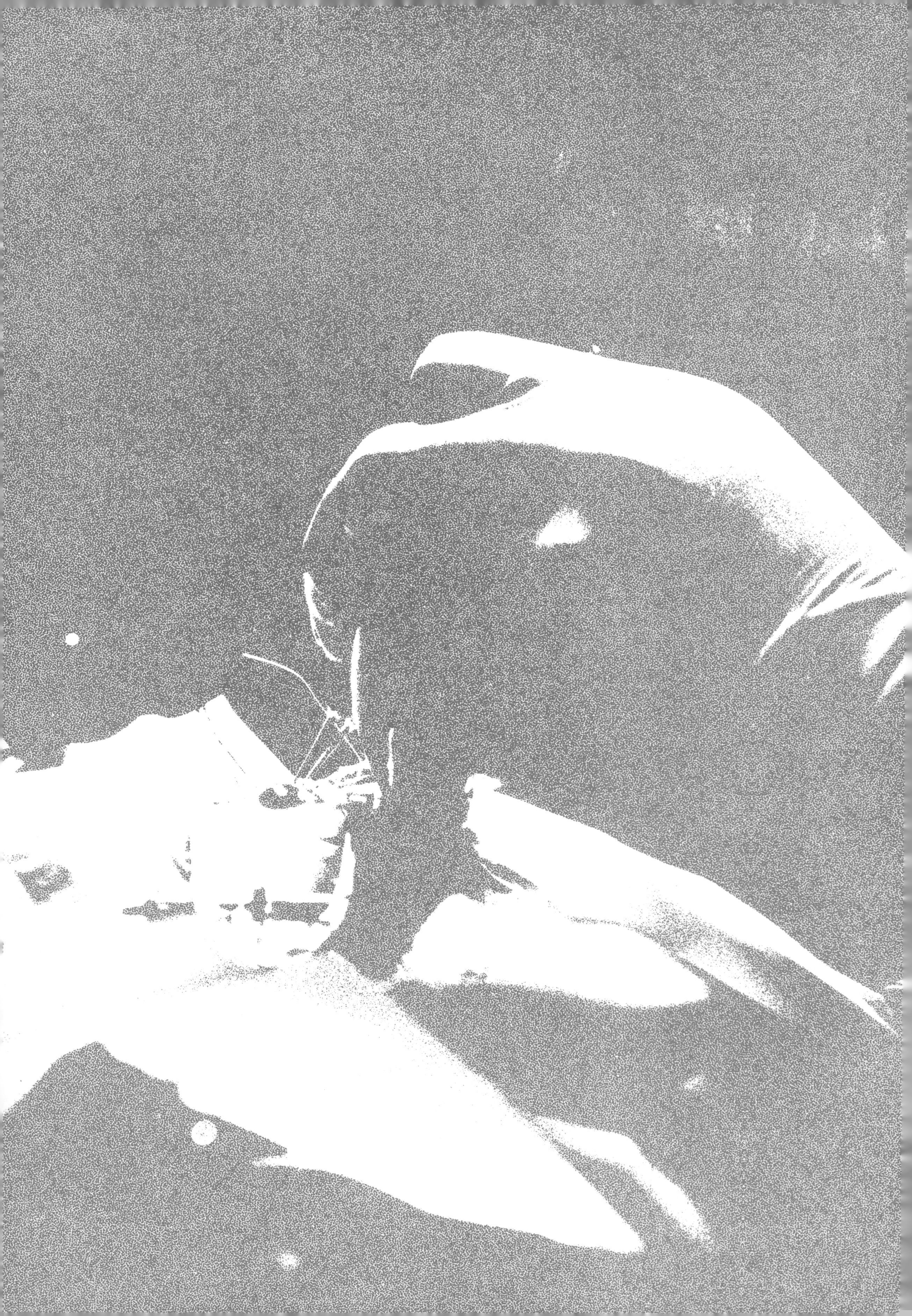

2
GLAUCOMA
SURGERY

EVALUATION OF THE ANTERIOR CHAMBER ANGLE

Frederick M. Kapetansky, M.D.

The ophthalmologist should have little trouble diagnosing an attack of acute angle-closure glaucoma. The patient usually reports pain, and the examination of the eye reveals ciliary injection, a cloudy cornea, and elevated intraocular pressure. By contrast, the appearance of intermittent or subacute angle-closure glaucoma is often subtle, and the diagnosis may easily be missed without meticulous attention to the history taking and the performance of painstaking gonioscopy. Using the Van Herick slit-lamp estimation of the anterior chamber depth, the clinician can readily identify those patients with occludable anterior chamber angles who should undergo thorough evaluation by gonioscopy. Under no circumstances is the Van Herick procedure a substitute for gonioscopy.

The Van Herick evaluation is simple, fast, and reliable, and is as important a part of routine ophthalmic examination as is the taking of an intraocular pressure. As the procedure becomes a routine part of practice, just as the observation of cup/disk ratio has, and the anterior chamber depth is graded and noted on each patient's chart, any change in the slit-lamp appearance of the angle may alert the ophthalmologist to anterior chamber narrowing, boding possible angle closure.

To perform the evaluation, the patient looks straight ahead while the examiner shines the incident light from the temporal side through the most peripheral transparent cornea at about a 45-degree angle from the examiner's line of view. The depth of the anterior chamber angle is measured by determining the distance between the corneal endothelium and the surface of the iris. This measurement is compared with the corneal thickness. Corneal abnormalities, such as corneal edema, bullous keratopathy, or prominent arcus senilis, may interfere with the reflection of the incident light on the iris and thereby compromise the reliability of this method.

The value recorded on the patient's chart is expressed as a fraction of the corneal thickness. If the anterior chamber depth measures greater than one-quarter the corneal thickness, the angle is probably not occludable [1] [2] . If the anterior chamber depth is one-quarter or less the corneal thickness [3] [4] gonioscopy is mandatory at this juncture in the examination because the angle is either occluded or occludable. Eyes with this angle depth may be dilated safely without marked risk of angle closure.

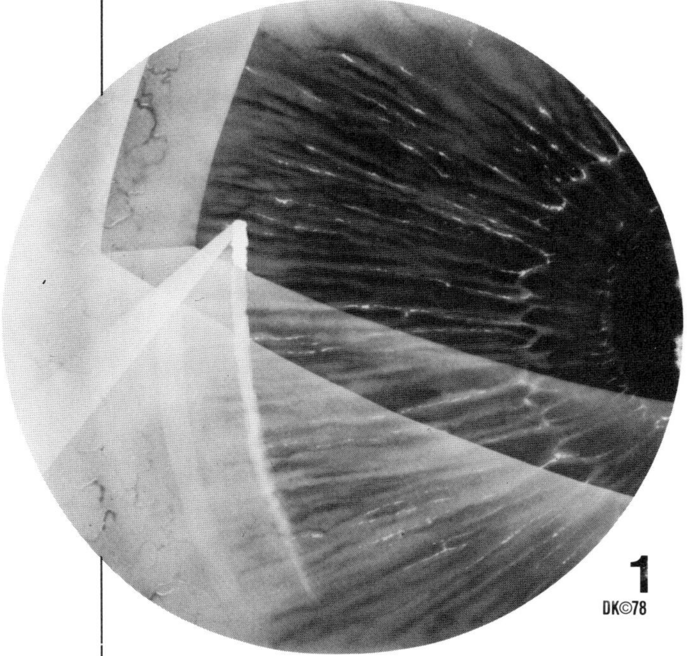

1
DK©78

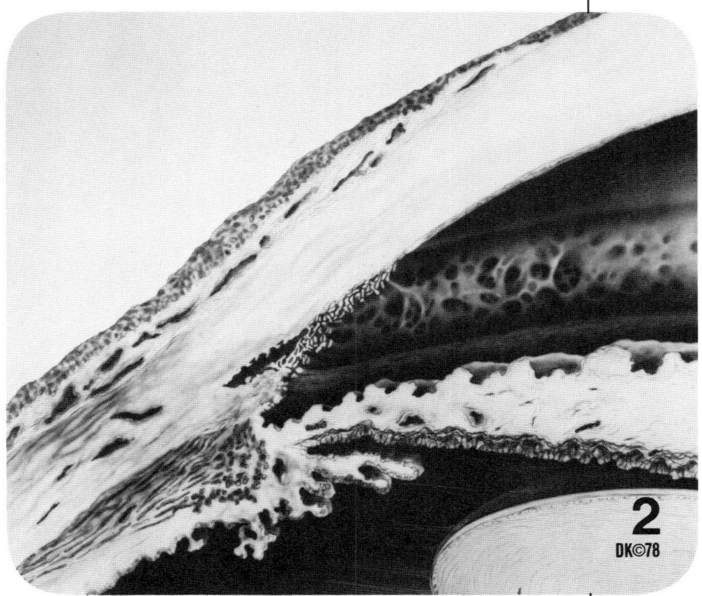

2
DK©78

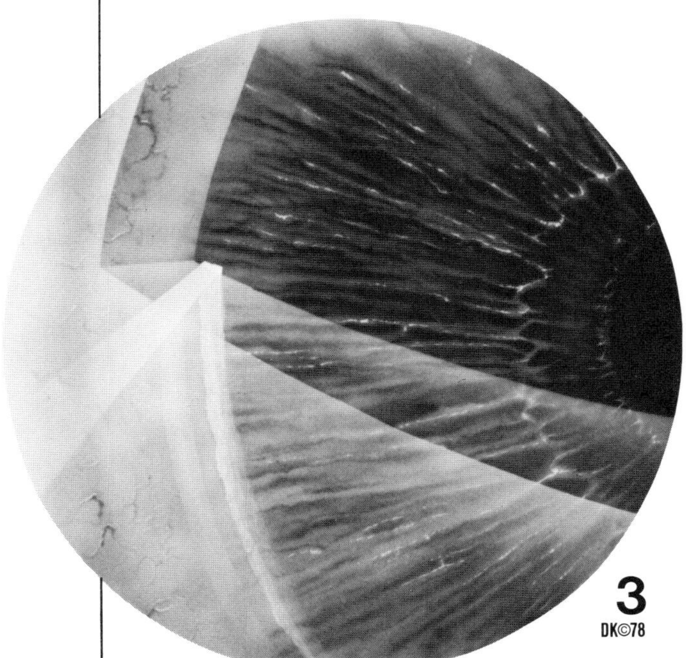

3
DK©78

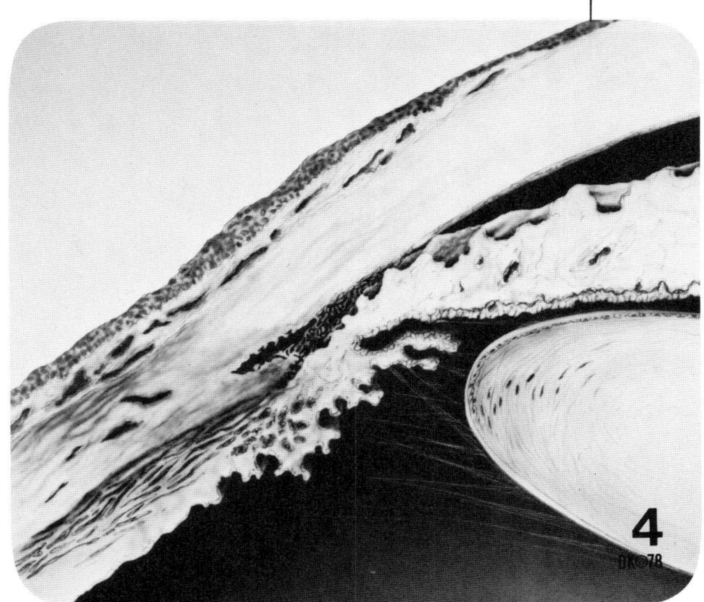

4
DK©78

The practicing ophthalmologist needs to be adept at both direct and indirect gonioscopy. Each instrument has its particular value in an office practice.

During indirect gonioscopy [5] with use of a Goldmann two- or three-mirror lens, the mirror reflects light into the angle, the angle image is reflected out, and a biomicroscope visualizes details. Slit-lamp magnification of the angle structures may reveal such subtleties as debris or fine vessels in the angle.

The observer's initial orientation is obtained by locating Schwalbe's line, SL [6], at the point where the anterior and posterior corneal light beams converge. Use of a narrow slit beam aids in the identification of this point, which also marks the beginning of the trabecular meshwork (TM). The meshwork is pale yellow and darkens somewhat when pigment is deposited on its surface. The canal of Schlemm (CS) lies behind the posterior portion of the trabecular meshwork and may appear as a discrete reddish-brown line when it is filled with blood.

Two additional landmarks need to be identified—scleral spur and ciliary body (SS and CB). The scleral spur is a bright-white, horizontal line just posterior to trabecular meshwork. It may be obscured to some extent by overlying iris processes (IP).

The ciliary body lies just behind the scleral spur in the deepest recess of the chamber angle. It is tan-brown, except in deeply pigmented irides, where it may be indistinguishable from iris. In normal angles, ballooning of the peripheral iris may obscure the view of the scleral spur and ciliary body.

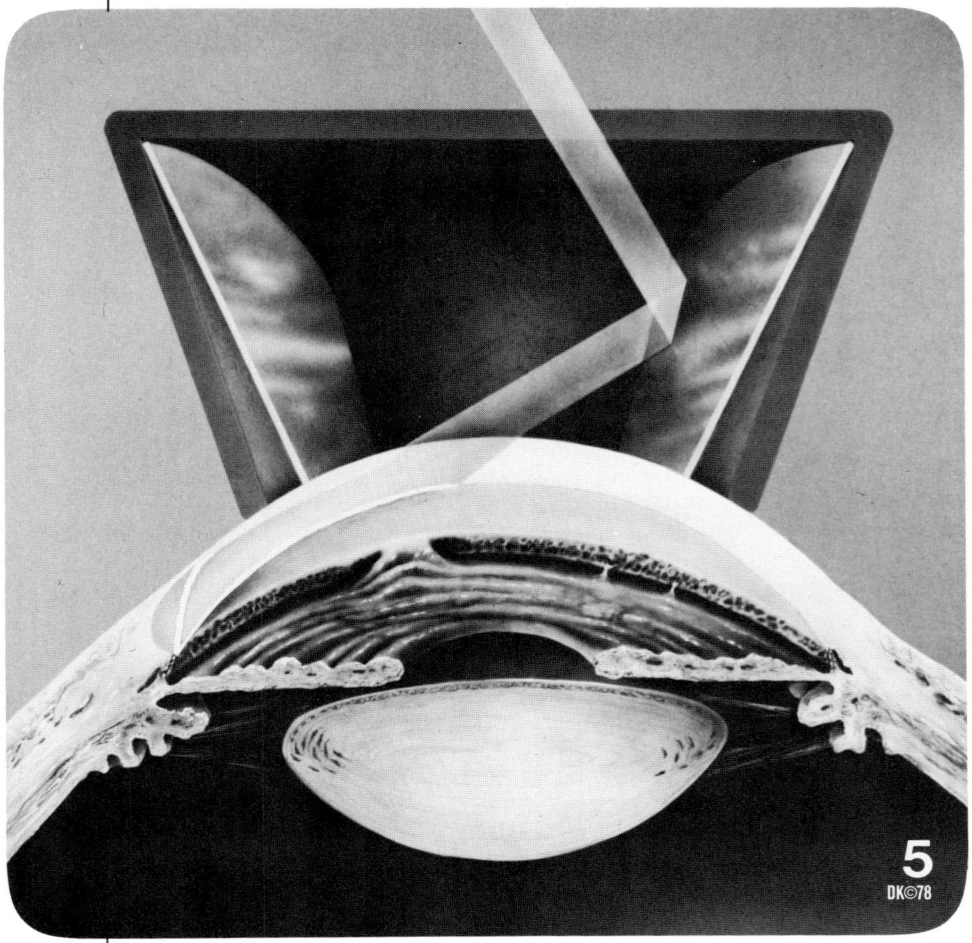

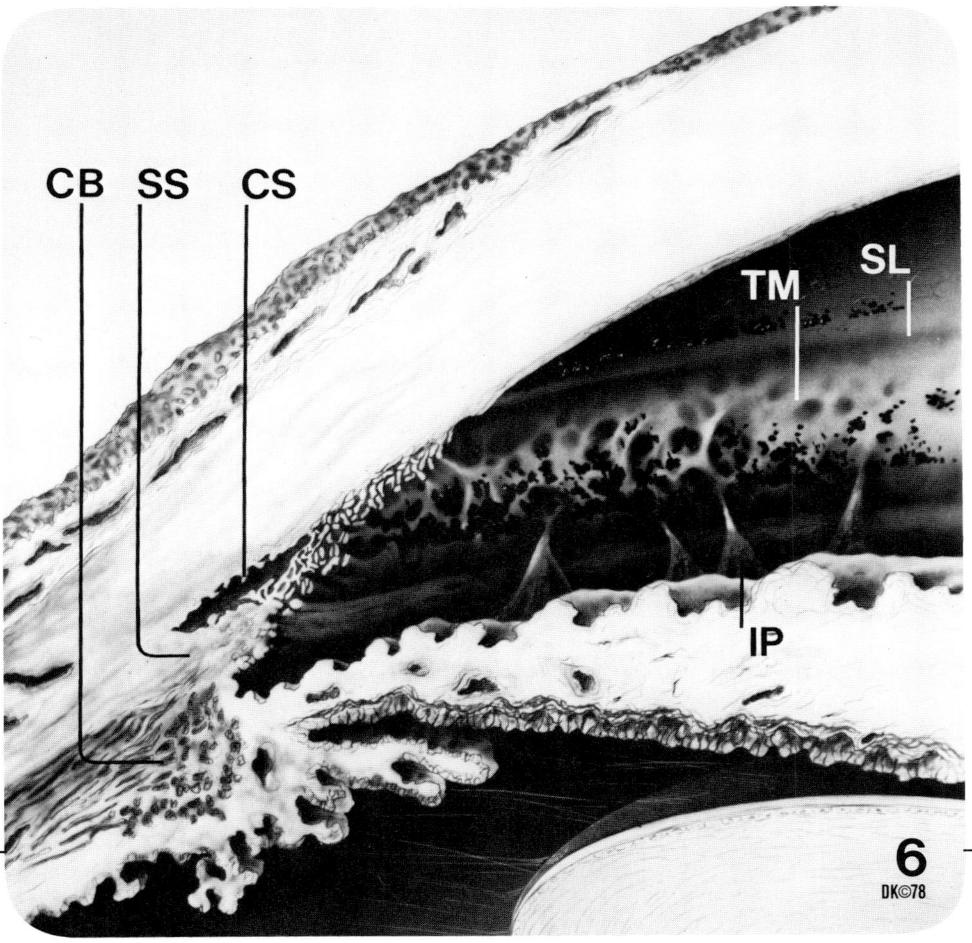

Donald A. Keller

The Zeiss four-mirror gonioscope [7], a special type of indirect gonioscopic lens, affords a quick screening evaluation of the chamber angle without the annoyance of application of gonioscopic gel between the lens and the cornea. Consequently, gonioscopy with a Zeiss lens permits other tests to be done immediately afterward because the patient's vision is not blurred, the cornea is not gummy, and the view into the eye is not obscured. These are obvious advantages when the physician is trying to evaluate an eye with a dangerously occludable angle before and after doing a darkroom provocative test for angle-closure glaucoma.

Indentation gonioscopy [8] is a technique whereby the examiner indents the central cornea with the tip of the Zeiss gonioscope, which forces the peripheral iris away from the chamber angle. This may be useful in situations where the angle is not readily seen, such as plateau iris or angle closure. This procedure permits better visualization of structures previously obscured by the iris, such as peripheral anterior synechiae, peripheral iris neovascularization, and inflammatory deposits. To achieve this visualization, the examiner aligns the central cornea, the Zeiss lens, and the slit-lamp oculars. The cornea is anesthetized, and the lens is gently centered on the cornea. Any deviation from this alignment—the moving of the patient's eye, for example—interferes with visualization of the chamber angle. Gentle pressure is then applied to the central cornea. This pushes the peripheral iris posteriorly, which provides for visualization of the previously obscured angle. In addition, the examiner cannot rotate the lens. The Zeiss lens is a valuable adjunct in gonioscopic evaluation but is not to be used to the exclusion of other instruments.

With direct gonioscopy (the Koeppe lens) [9], the observer views the angle directly through the smooth-domed lens, using a direct light source and a simple magnifying system, such as a hand-held binocular microscope. The examiner may sacrifice visualization of some fine intraocular details for a broad view of the chamber angle. The direct gonioscopic lens allows visualization of the chamber angle even in the face of central corneal opacities. This panoramic view helps orient the observer to important angle landmarks—the trabecular meshwork, scleral spur, and ciliary body, TM, SS, and CB [9]. With the use of sclerotic scatter, trabecular meshwork, iris processes, IP [9], and a portion of the ciliary body usually stand out vividly. Moreover, the extent of peripheral anterior synechiae, PAS [9] is easily appreciated by this technique. When the examiner is dealing with a recessed or traumatized angle, both eyes can be compared effectively, and differences between the injured and the noninjured eye become readily apparent.

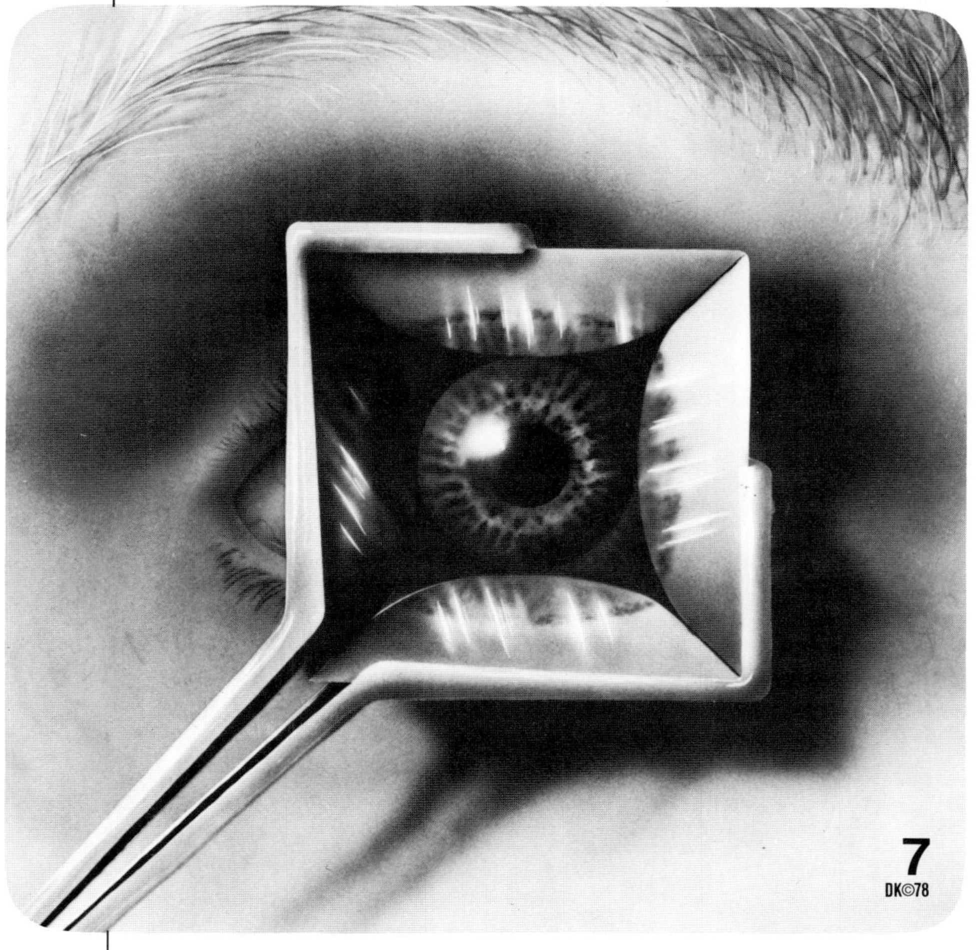

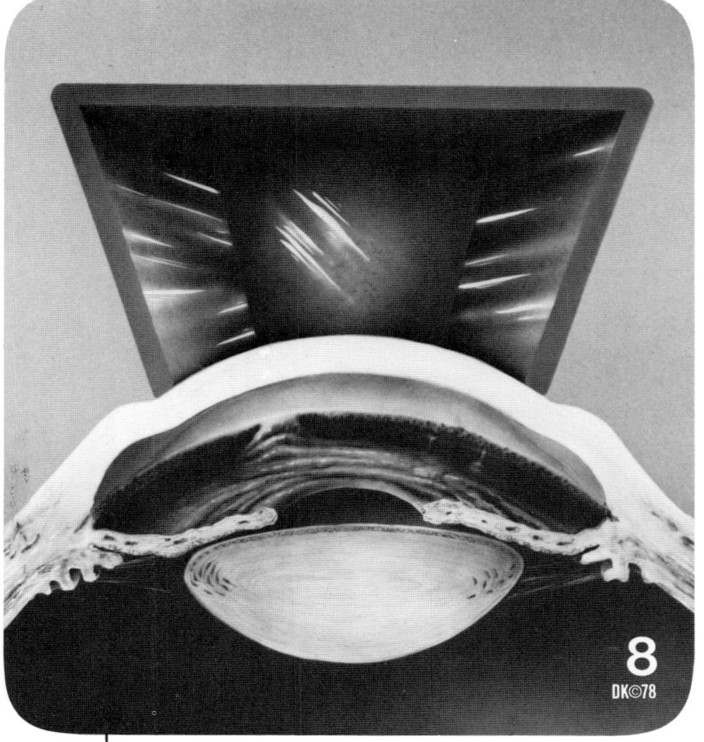

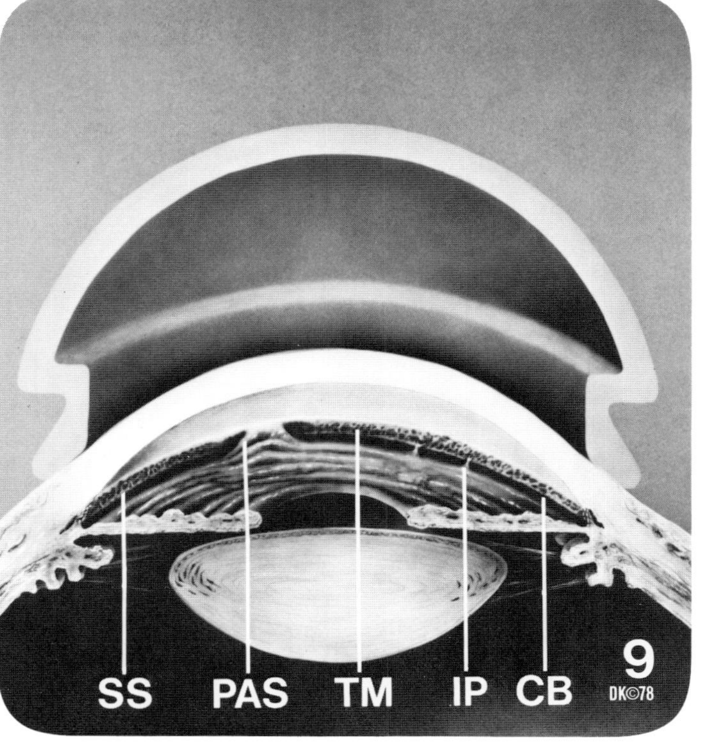

Donald A. Keller

PERIPHERAL IRIDECTOMY

Frederick M. Kapetansky, M.D.

In an eye afflicted with acute angle-closure glaucoma, the normal flow of aqueous humor from the ciliary processes, where it is produced, through the pupillary aperture into the anterior chamber, where it is absorbed through the trabecular meshwork, is interrupted or halted altogether. This interruption of aqueous flow at the pupillary border results from the iris sphincter pressing posteriorly against the anterior lens surface, thereby creating a pupillary block. When this pupillary block inhibits the flow of aqueous sufficiently, the peripheral iris is pushed against the trabecular meshwork producing iris bombé. As a direct consequence of this iris-trabecular meshwork contact, the intraocular pressure rises. Excision of any portion of the iris permits the aqueous humor to leave the posterior chamber and enter the anterior chamber by a route other than via the pupillary area. This rerouting of aqueous flow prevents both the development of an iris bombé and the subsequent contact of the peripheral iris with the cornea and trabecular meshwork. In many ways, the peripheral iridectomy, when performed for primary angle-closure glaucoma, represents one of the most successful operations in ophthalmology.

Before an iridectomy can be performed, intraocular pressure is lowered to normal or below normal levels. Instillation of a drop of pilocarpine 1 percent or 2 percent every 15 to 30 minutes opens the anterior chamber angle by pulling the iris away from the cornea. As a practical matter, an osmotic agent such as glycerol or mannitol is usually necessary to lower the intraocular pressure to a level at which the iris sphincter responds to pilocarpine. Preoperative gonioscopic confirmation that the anterior chamber angle has indeed been opened helps insure a satisfactory surgical result.

When the need for peripheral iridectomy has been determined, the surgeon may decide to proceed immediately to the operating room or to defer operation until the eye is less inflamed (usually not more than 24 to 48 hours). I recommend that surgery be done as soon as the operating room is available with its regular staff of trained personnel. There seems to be little indication or advantage in the performance of an "emergency" iridectomy.

The use of a conjunctival flap is optional when performing an iridectomy. If the surgeon prefers a conjunctival flap, a 4-mm peritomy at the 12-o'clock meridian permits direct visualization of the surgical limbus [1].

While a fine-toothed forceps stabilizes the sclera just posterior to the surgical limbus, an ab externo incision is made into the anterior chamber with either a No. 69 Beaver blade [2] or a razor blade, or both may be used. The exact placement of this incision is extremely important. Care must be taken to place the incision in the anterior, A [3] or middle, M [3] region of the surgical limbus, thereby avoiding the posterior reaches of the limbus, P [3]. In addition, the incision is made

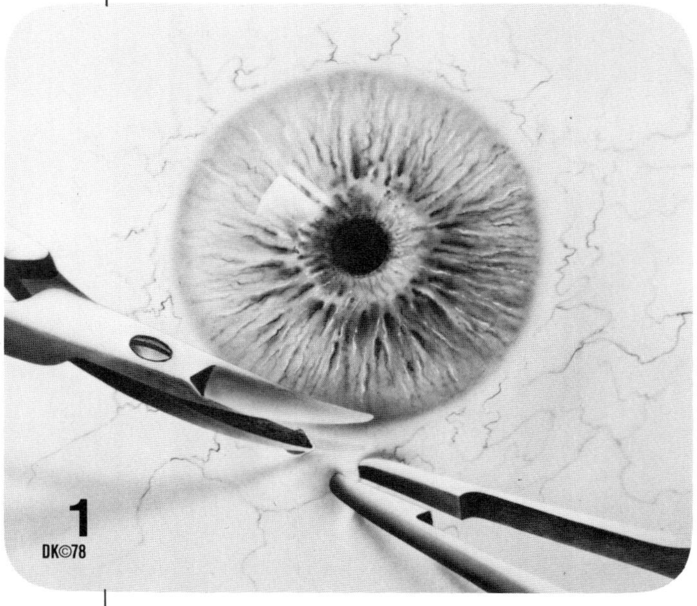

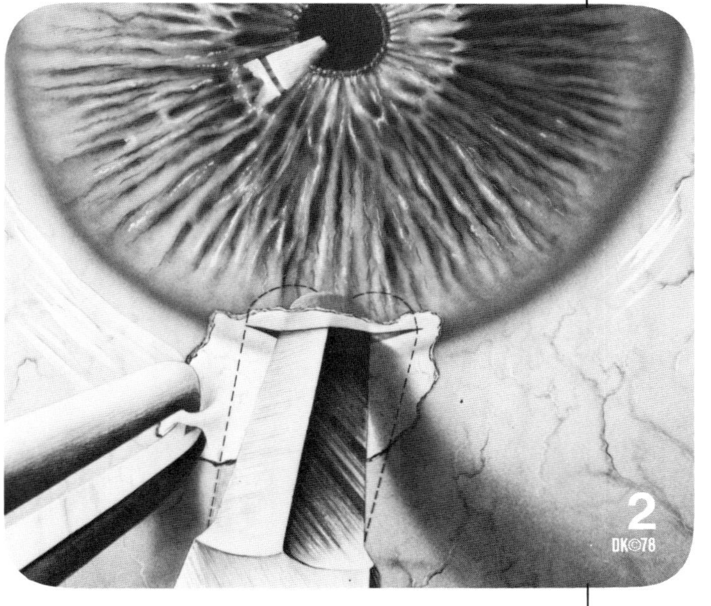

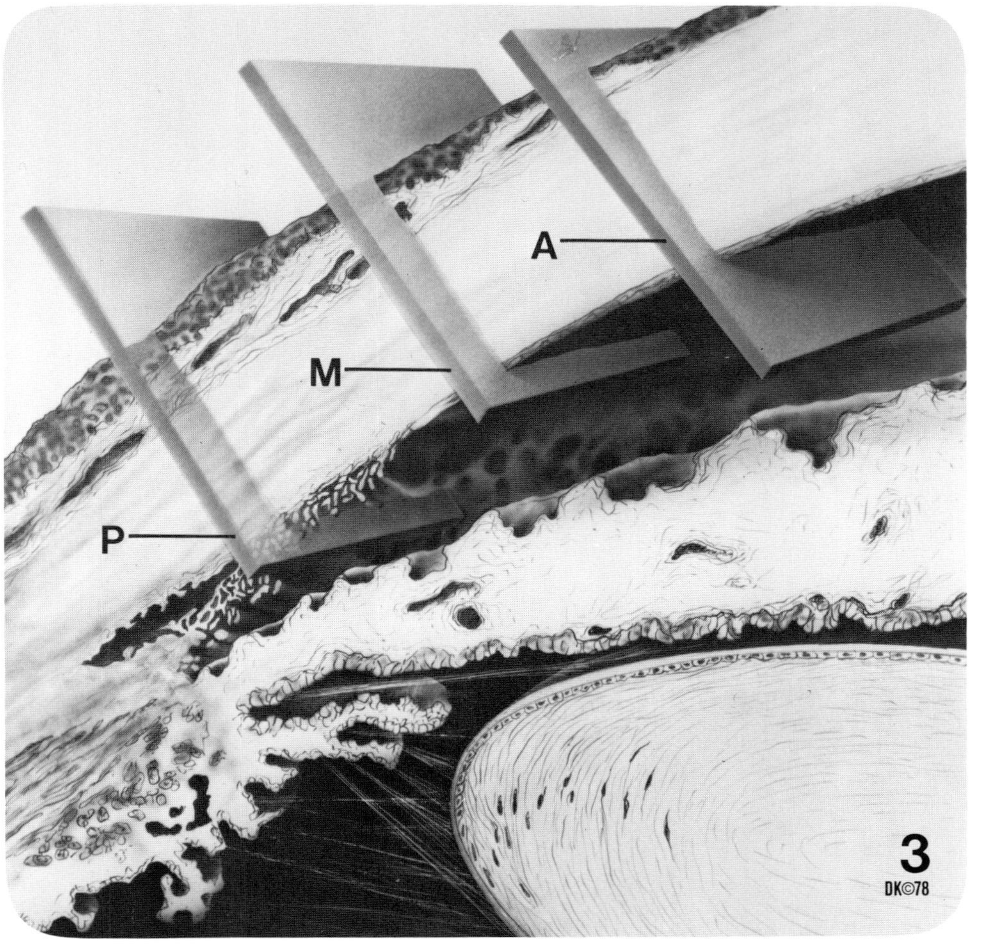

Donald A. Killar

perpendicular to the surface of the cornea, P [4] to avoid shelving. The posterior corneal flap produced by a shelving incision, S [4] tends to interfere or may even prevent subsequent iris prolapse.

The limbal incision is at least 3 mm long as measured with calipers, since estimates of length, when viewed through the operating microscope, tend to be inaccurate. The internal corneal incision measures the same 3 mm as the external corneal incision [5]. To achieve this squaring off, the surgeon makes the first full-thickness cut with a razor blade from left to right. Then the surgeon inverts the blade to complete the incision to the left [6]. An inadequate internal opening may interfere with iris prolapse.

With the anterior edge of the incision held with a fine-toothed (0.12-mm) forceps in one hand and the posterior edge with a similar forceps in the other hand, the surgeon may gently separate the wound edges to permit iris prolapse [7]. Alternatively, the surgeon may press on the posterior lip of the wound to cause iris prolapse. If the iris does not prolapse readily, the internal extent of the wound may not be the necessary 3 mm. If this is determined, it should be corrected. If either of these methods fails to prolapse the iris, the surgeon may reach inside the wound to extract the iris with forceps.

A fine-toothed (0.12-mm) forceps withdraws the prolapsed iris further from the incision, and with a small scissors, a piece of the iris is excised tangential to the limbus.

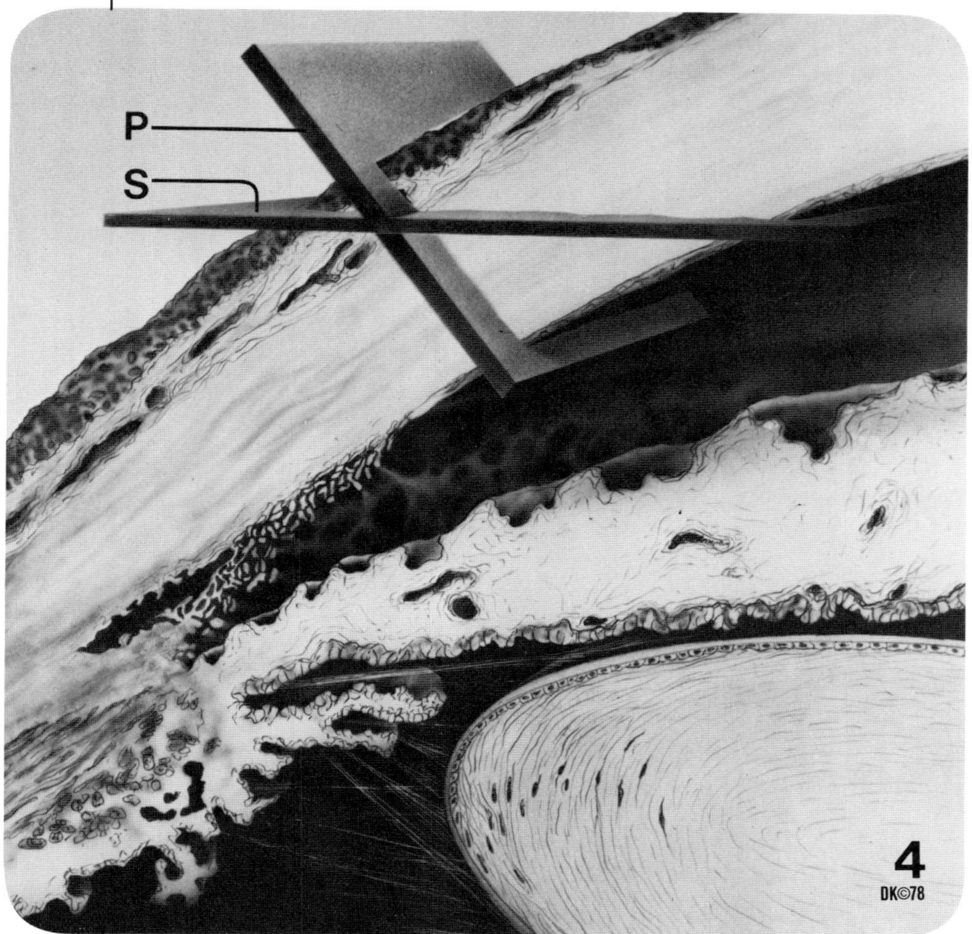

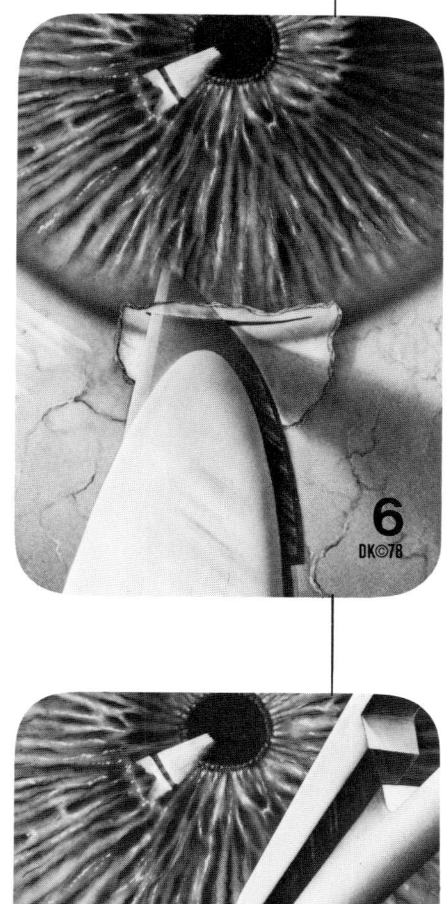

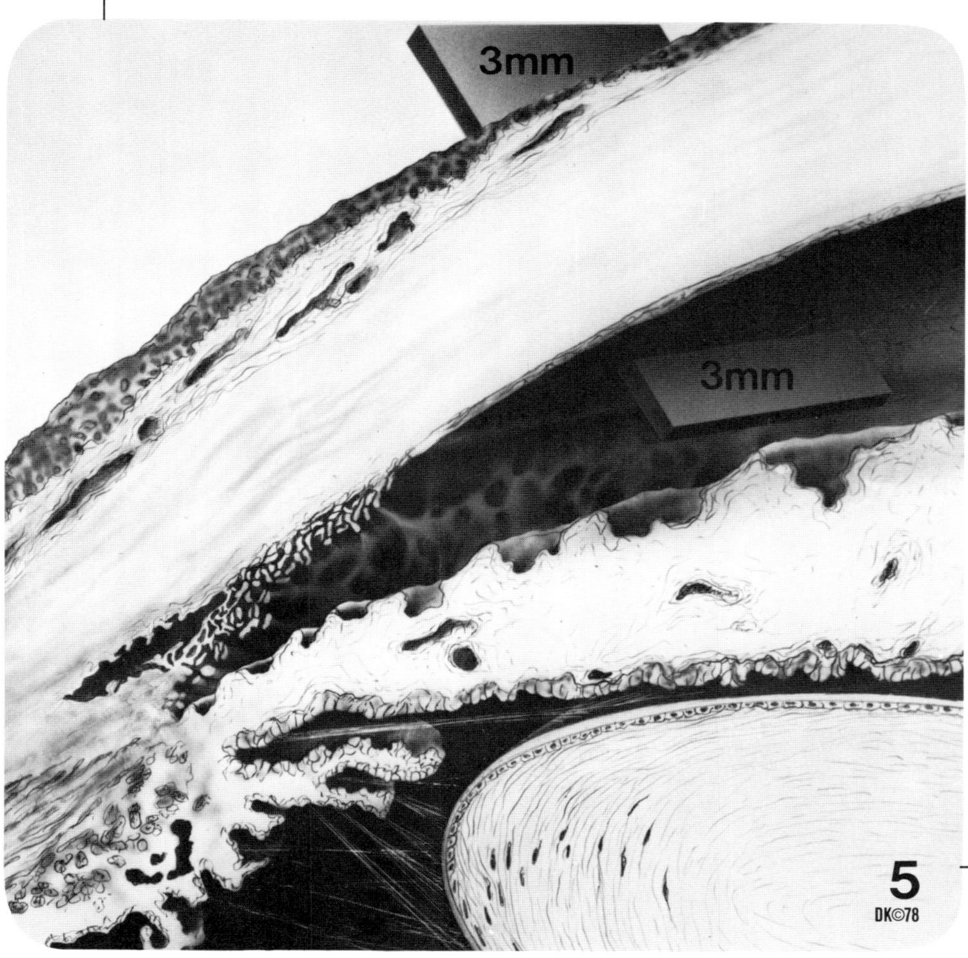

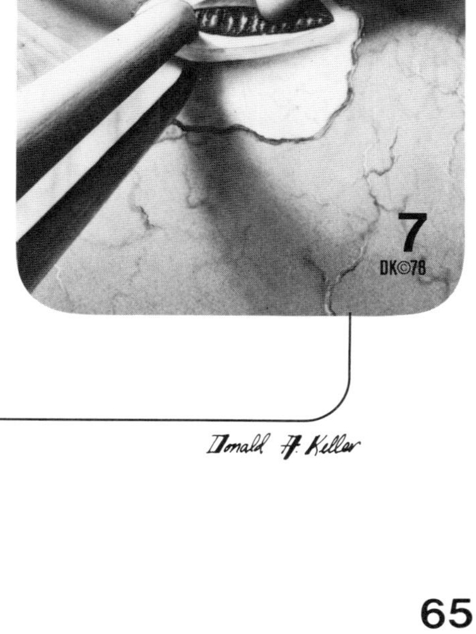

Donald A. Keller

This tangential cut insures a broad peripheral iridectomy [8]. If the iris pillars do not reposit spontaneously, the surgeon may lift the anterior edge of the incision with a fine-toothed forceps and irrigate the wound with balanced salt solution using a 27- or 30-gauge irrigating cannula [9]. An iridectomy larger than the corneal incision tends to avoid the problem of repositing the iris, since the edges of the iridectomy extend beyond the length of the corneal incision.

At the surgeon's option, a solution of acetylcholine 1 percent may be irrigated into the anterior chamber through a 27- or 30-gauge cannula to induce rapid miosis.

To ascertain that the iridectomy penetrated the iris completely, the surgeon should inspect the undersurface of the excised iris for jet-black uveal pigment, or the surgeon may shine the coaxial light of the operating microscope directly through the pupil and observe the red reflex through the iridectomy.

Two interrupted 10-0 nylon sutures on a half-circle needle are placed 1 mm apart at a depth of one-half the corneal thickness to reappose the anterior and posterior edges of the wound [10]. Although the conjunctival flap does not require a suture, the surgeon may choose to close the conjunctiva with a single 10-0 nylon suture knotted on the conjunctiva's underside [10].

A watertight seal [11] is important because wound leakage after an iridectomy has disastrous consequences. It leads to a flat anterior chamber with the inevitable formation of permanent peripheral anterior synechiae.

Postoperatively, the pupil is dilated with mydriatic (phenylephrine hydrochloride) or cycloplegic (cyclopentolate hydrochloride) drops daily until all postoperative reaction subsides. The use of steroid eye drops is optional. Caution should be exercised in the prolonged use of topical corticosteroids since steroid glaucoma may develop in a genetically predisposed eye. Although there may well be a transient elevation of intraocular pressure during the first 24 to 48 hours after a successful iridectomy, this occurrence should not prompt the surgeon to institute glaucoma therapy. Allowing the eye to respond over time appears to be the prudent course to follow.

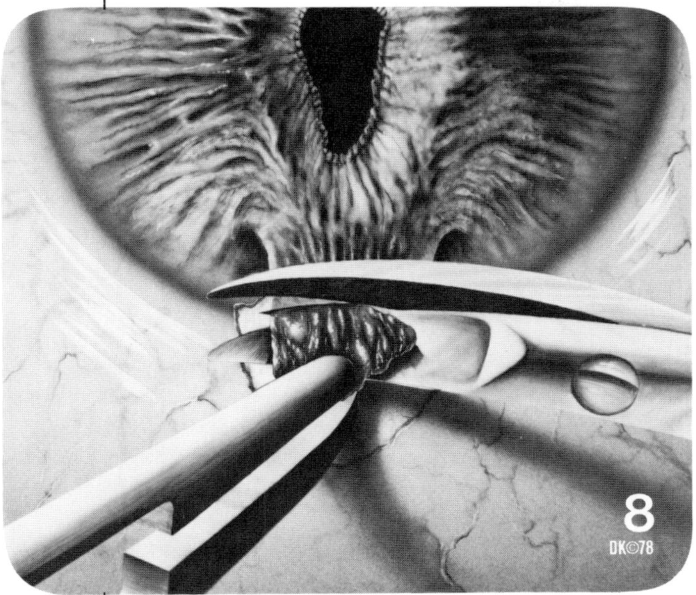

8
DK©78

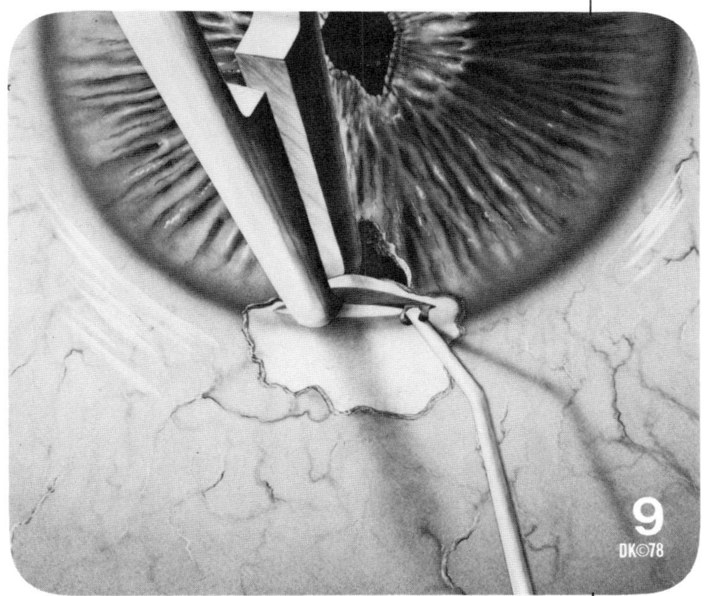

9
DK©78

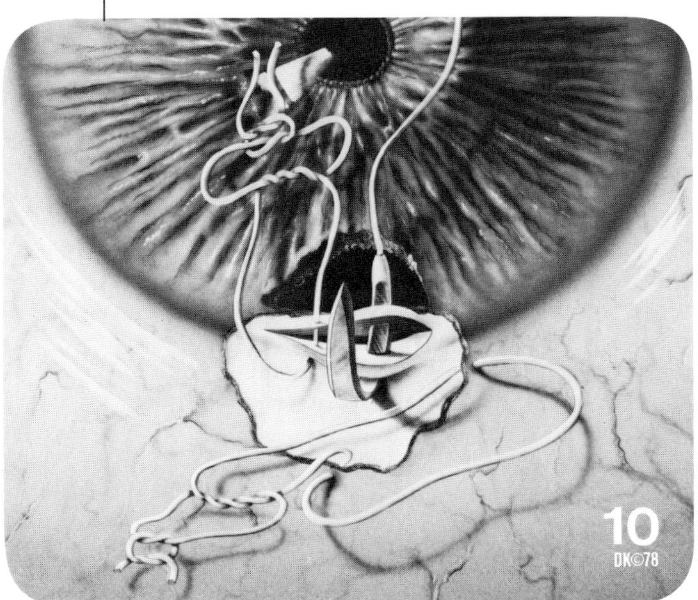

10
DK©78

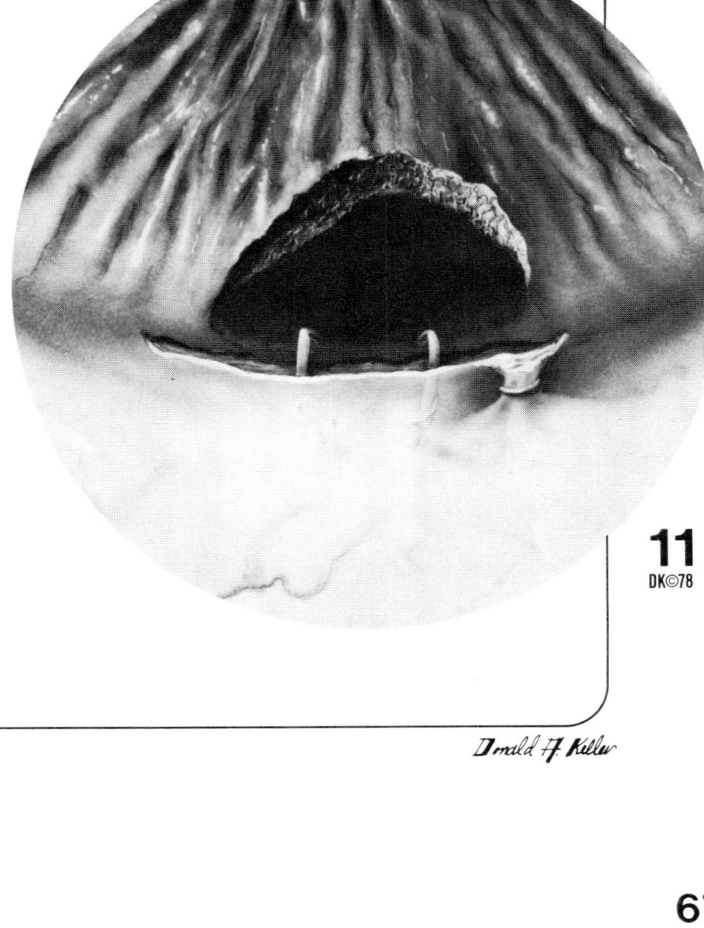

11
DK©78

Donald A. Keller

TRABECULECTOMY

Frederick M. Kapetansky, M.D.

If chronic simple glaucoma is an insidious, ischemic assault on the structures of the optic nerve head, then lowering the intraocular pressure is certainly a reasonable method of minimizing this ischemic process. Chronic simple glaucoma, in which the anterior chamber angle appears open, presents some obstruction to the flow of aqueous humor through the area of the trabecular meshwork and canal of Schlemm. Only in the face of an optic nerve that is susceptible to an ischemic process is the build-up of intraocular pressure significant. Many healthy eyes experience an increase in pressure, but only those eyes that are predisposed to an ischemic process will succumb to the effects of this elevated pressure.

When maximum medical therapy (i.e., miotics, epinephrine, and carbonic anhydrase inhibitors) fails to normalize the intraocular pressure and prevent progression of damage to the optic nerve and the further loss of vision, then surgical intervention represents a reasonable alternative. The goal of every operation for chronic simple glaucoma is to establish an aqueous outflow channel that will bypass the trabecular meshwork and canal of Schlemm and permit aqueous to drain from the anterior chamber to the subconjunctival space. Minimal disruption of the anatomy and physiology of the eye by the surgical procedure will preserve as much undistorted vision as possible.

Trabeculectomy is the operation I prefer to treat this disease. Many other types of filtering procedures are known to the ophthalmic surgeon—sclerectomy, thermal sclerostomy, trephination, and iridencleisis—and each has its advocates. I prefer the newer technique of trabeculectomy because it is the least traumatic, is easy to teach, and is easy to do, especially by the general ophthalmologist who may perform only one or two each year. It also has a lower complication rate than other glaucoma procedures. Most procedures seem to achieve about 90 percent success of lowering intraocular pressure.

There are additional advantages of trabeculectomy. The scleral flap covering the opening controls the rate of aqueous flow from the eye, and with gradual aqueous outflow, the anterior chamber is less likely to collapse during the immediate postoperative period. Due to the atraumatic nature of this procedure, postoperative morbidity is minimal. It is too early in the history of the procedure to ascertain the risk of cataract formation after a trabeculectomy.

General anesthesia circumvents the use of orbital injection of an anesthetic solution, with its attendant risk of hemorrhage, although local anesthesia may be the preference of some surgeons. Just prior to the incision, the anesthesiologist should inject 50 ml of 25 percent mannitol intravenously over a five-minute period. This gradually lowers the intraocular pressure.

Under low magnification, lidocaine with epinephrine is injected under the conjunctiva [1] through a 25-gauge needle to outline the area for dissection and to constrict the blood vessels that have been dilated by the constant use of glaucoma medication. A Castroviejo 0.12-mm forceps lifts the conjunctiva to prevent injection into the superior rectus muscle. The fluid dissects down to the limbus. In a previously operated eye, the blister that forms on the conjunctiva is the area with the least scarring and the most potential for effective drainage.

The conjunctival incision, made with microscopic corneal scissors, extends from the 11- to 1-o'clock positions at a distance of 10 mm from the corneoscleral limbus [2]. A 7-0 chromic catgut suture retracts the conjunctival flap. If the surgeon directs the scissors toward the limbus during the subconjunctival dissection, Tenon's capsule drops down out of the way [3]. A section of the underlying free Tenon's capsule is excised with corneal scissors in a shape that roughly approximates the size of the scleral flap to be made [4].

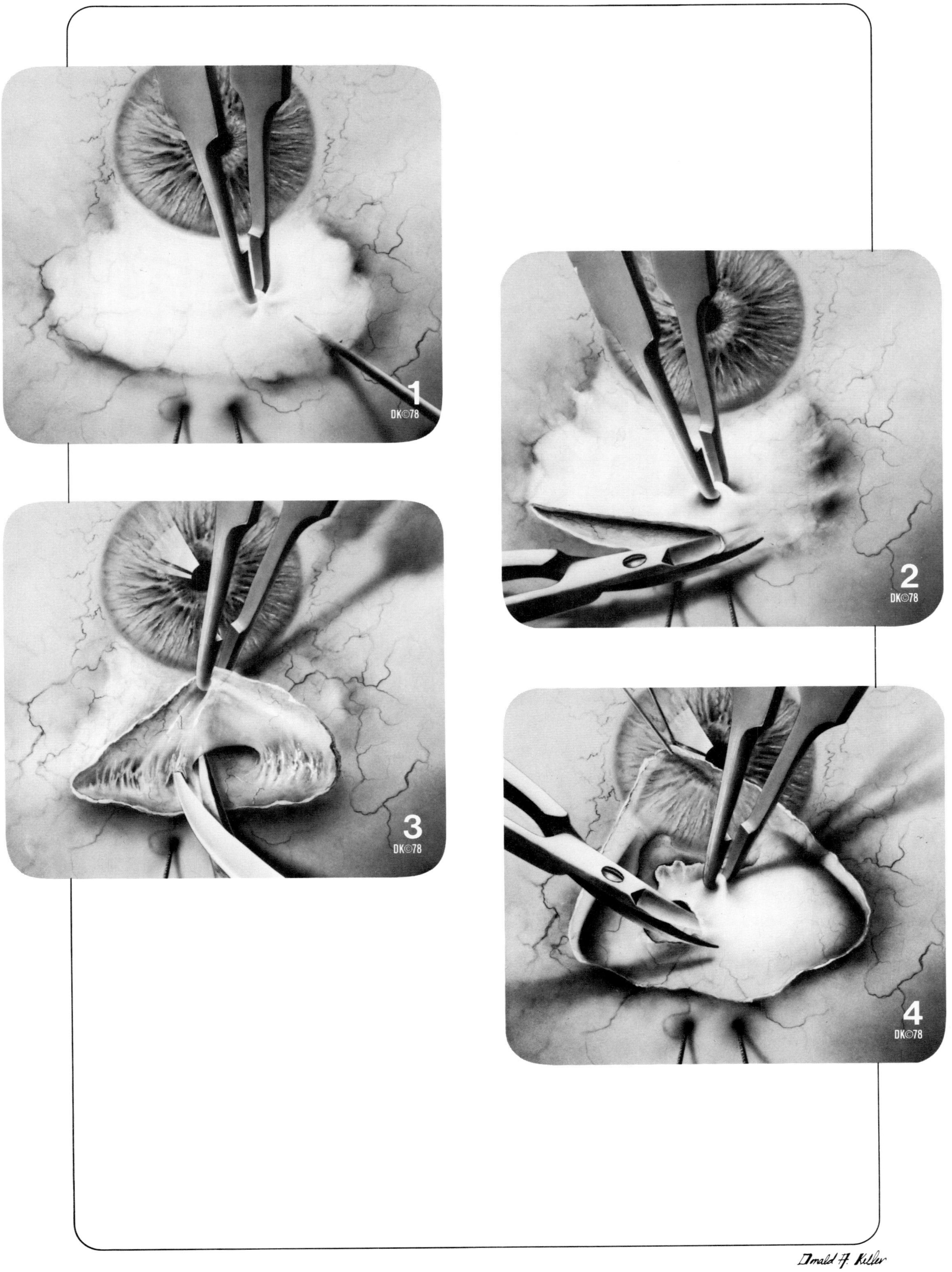
1
DK©78
2
DK©78
3
DK©78
4
DK©78

This partial excision of Tenon's capsule may prevent scarring and obliteration of the drainage opening to be created. There is a risk that the removal of too much Tenon's capsule will compromise the eye's ability to ward off infection. Nevertheless, I believe that the risk is worthwhile because intraocular pressures have not been as low as expected after trabeculectomy, possibly because Tenon's capsule compromised aqueous outflow.

Calipers set at 5 mm measure the size of the scleral flap [5] . Cautery points demarcate the corners of the square. Under higher magnification, a sharp, No. 69 Beaver blade penetrates half the scleral thickness [6] [7] . A Pierse forceps grasps the tissue without tearing it and raises the corner of the flap, while a dull Beaver blade separates the lamellae of the sclera [8] . The action of the surgeon is a combination of steady traction with the Pierse forceps and pressure with the dull Beaver blade.

The scleral flap, hinged at the limbus, is retracted lightly with a 7-0 chromic catgut suture. To remove the inner sclera, the surgeon makes two radial incisions with a razor blade, 3 mm long and 0.5 mm inside the trap door incision, through the remaining half-thickness of sclera. At this point, the eye begins to decompress, and the intraocular pressure lowers slowly. A circumferential razor blade cut through clear cornea connects the radial incisions [9] . Bulging iris fills the opening and prevents aqueous from

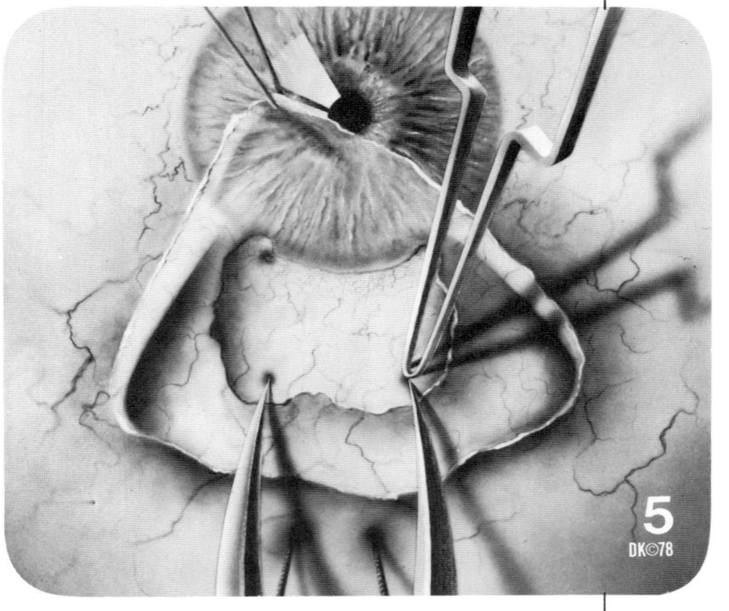

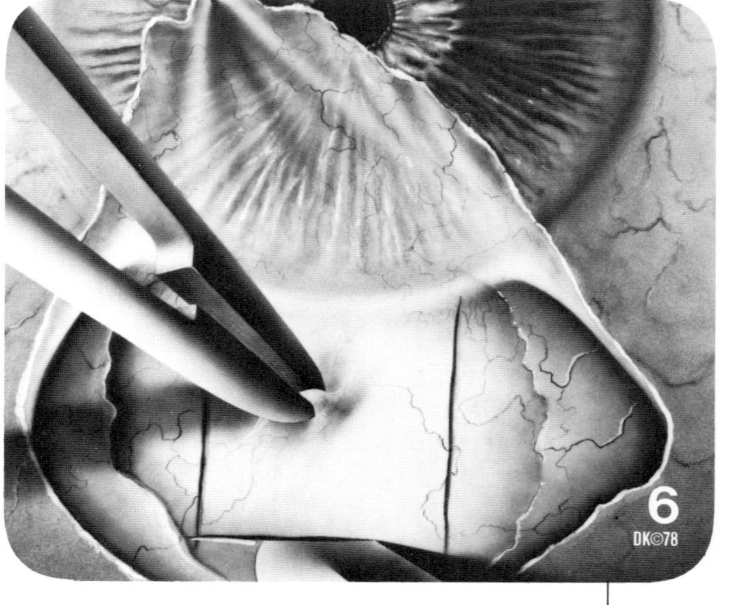

Donald F. Kilder

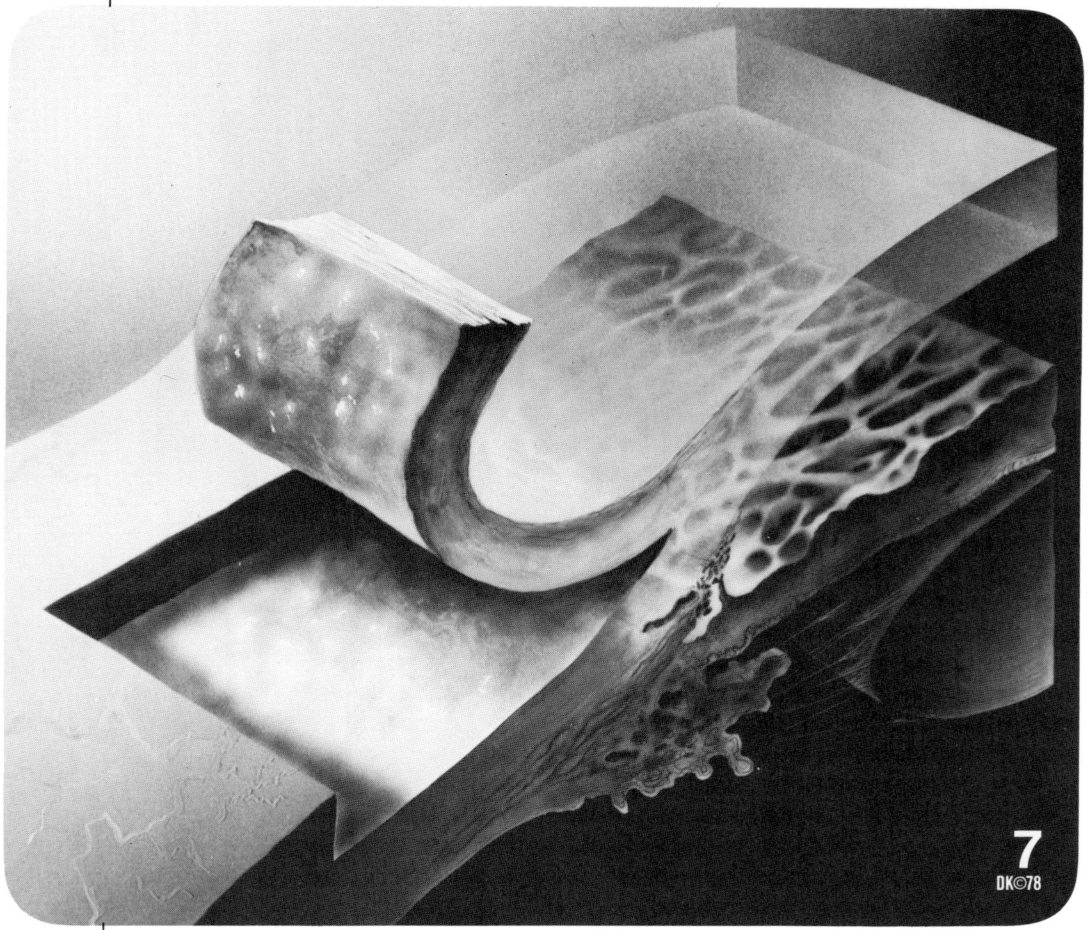

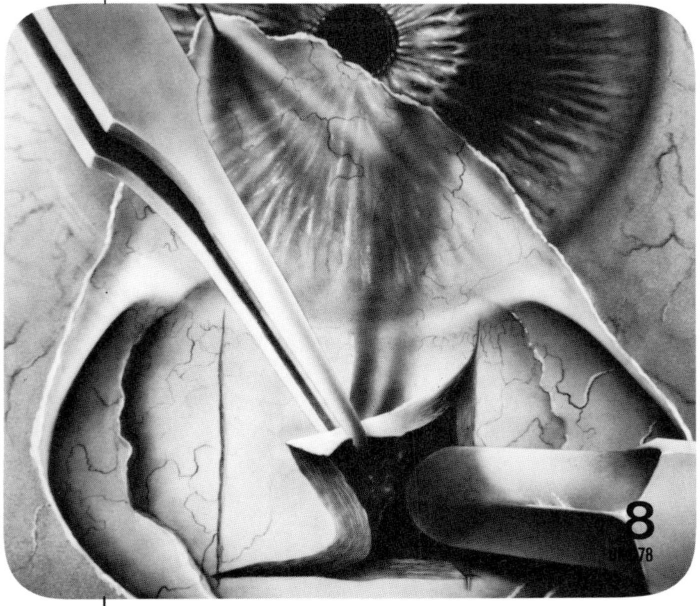

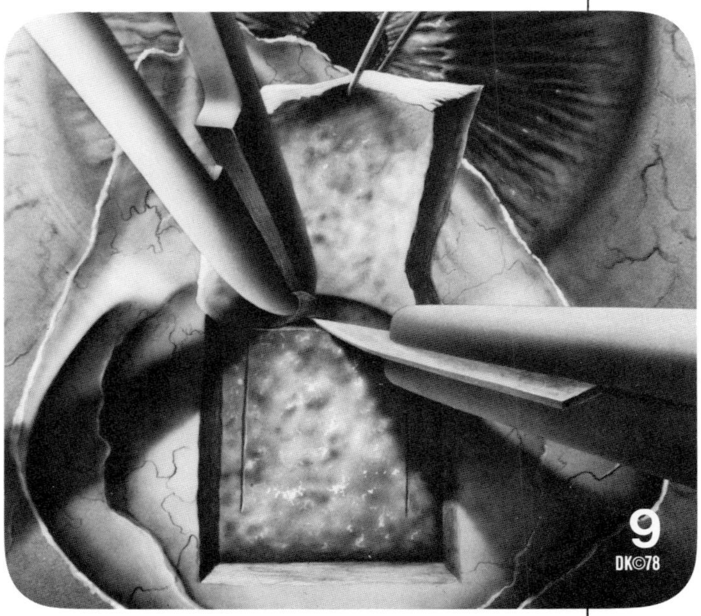

Donald F. Keller

gushing out of the eye. If the iris prolapses into the wound, a 25-gauge needle deflates the iris, aqueous trickles from behind it, and the iris recedes [10]

The inner sclera is retracted with 0.12-mm forceps and dissected free from the underlying ciliary body by dividing the scleral spur with fine microscopic scissors [11] [12] .

The 0.12-mm forceps grasps the iris, and a peripheral iridectomy is done [13] . Care is taken to withdraw the iris slightly to avoid damage to the underlying lens. The iridectomy must be larger than the 3-mm incision into the anterior chamber so as not to interfere with the subsequent aqueous flow. The iridectomy eliminates pupillary block and prevents iris prolapse into the trabeculectomy site.

The scleral flap is replaced, and the corners are sutured loosely with 10-0 nylon [14]. The conjunctival flap, closed tightly with a running, locking 7-0 chromic catgut suture, covers the scleral dissection [15]. The locking conjunctival suture prevents aqueous from leaking out from under the conjunctiva. While still in the operating room, the patient receives 10 percent phenylephrine hydrochloride drops to induce immediate pupillary dilatation. Antibiotic ointment, a patch, and shield are applied.

On the first postoperative day, infection must be ruled out. The patient receives 10 percent phenylephrine hydrochloride, 1 percent atropine sulfate, and possibly 1 percent cyclopentolate hydrochloride, as well as a steroid-antibiotic eye drop. A six-week course of high doses of steroids delays the healing process and keeps the scleral flap open to simulate a normal outflow channel. If the patient develops steroid glaucoma after several weeks' treatment, steroids may be stopped as long as drainage is evident. Pressure will lower with tapering or cessation of steroids. As soon as the reaction in the eye subsides, dilation of the pupil may be stopped (one to two weeks' course).

Eyes restore themselves to their normal shape very quickly after surgery. Collapse of the anterior chamber is a rare complication of this procedure. The postoperative incidence of cataract with this procedure remains to be determined.

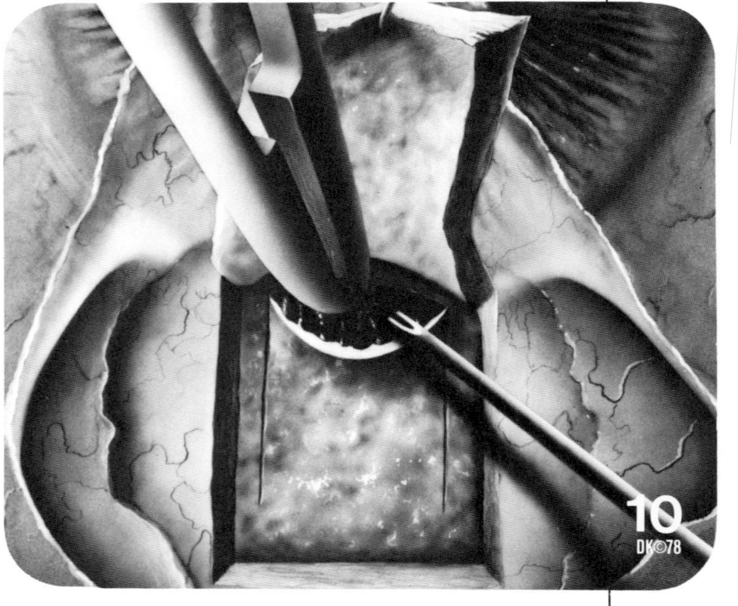

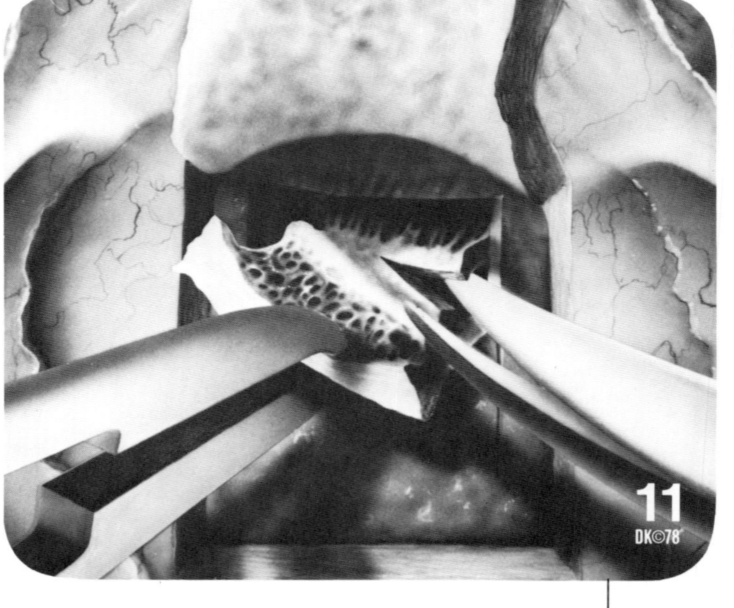

Donald A. Keller

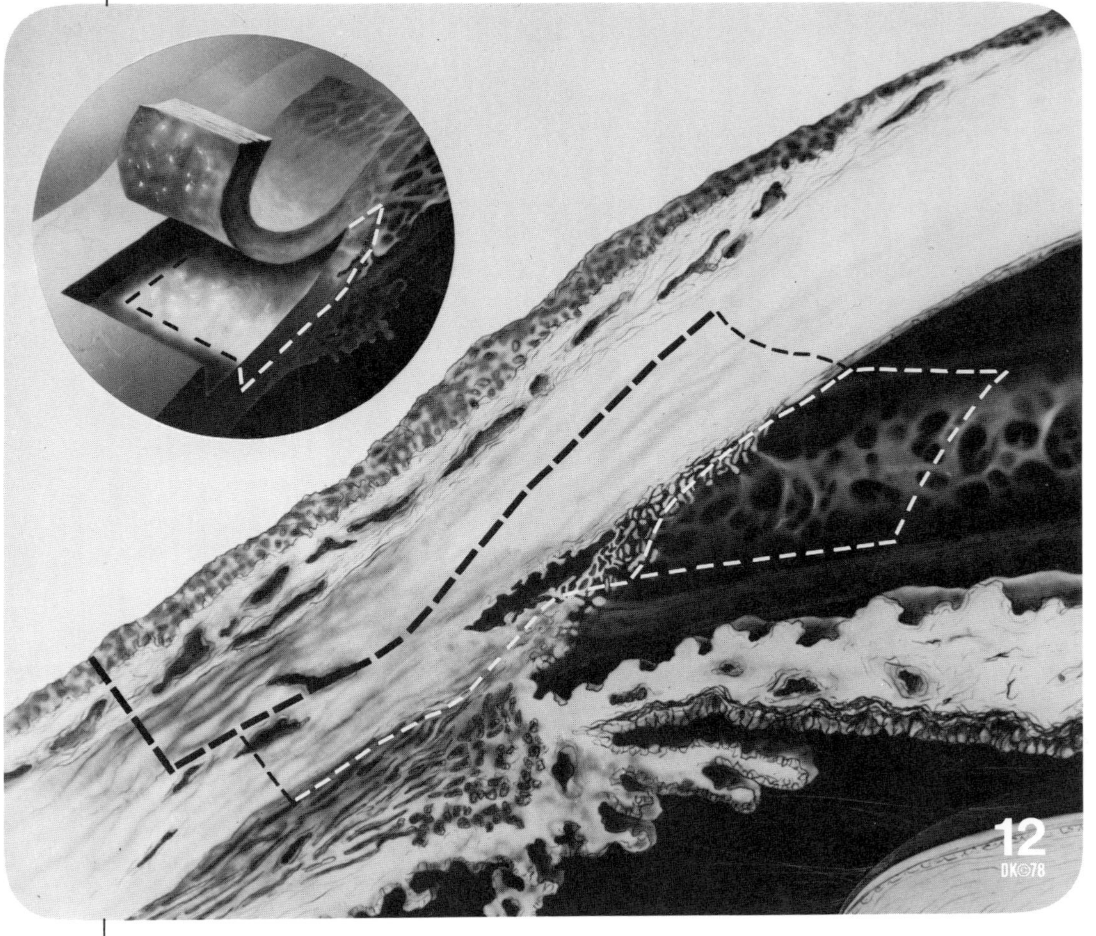

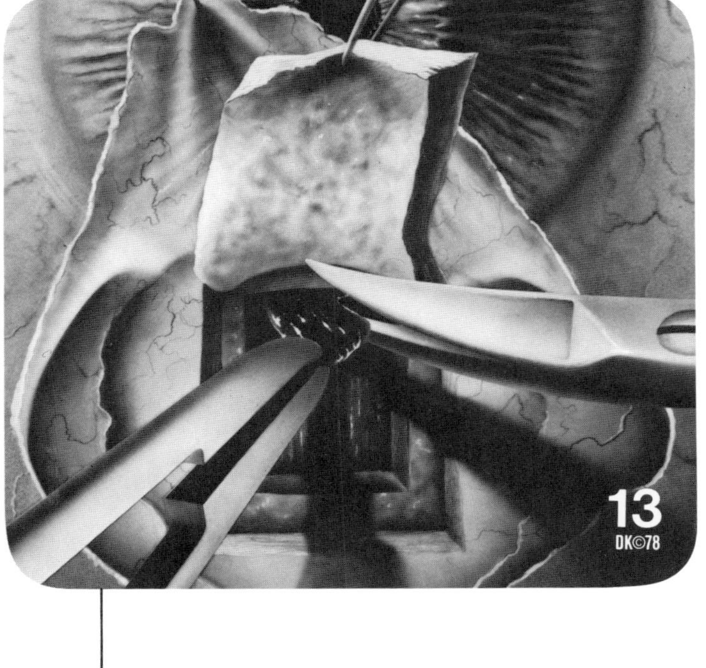

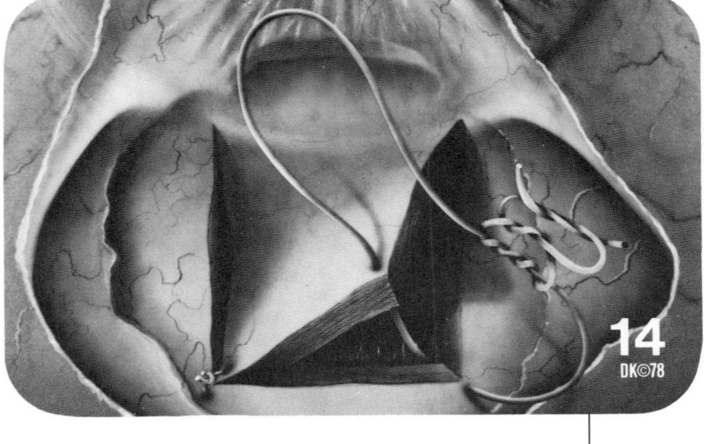

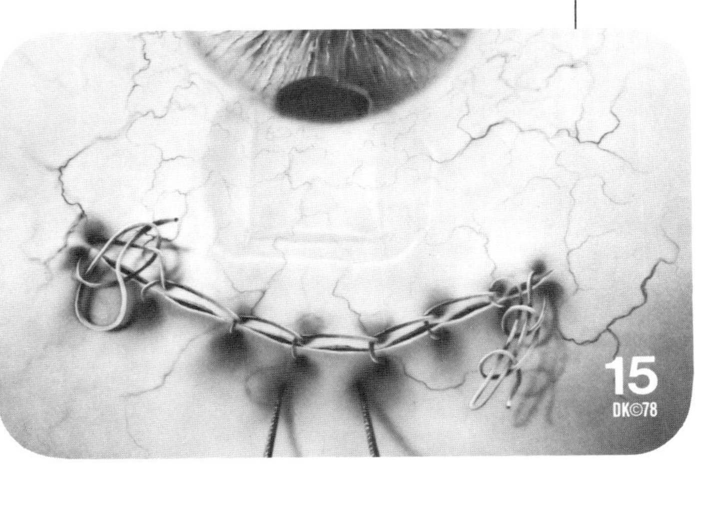

Donald A. Kelber

CYCLOCRYOTHERAPY

Frederick M. Kapetansky, M.D.

The surgical correction of glaucoma focuses on either improving aqueous outflow through filtering operations or reducing aqueous production through ciliary body destruction.

The destruction of the ciliary body epithelium by heat has been used for decades to reduce aqueous production. The discovery that hypothermia also was effective was a major therapeutic breakthrough. Since diathermy was destructive to the sclera and ciliary body, many eyes became phthisical following treatment. Cyclocryotherapy is much more easily controlled and safer than cyclodiathermy. The operative technique is quite simple. Akinesia and anesthesia are obtained with a retrobulbar block. A sterile field is not necessary. Before the probe is applied, the surface of the limbal area must be dried thoroughly with a cotton-tipped applicator to prevent the spread of the cold across the surface which helps to prevent an excessively large ice ball.

Cryotherapy machines commonly used in retinal surgery are quite suitable for use in cyclocryotherapy. Liquid nitrogen serves as the coolant. We recommend the use of a 2-mm retinal probe since it can be precisely applied, and the temperature of the tip is both controllable and measureable. Cold is transmitted through the sclera to the ciliary body to involve eventually the pigmented epithelial layer of the ciliary body.

Cyclocryotherapy is best applied when the glaucoma is recalcitrant to other forms of medical management. When a blind, painful eye is involved, cyclocryotherapy can be used to relieve pain and frequently avoid enucleation.

A tendency exists to place the probe too far posteriorly in order to avoid freezing the cornea; consequently, the ciliary body is not frozen. It must be remembered that the ciliary body extends from the limbus 3.5 mm posteriorly, and the ciliary body epithelium lies 1.5 mm below the scleral surface [1]. Therefore, if the ciliary body is to be adequately frozen, the probe should be placed approximately 1.5 mm from the limbus. It is impossible to avoid freezing some of the peripheral cornea. Since the radius of the ice ball is slightly greater than 1.5 mm, the area frozen by the probe extends posteriorly approximately 3 mm from the surgical limbus to a depth of 1.5 mm.

The surgeon holds the probe on the surface of the eye for one full minute at each point to achieve maximum freezing [2]. The temperature of the probe is adjusted between -70° C to -80° C. Immediately after the probe is removed, the treated area is stark-white, frozen, avascular, and has a slight dimple where the probe was located. The sclera defrosts within one minute. After thawing, the frozen area is indistinguishable; therefore, the surgeon must establish a systematic pattern of freezing. Twelve applications of the cryoprobe are spaced uniformly around the globe [3].

To minimize postoperative inflammation, we recommend a subconjunctival injection of 0.5 ml of an aqueous solution of corticosteroids in the two inferior quadrants. In addition, topical atropine should be applied once a day and corticosteroid four times a day until postoperative inflammation subsides.

The effect of freezing the ciliary body is variable. In those instances where only transient lowering of the pressure is obtained, the procedure may be repeated.

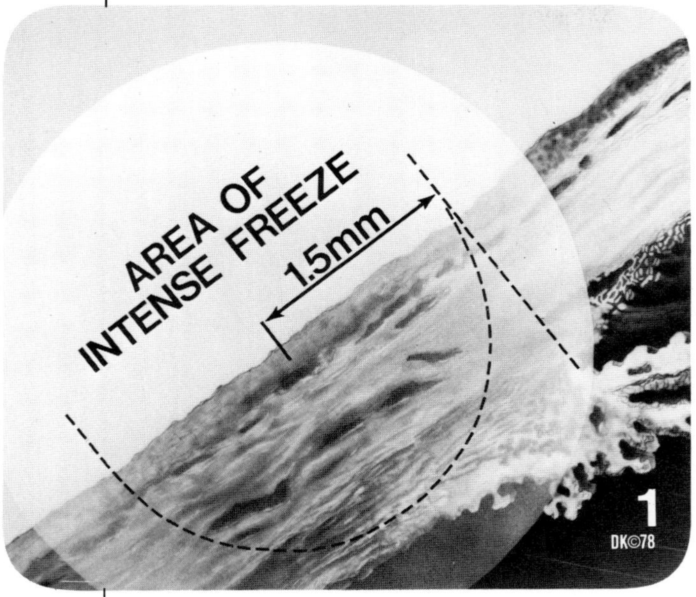

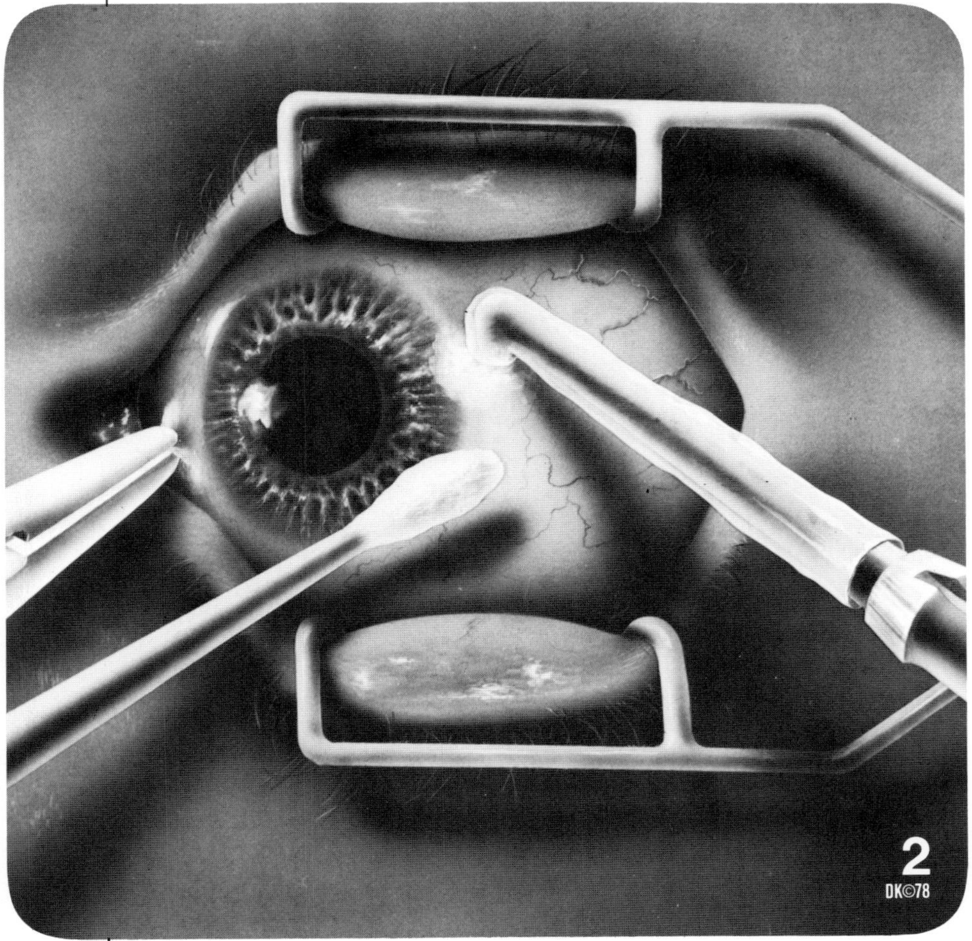

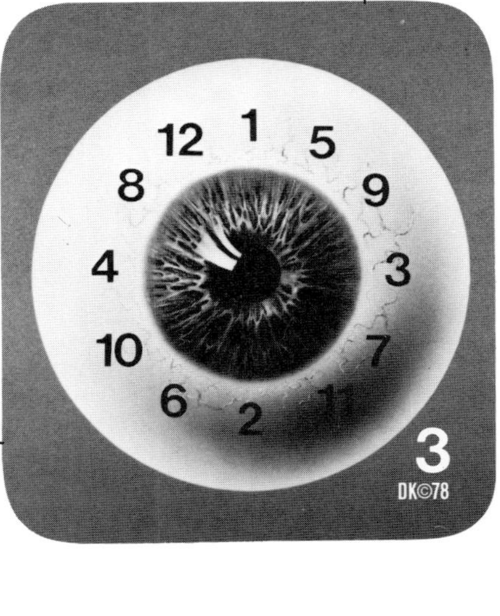

Donald A. Keller

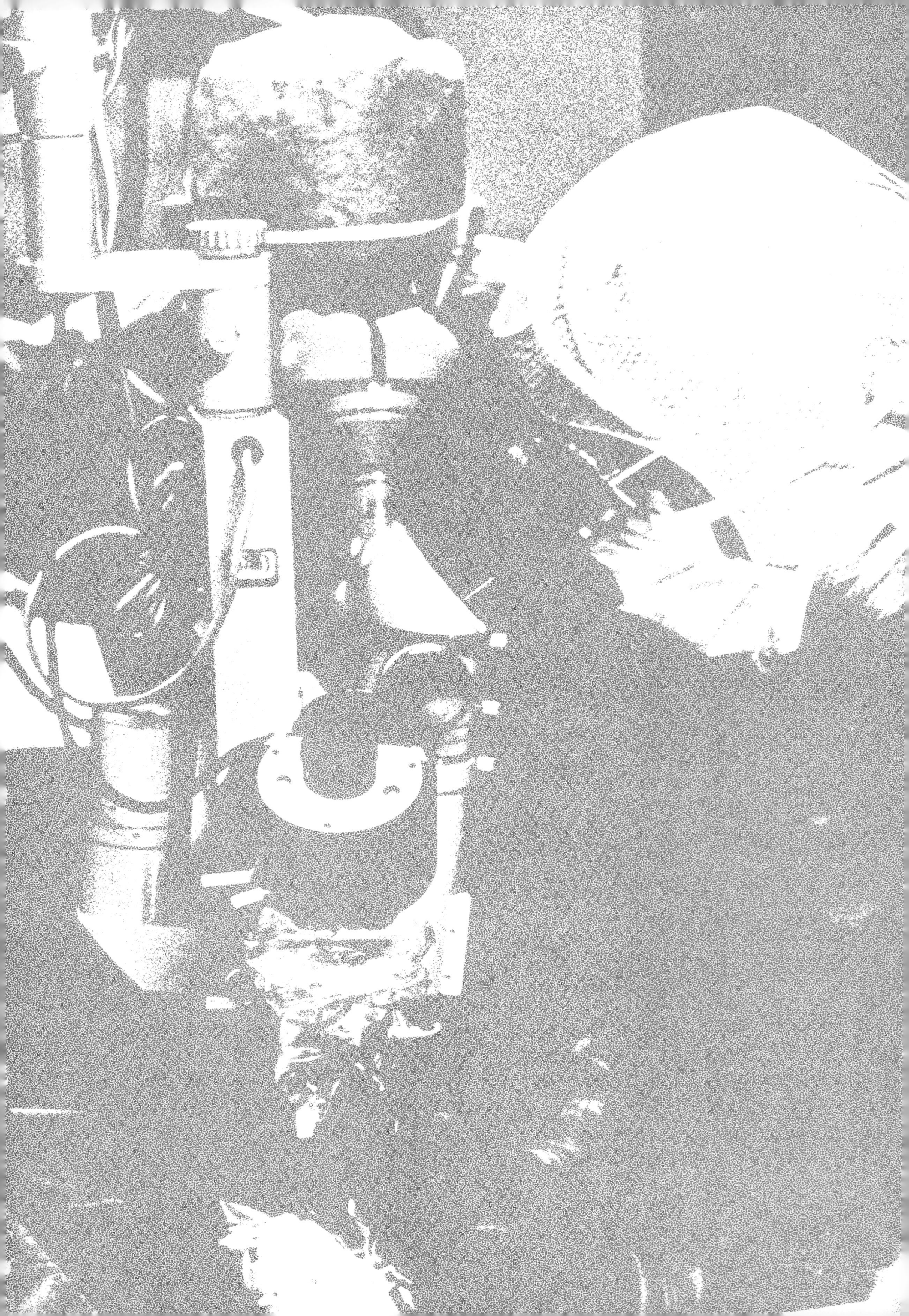

3
CORNEAL
SURGERY

ANATOMY OF THE CORNEA

Frederick H. Davidorf, M.D.

The transparency of the cornea is largely a result of the special organization of the corneal tissue. The principal refracting surface of the eye, the cornea originates from the mesodermal tissue and is composed primarily of collagen fibrils, ground substance, and water. Unlike collagen fibers elsewhere in the body, corneal collagen fibrils are parallel, thinner, and more uniform in diameter.

The cornea's state of detergescence also is responsible for its transparency. The exact mechanism by which detergescence is maintained is not known, but the endothelial and epithelial layers play an important role. Endothelial cells function as a pump mechanism that uses aerobic glycolysis. Glucose and oxygen are necessary for this metabolic process. The epithelium probably participates in this process as well. The aqueous humor provides the primary source for glucose. Oxygen is derived from the air and passes through the tear film and epithelium to the stroma. Oxygen also comes from the aqueous humor and passes through the endothelium.

The cornea is supplied with rich sensory nerves which are derived from the ophthalmic division of the fifth cranial nerve. The long ciliary nerves reach the cornea through the sclera. These nerves are myelinated in 2 to 3 mm of peripheral cornea. As they extend centrally, they lose myelin, branch, and become smaller. These unmyelinated nerves supply the epithelium, Bowman's layer, and anterior stroma.

The corneal depth measures approximately 0.5 mm centrally and is slightly thicker in the periphery. It consists of five layers: 1) epithelium (EPI), 2) Bowman's layer (BL), 3) stroma (S), 4) Descemet's membrane (DM), and endothelium (END) [1] .

The epithelium is very active metabolically, and the cells are replaced every seven days. This layer occupies approximately 10 percent of the corneal thickness and is composed of three groups of cells: basal (BC), wing (WC), and superficial, SC [2] . The basal layer consists of a single row of tall, polygonal cells and rests on a basement membrane that blends into Bowman's layer. The basal cells interdigitate with the intermediate layer, the wing cells. These cells occupy two to three layers and consist of basal cells that have divided and migrated anteriorly. These lateral extensions are thin and wing-like, giving the cell its name. Long, thin cells with flattened nuclei characterize the superficial group. These cells compose two layers of the cornea. Many microplicae and microvilli extend from the surface of the most superficial layer and are intimately associated with the precorneal tear film.

Bowman's layer is composed mainly of collagen and ground substance. Therefore, it is not a true membrane as once defined. No cells are present in this layer, with the exception of the extensions of Schwann cells, which surround the nerves that course through the layer to reach the epithelium. While the anterior surface of Bowman's layer is smooth, posteriorly it blends into the corneal stroma.

The stroma accounts for 90 percent of the corneal thickness. The collagen fibers are arranged in regular parallel lamellae. Keratocytes, which can be seen throughout the stroma, are morphologically nearly identical to fibroblasts found elsewhere. These cells are thin and have long processes that parallel the corneal lamellae. The space between the collagen fibrils and keratocytes is occupied by ground substance that is responsible for the even spacing between the individual collagen fibrils.

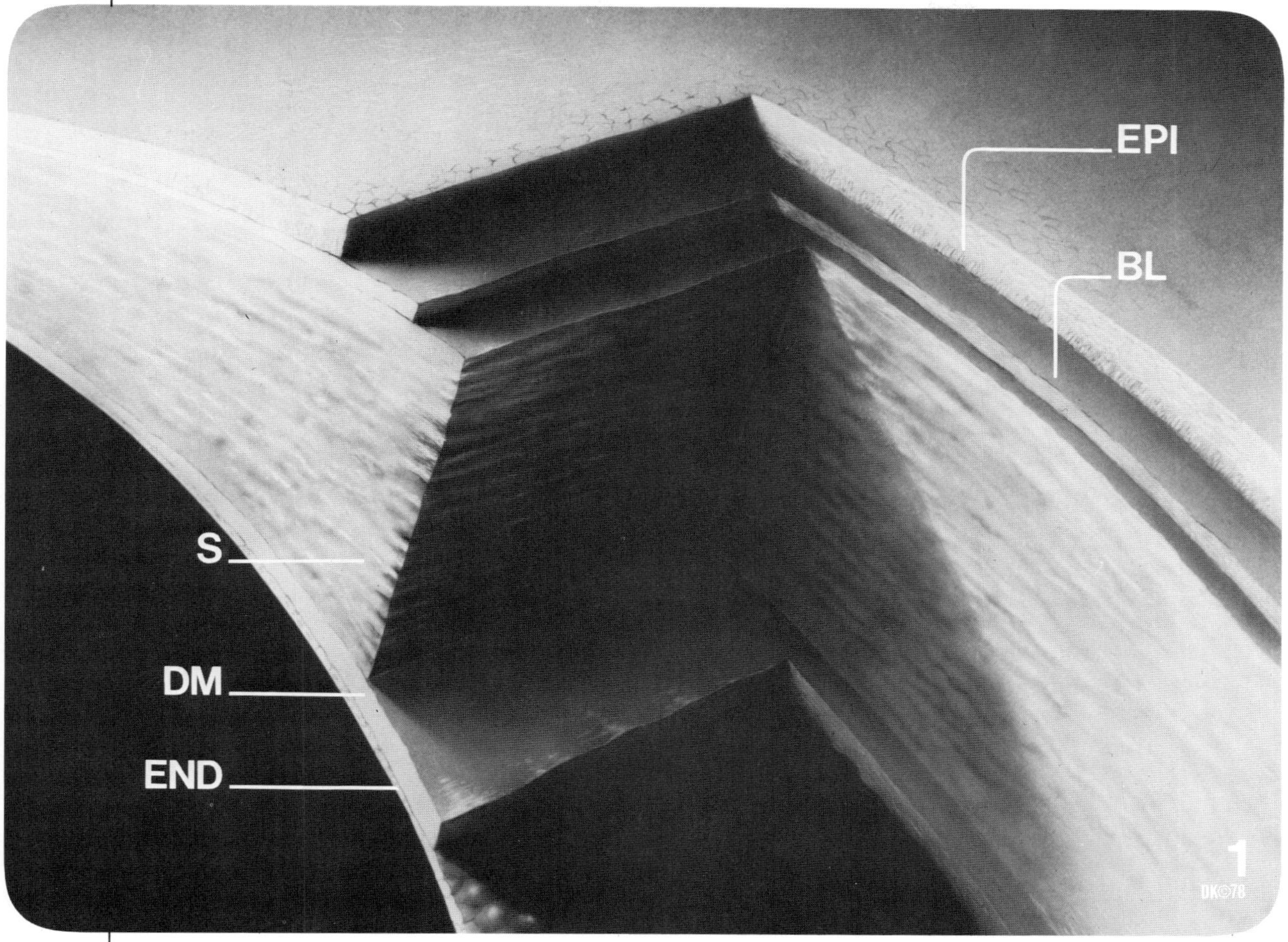

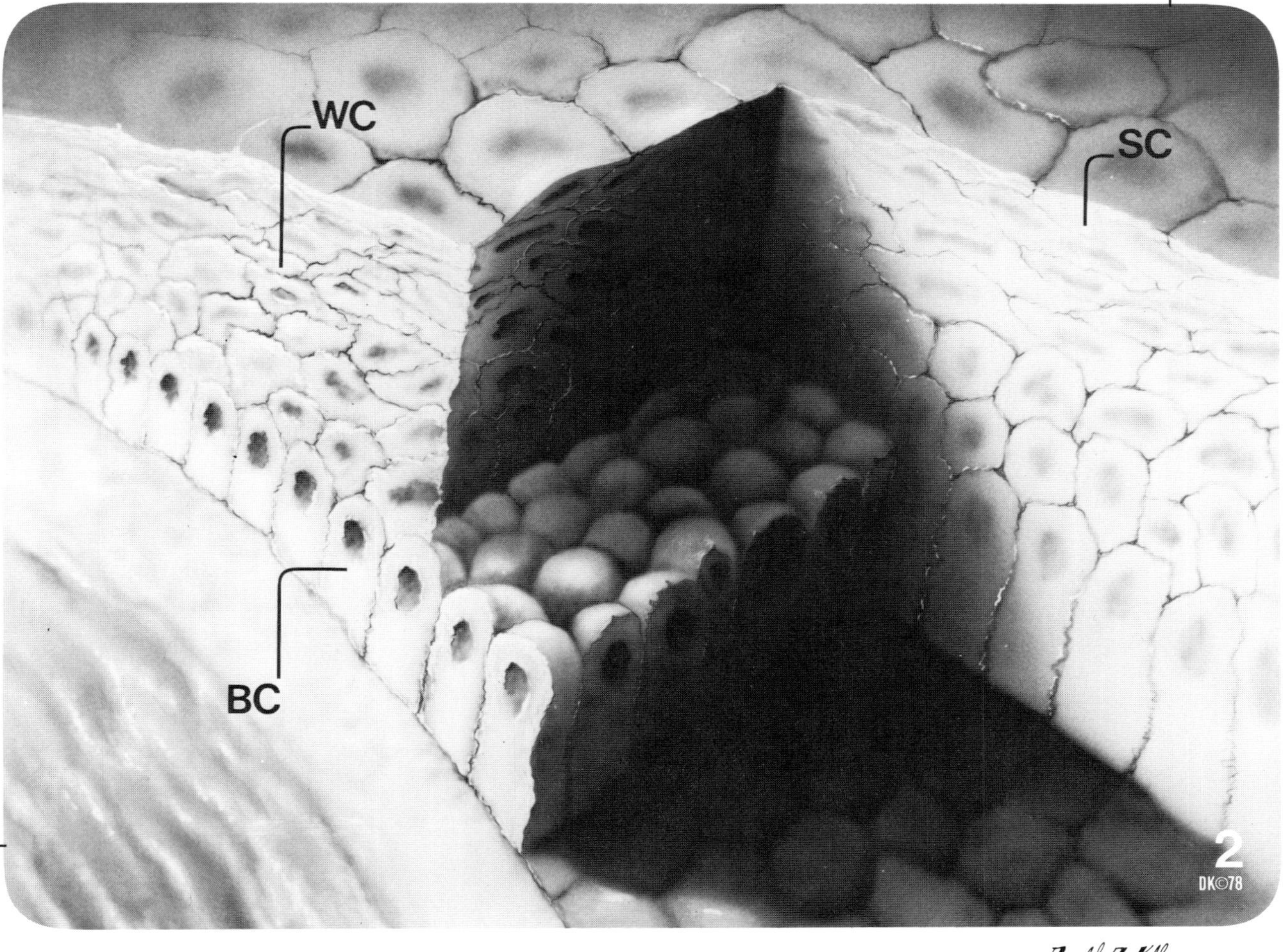

Donald A. Keller

Descemet's membrane, DM [3], the basement membrane of the corneal endothelial cells, gradually thickens throughout life and is composed of very uniformly arranged stratified layers.

The endothelial layer, EL [4], consists of a single layer of hexagonal cells. In young individuals, the endothelial cell nuclei exhibit a regular arrangement that becomes more irregular as the nuclei degenerate with age. This layer is very active metabolically, and electron microscopic studies have identified the presence of organelles characteristic of cells engaged in active transport and protein synthesis. Adjacent cells show complex interdigitation with each other. On both the anterior and posterior surfaces of the cell, numerous pinocytotic vesicles are present. Microvilli can be seen projecting from the posterior cell membrane into the anterior chamber.

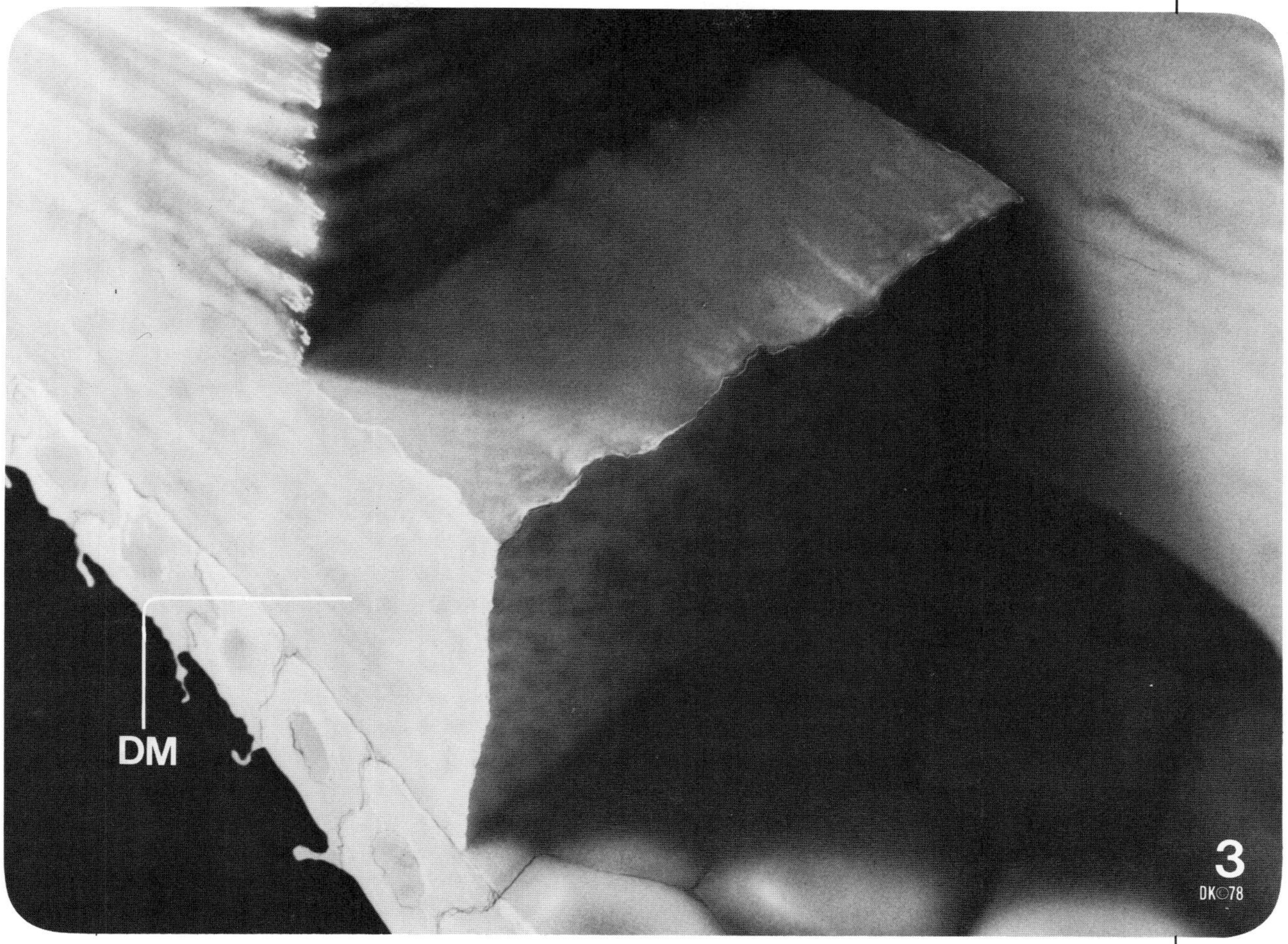

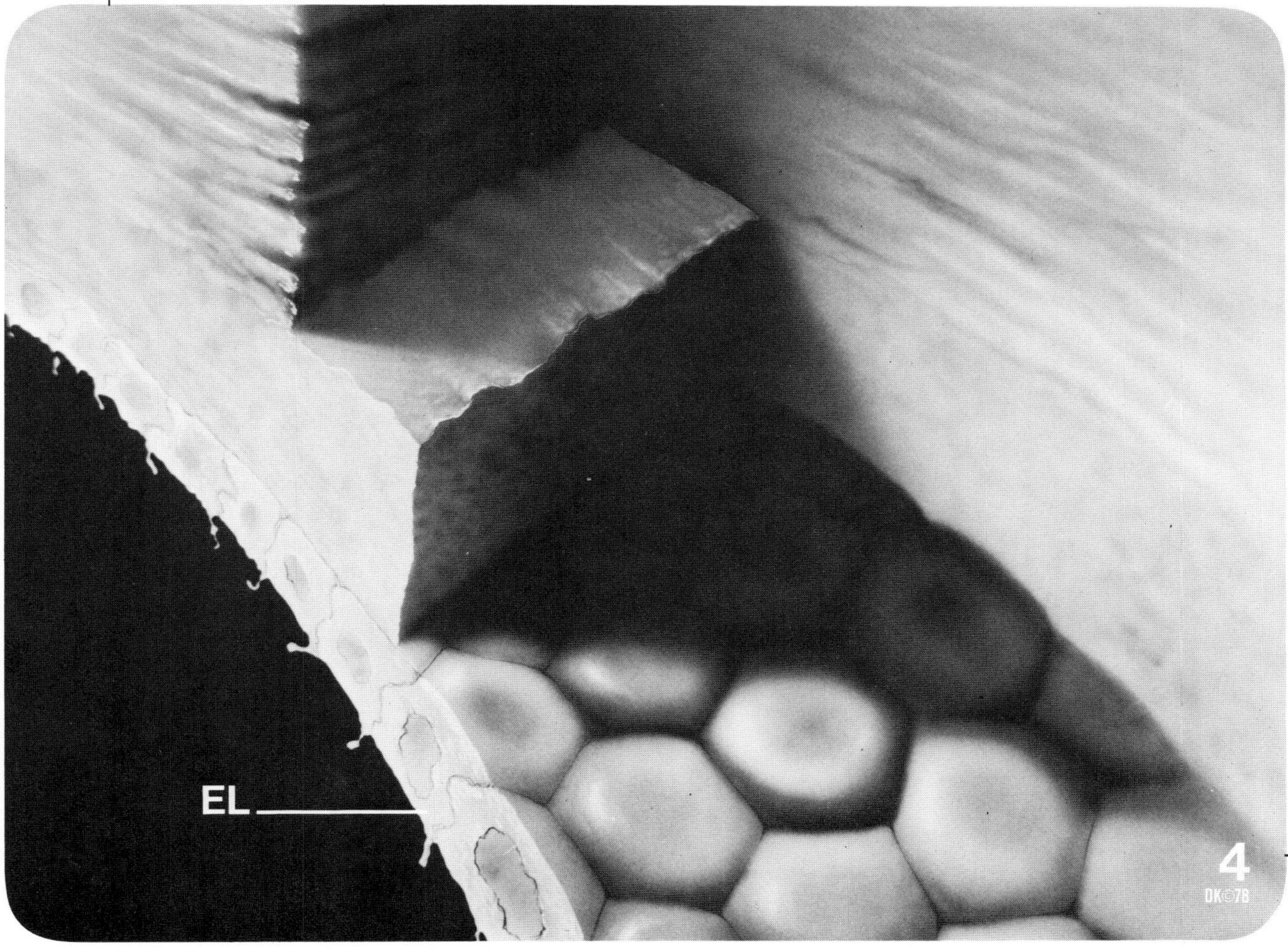

Donald H. Keller

PENETRATING KERATOPLASTY

Richard H. Keates, M.D.
Richard G. Lembach, M.D.

The indications for performing penetrating keratoplasty have not changed markedly over the years. The most common causes for corneal opacities include edema of endothelial dysfunctions, keratoconus, scarring after infection, and trauma. Thanks to technologic advances in the manufacture of fine suture material and needles, the widespread use of the operating microscope, and improved medical management, the success rate of penetrating keratoplasty has dramatically increased. The recent improvements in tissue storage have also contributed to improved prognosis in these patients. This chapter describes the surgical technique for this operation.

To decrease the chance of vitreous loss in an aphakic eye, the patient should be positioned on the operating table so that the neck is not hyperextended. Better access to the globe is achieved if the surgeon turns the patient's head slightly to the side opposite the eye to be operated. This maneuver facilitates cutting and suturing the graft. After routine retrobulbar anesthesia, at least three minutes of ocular massage is recommended to insure a soft eye for surgery. We also recommend a wire speculum for lid retraction. Placement of a 4-0 black suture through the tendon of the superior rectus muscle is performed with forceps grasping the limbus at the 6-o'clock position and rotating the eye down [1]. This maneuver exposes the superior rectus tendon. The tendonous insertion is grasped with Elschnig forceps. The suture is passed through the tendon, with care taken always to point the needle tip away from the globe. Traction applied to the suture confirms its location in the superior rectus tendon. A traction suture is placed through the insertion of the inferior rectus tendon in a similar manner.

The approximate size of the graft can be determined preoperatively, based on the location of the corneal opacities [2]. The average corneal transplant is 7.5 mm in diameter. It is desirable to confirm the adequacy of the size of the graft by measuring it with calipers. Once the surgeon has determined the size of the graft, the cornea is marked for graft placement. We recommend use of a disposable Castroviejo trephine. The guard plate is set so that it penetrates three quarters of the cornea's thickness [3]. This requires approximately 0.3 mm of exposed cutting surface. The first assistant grasps the superior and inferior rectus traction sutures to stabilize the globe during marking and trephination [4]. The tendon of the medial rectus muscle or the horizontal limbal tissue is grasped with a 0.3-mm Castroviejo forceps, and the eye is rotated temporally so that a tangential view of the cornea is possible. The visual axis is slightly down and nasal from the anatomic center of the cornea; therefore, the surgeon must visualize the inferior nasal quadrant to insure that the trephine blade is centered correctly.

The surgeon places the guarded trephine on the corneal surface and rocks and spins the trephine in a circular motion trying to apply equal pressure on all edges of the cutting surface so that uniform depth is obtained [5]. Proper setting of the trephine guard insures that the anterior chamber is not entered during this maneuver. Once the trephination is complete, the surgeon turns his attention to preparation of the donor button. The donor cornea should be examined with a slit lamp to be sure that it is clear and free of any considerable endothelial abnormality. We recommend obtaining the specimen as soon as possible after death of the donor, and we generally avoid the use of corneas removed over 24 hours after donor death.

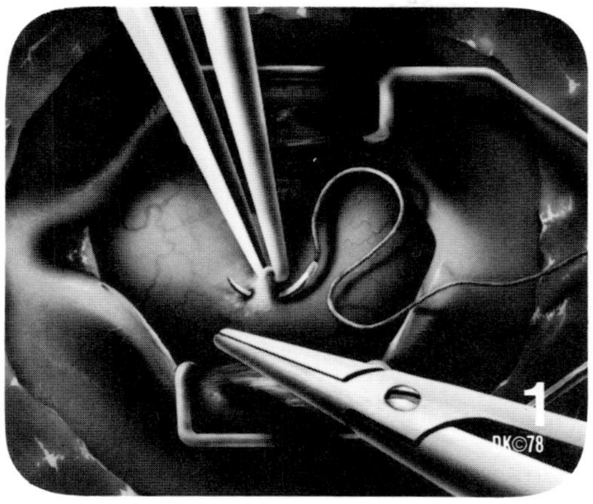

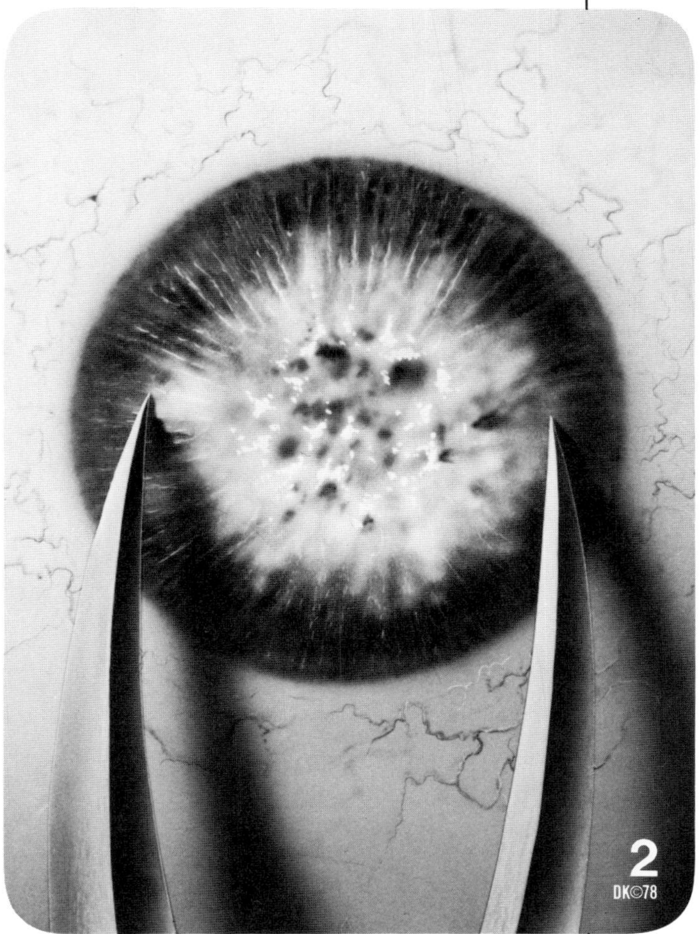

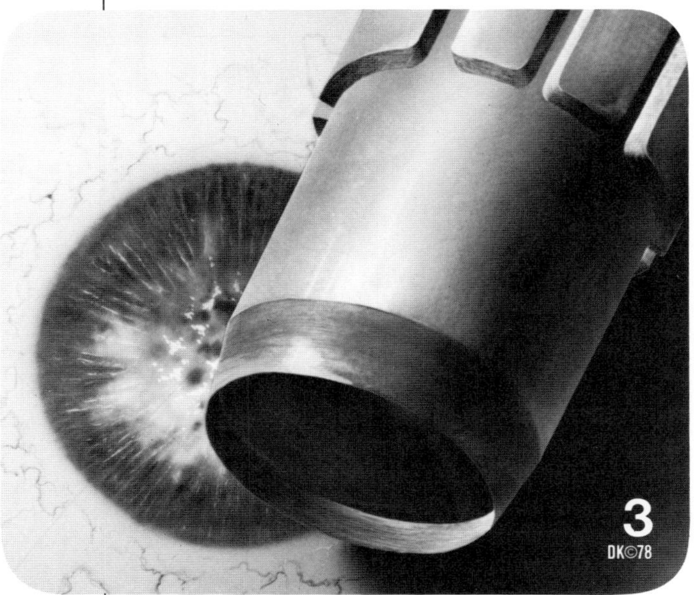

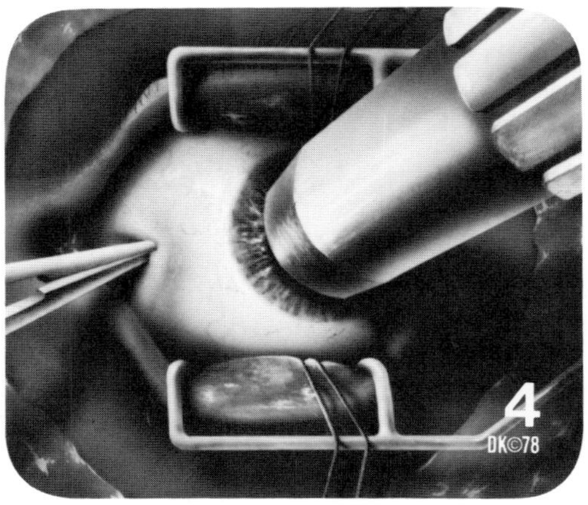

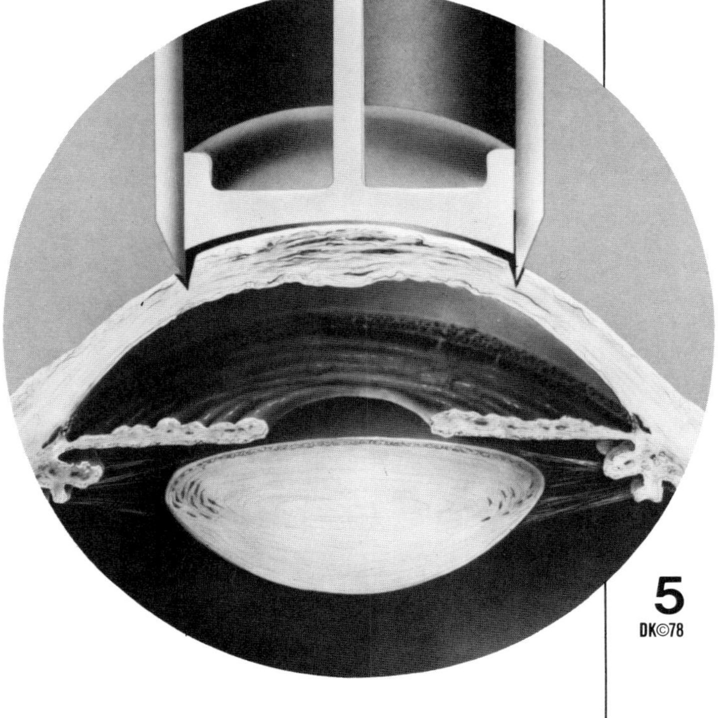

5
DK©78

Donald A. Keller

To prepare the donor cornea, the entire cornea and a rim of sclera are removed from the globe. During the removal, the globe may be stabilized by wrapping it with a square of sponge. Several millimeters from the limbus, a razor blade knife penetrates full-thickness sclera to expose the underlying uvea. The tips of a Westcott scissors are inserted into the scleral opening, and the incision is extended circumferentially. With a 0.12-mm Castroviejo forceps, the surgeon grasps the edge of the sclera and lifts the cornea by its scleral ring from the globe. When transferring the tissue to the storage bottle, the surgeon must exercise extreme care to avoid damage to endothelial cells. The tissue is refrigerated until its use, usually within 48 hours of its removal.

At the time of surgery, the donor cornea is transferred from the storage bath to a metal cup with the McCarey-Kaufman medium solution. When the surgeon is ready to prepare a donor button, a fine Castroviejo forceps lifts the graft from the metal cup by the scleral ring and places it on the Teflon cutting block with the epithelial surface down [6]. Extreme care must be exercised in the cutting of the donor material to minimize trauma to the endothelial cells. It is mandatory that the trephine be centered directly over the donor tissue to avoid an oval button or shelved edge [7]. The same trephine is used with the guard fully retracted. It is placed on the donor material directly perpendicular to the surface of the endothelium. Firm pressure is applied to the trephine so that it passes through the donor tissue into the Teflon block. This effects a clean cut with uniform edges. When the trephine passes completely through the cornea, the surgeon can feel the difference in the resistance of the tissue as compared to the Teflon block. If the tissue has been cut cleanly, the graft button will remain on the block as the trephine is removed. The remainder of the cornea may be sent to the laboratory for endothelial analysis.

The donor button is removed from the block with a lens loop. This is slid under the donor button. A 0.12-mm Castroviejo forceps stabilizes the button during this maneuver. The tissue is lifted from the block and placed in a Petri dish where a drop of balanced salt solution is placed on the endothelium. The epithelium is always down, protecting the endothelium from contact with the container. The Petri dish containing the donor material is placed on the surgical stand for later use.

After preparing the donor material, the surgeon begins to remove the diseased cornea [8] [9]. The edge of the cornea is grasped with a fine Colibri forceps. The razor blade is inserted perpendicularly to a depth

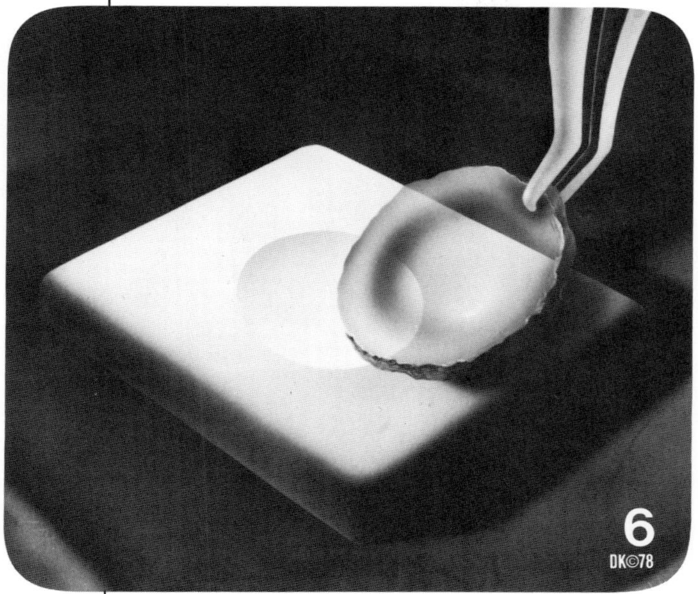
6
DK©78

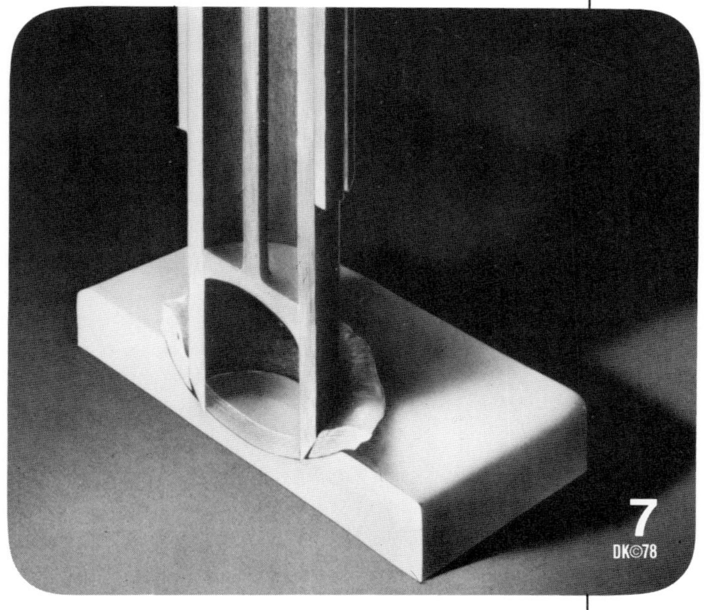
7
DK©78

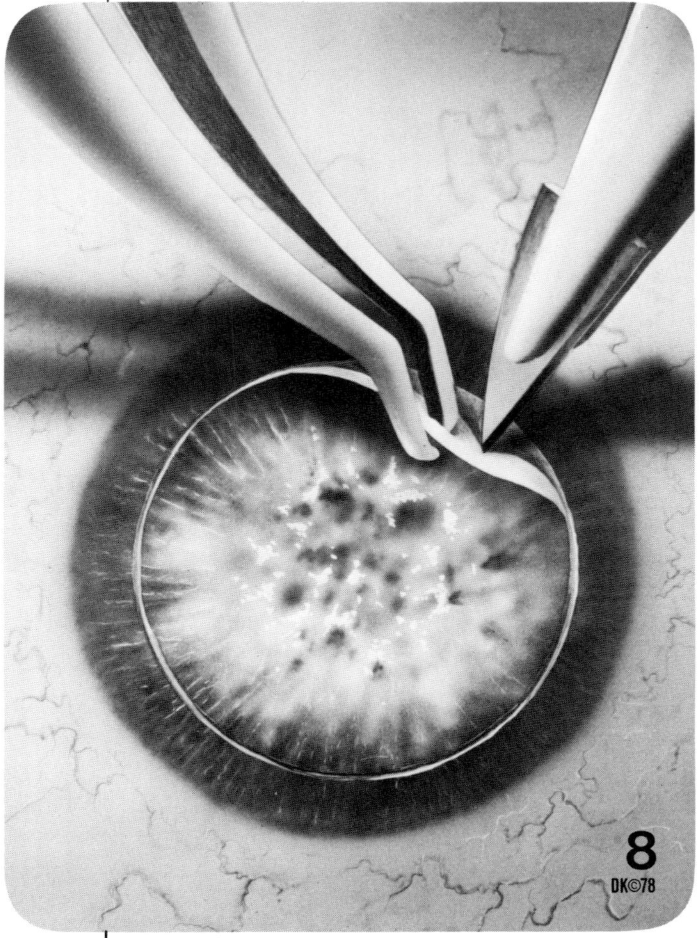
8
DK©78

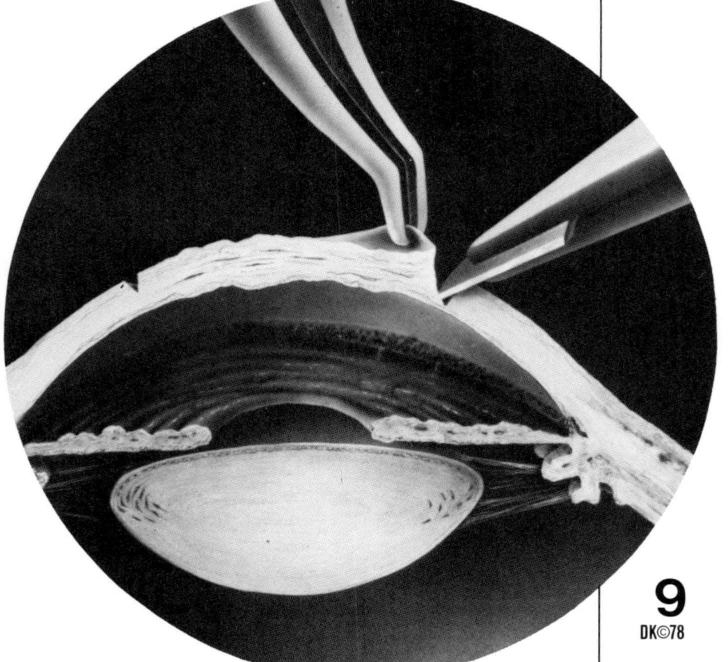
9
DK©78

just superficial to Descemet's membrane and advanced approximately 1 cm. The cornea is then regrasped, and the deepening procedure is continued 360 degrees. Descemet's membrane appears as a translucent layer as it is approached. The edges of the wound are perpendicular, while the entrance into the anterior chamber is slightly shelved. This entry into the anterior chamber is usually most convenient in the superior temporal or nasal position [10]. The razor blade is used to make a 3- to 4-mm incision into the anterior chamber. An incision of this size provides easy entrance for the corneal scissors. Fine corneal Castroviejo right- and left-handed scissors are used to complete the incision for removal of the host corneal button [11] [12]. In aphakic eyes, the surgeon frequently encounters vitreous prolapse while developing the corneal incision. Should this occur, a liberal vitrectomy is performed with use of cellulose sponges to decompress the vitreous, as described in microscopic intracapsular cataract extractions. It is important that the iris diaphragm in aphakic eyes fall back so that there is no vitreous in the anterior chamber. The vitrectomy reduces the chance of vitreous contact with the new graft and subsequent graft failure.

When the diseased cornea has been completely incised, it is left in place until the new donor corneal button is transferred. The method of transfer is extremely important and is designed to protect the delicate endothelium of the donor graft. The Petri dish containing the donor tissue is handed to the surgeon. The lens spoon is used to lift the donor button with the epithelial surface in contact with the spoon [13]. The diseased cornea is then removed. The donor button is placed at the inferior edge of the wound perpendicular to the edge. The lens spoon helps rotate the donor tissue so that it falls into place in the recipient bed. Care must be taken to prevent the graft from falling through the bed.

Once the donor corneal button is properly positioned, the surgeon begins suturing the graft [14]. A fine-toothed Colibri forceps is used to grasp the donor button firmly for placement of the initial cardinal suture at 12 o'clock. Since the first suture has no anchoring other than the one point fixation of the Colibri forceps, the needle is passed deeply into the stroma directly underneath the forceps to avoid rocking of the button. Any misalignment of the first suture may interfere with subsequent suture placement and increase the danger of scraping the endothelium against the graft edge. The tip of the needle engages the host stroma with a lifting motion that facilitates the Colibri grasp of the host edge. Once the host tissue is firmly grasped, the surgeon elevates it slightly, facilitating placement of the suture [15]

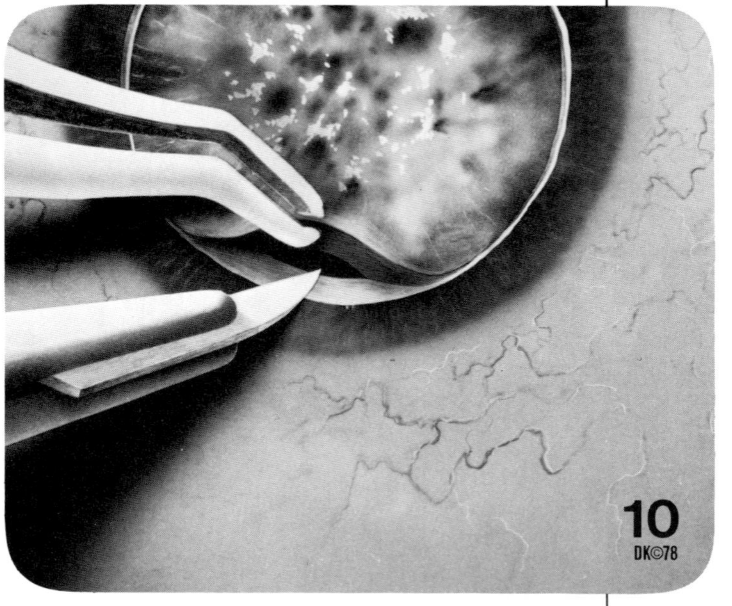

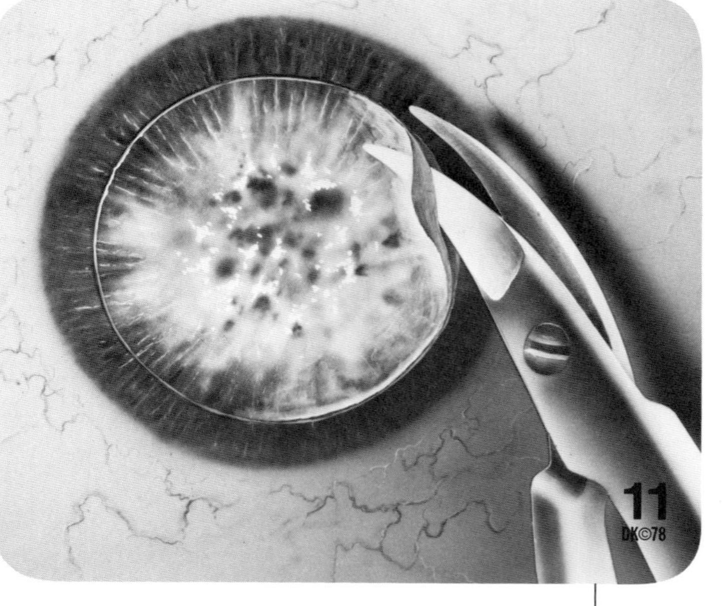

Donald A. Keller

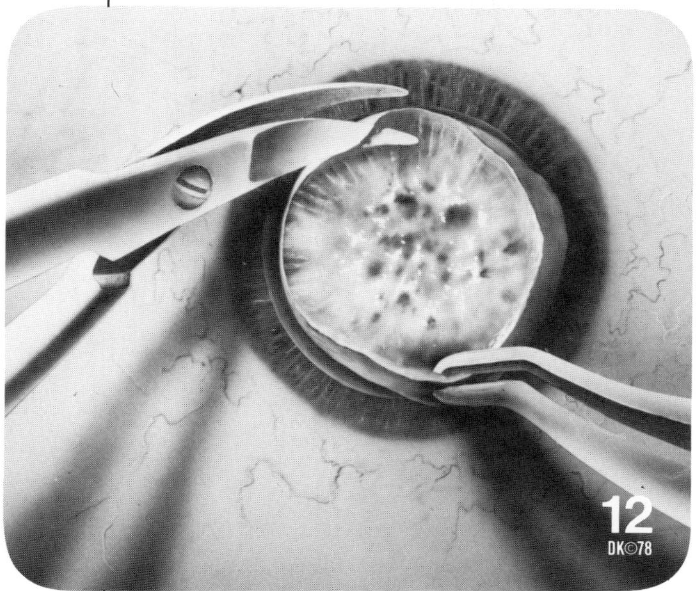

12
DK©78

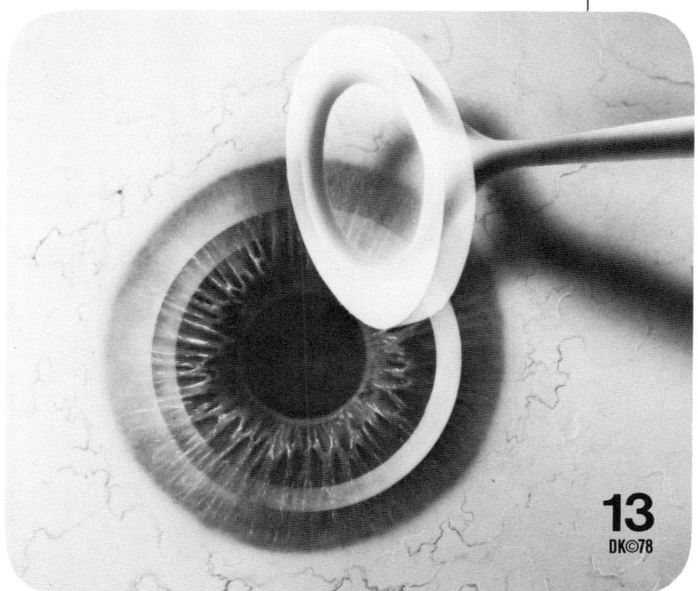

13
DK©78

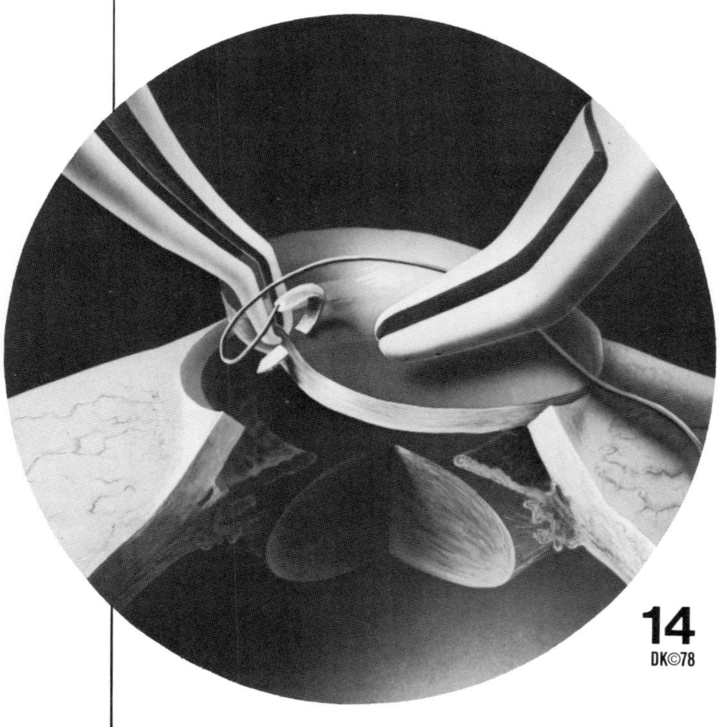

14
DK©78

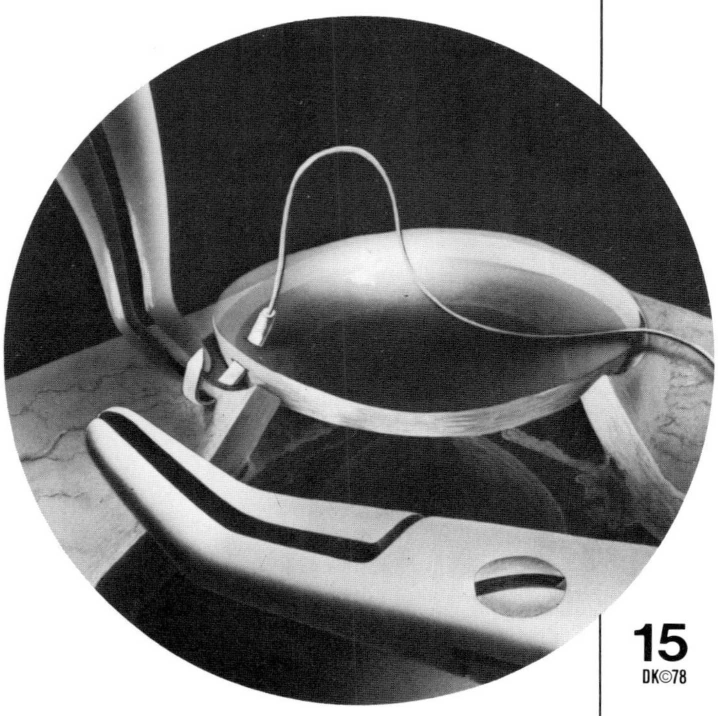

15
DK©78

Donald F. Keller

The needle is passed through the corneal edge of the host. The suture is tied but not cut until the 6-o'clock suture is placed in a similar manner and tied. The remaining 3-o'clock and 9-o'clock quadrants are sutured in a similar fashion **16**. The surgeon should now be able to restore the anterior chamber with use of balanced salt solution. In aphakic eyes, the anterior chamber may be re-formed with air. We recommend either four or eight cardinal sutures followed by a running suture technique to secure the graft **17**. This is performed with a double-armed 15-cm 10-0 nylon suture. In corneas with marked vascularization, we recommend use of only interrupted sutures with buried knots. For a right-handed surgeon, it is more convenient to begin the suture in the superior temporal quadrant. The needle is placed deeply into the stroma just above Descemet's membrane in the donor tissue as well as the recipient bed. As the needle engages the cornea, the Colibri forceps is used to gently lift the tissue, which provides for maximum accuracy in the placement of the needle **18**. It requires approximately 16 bites, or two to four passages per quadrant, to complete the running suture. The surgeon should leave approximately 5 cm of suture initially. Should the suture break during its placement, it may be necessary to use this end to complete the running suture **19**. With fine tying forceps the running suture is tied, and the ends of the sutures are cut as close to the knot as possible.

The surgeon may use subconjunctival antibiotics and topical corticosteroids at the completion of the procedure.

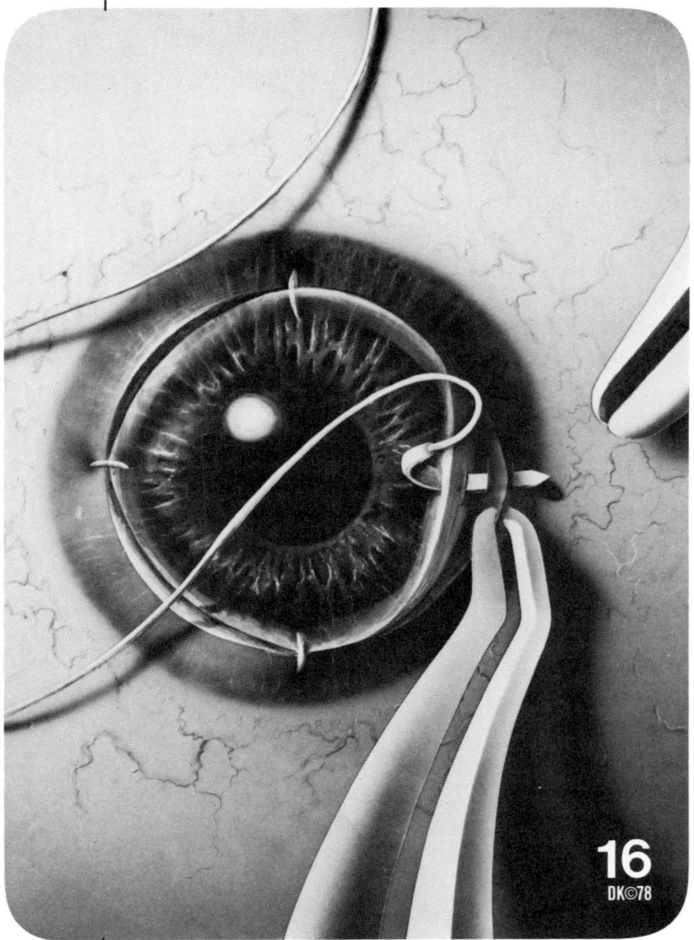
16
DK©78

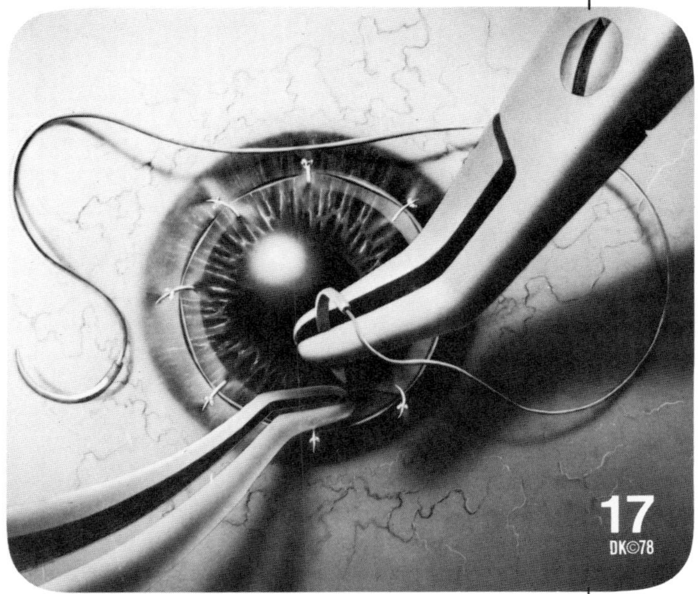
17
DK©78

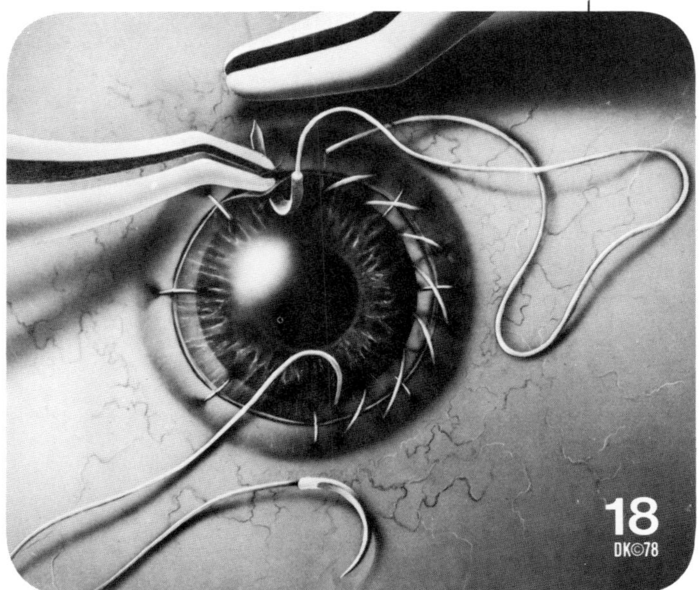
18
DK©78

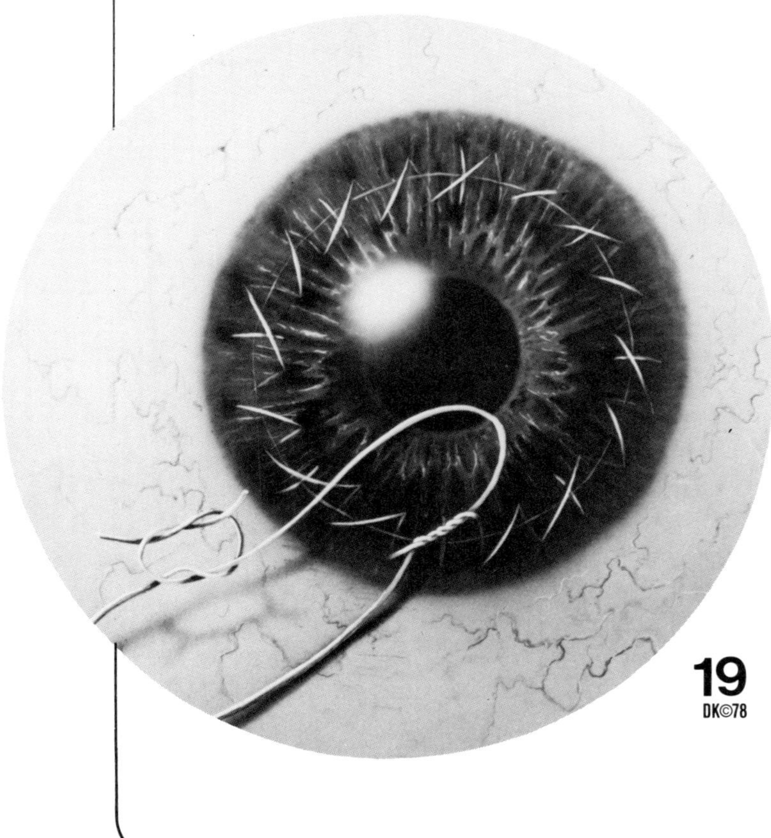
19
DK©78

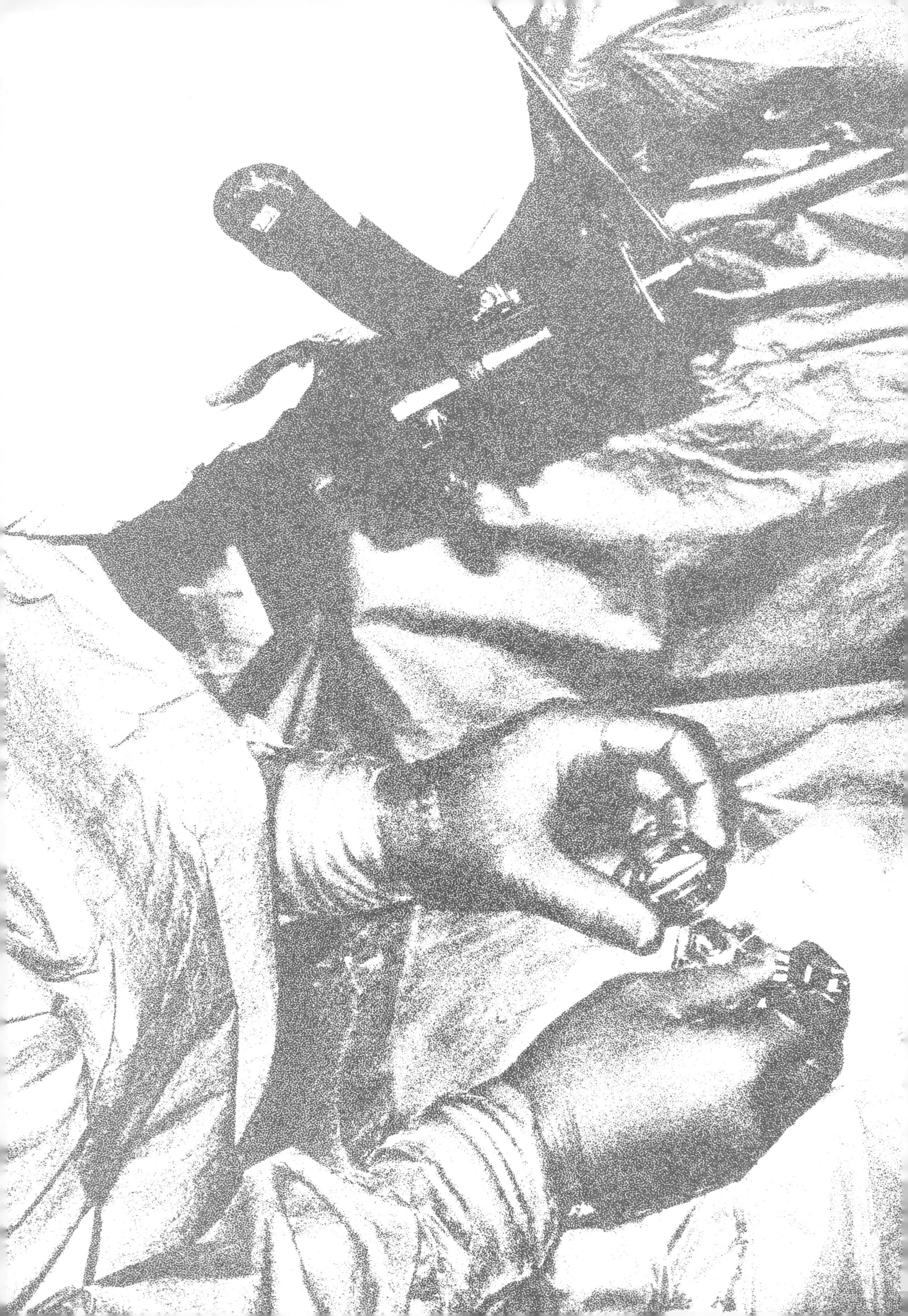

4

RETINAL

SURGERY

ANATOMY OF THE RETINA

Frederick H. Davidorf, M.D.

The retina is a complex and highly ordered neural structure, and a complete understanding of its organization and function awaits further investigation and new research tools. Nevertheless, the morphologic appearance of the retina has been well defined through light and electron microscopic studies. The retina may be divided into peripheral and central portions. The peripheral retina contains ten layers which can be viewed with the light microscope. These are 1) retinal pigment epithelium (PE); 2) rod and cone layer (RC); 3) outer limiting membrane (OLM); 4) outer nuclear layer (ONL); 5) outer plexiform layer (OPL); 6) inner nuclear layer (INL); 7) inner plexiform layer (IPL); 8) ganglion cell layer (GCL); 9) nerve fiber layer (NFL); and 10) inner limiting membrane (ILM). A more accurate study of retina can be made with both scanning electron microscopy [1] and transmission electron microscopy [2].

The retinal pigment epithelium (RPE) consists of a single layer of hexagonally shaped cells of uniform size. The photoreceptors consist of outer and inner segments (OS and IS). An intimate and dynamic relationship exists between the outer segments of the photoreceptors and the villi (V) of the pigment epithelial cells. Microvilli, which extend from the apexes of the RPE cells, encompass the tips of the outer segments of the rods and cones. The size and shape of the rods and cones vary considerably throughout the retina.

The outer limiting membrane is not a true membrane, as histologists once believed, but consists of the terminations of the Müller cells (MC), which form fiber baskets. These simulate a membrane.

The extensions of the inner segments of the photoreceptors pass through this fenestrated outer limiting membrane to their respective cell bodies. These cell bodies compose the outer nuclear layer. The thickness of this layer varies considerably, from the very thin periphery to the thickest region posteriorly. Müller cell processes fill the intracellular spaces.

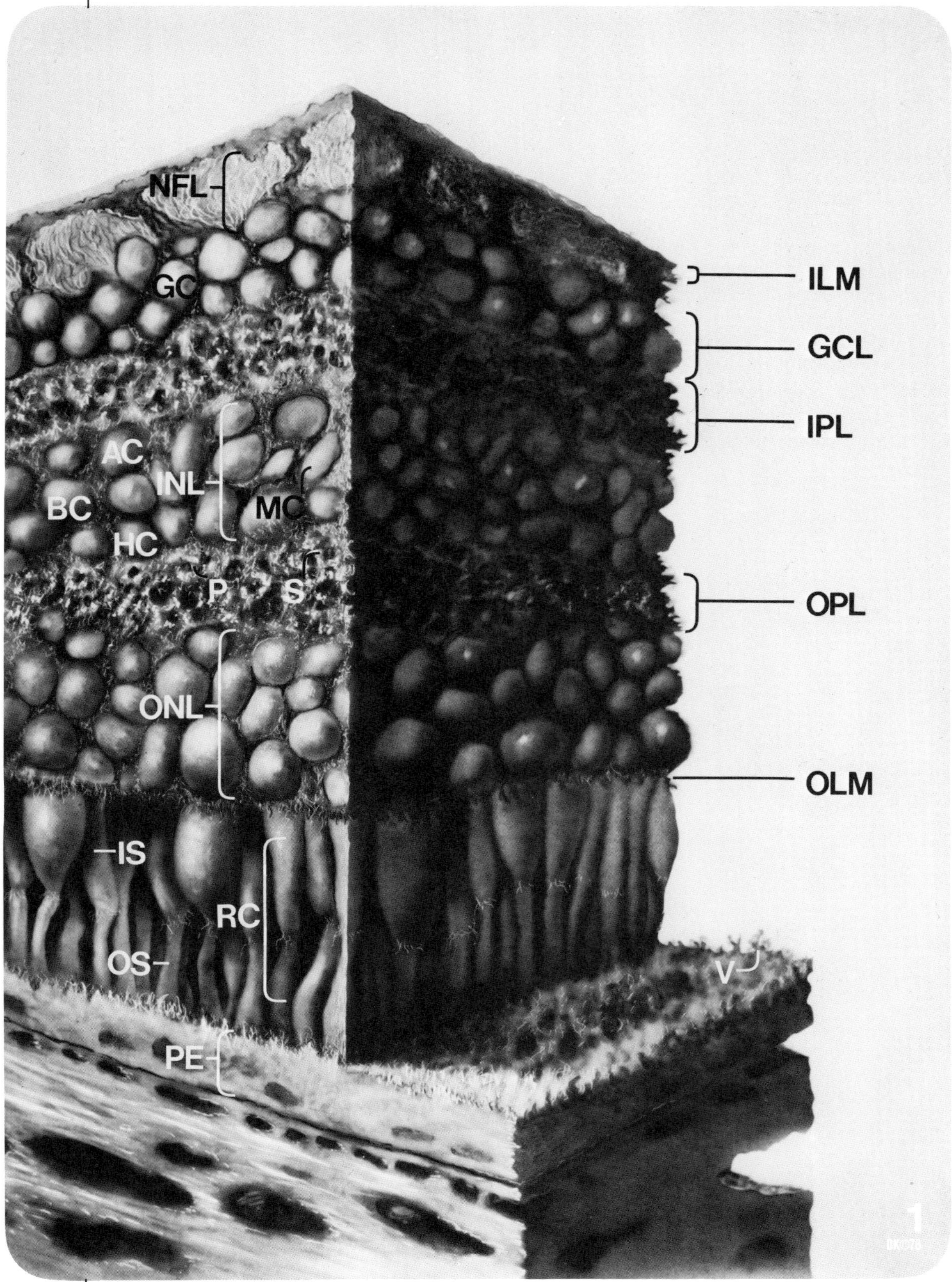

Donald A. Keller

In the outer plexiform layer, the axon of the rod synapses with the bipolar cell to create a round structure known as a spherule (S). The axon of the cone forms a broader synaptic juncture called a pedicle (P).

The inner nuclear layer contains the cell bodies of bipolar cells (BC). Three additional cell bodies found in this layer are horizontal cells (HC), Müller cells (MC), and amacrine cells (AC). The bipolar cell, the first order neuron, lies completely within the retina and synapses with the second order neuron, the ganglion cell (GC). The horizontal cells are found in the outer portion of the outer nuclear layer and probably are involved in the integration of impulses from adjacent cells. Horizontal cell processes, which connect adjacent spherules and pedicles, have been identified also. Müller cells extend from the outer limiting membrane to the inner limiting membrane and are thought to supply the major structural support for the retina. Additionally, they probably function in the transport of nutrients and may also aid in the conduction of electrical impulses. Amacrine cells are located primarily in the innermost portion of the inner nuclear layer. These function similarly to horizontal cells; that is, they integrate electrical activity between adjacent cells. The amacrine cell processes extend into the inner plexiform layer and synapse with adjacent bipolar and ganglion cells.

The inner plexiform layer is very complex and represents synapses between amacrine, bipolar, and ganglion cells. Numerous intertwining cell processes give its cut surface a sponge-like appearance when viewed with the scanning electron microscope.

The ganglion cell layer varies greatly throughout the retina. The cells are most populous and closely spaced posteriorly and become less dense peripherally. Throughout most of the retina, they form a single row of cells, but in the macular region, as many as eight to ten layers may exist. The cells generally are spherical and varied in size.

The nerve fiber layer is composed of the axons of the ganglion cells. The axons are oriented in bundles surrounded by Müller cell processes.

The inner limiting membrane appears homogenous. Müller cell footplates are contiguous with the membrane. The retinal surface is smooth peripherally where nerve fiber bundles are sparse and Müller cell processes are abundant. Posteriorly, however, ridges appear on the retinal surface which correspond to individual nerve fiber bundles.

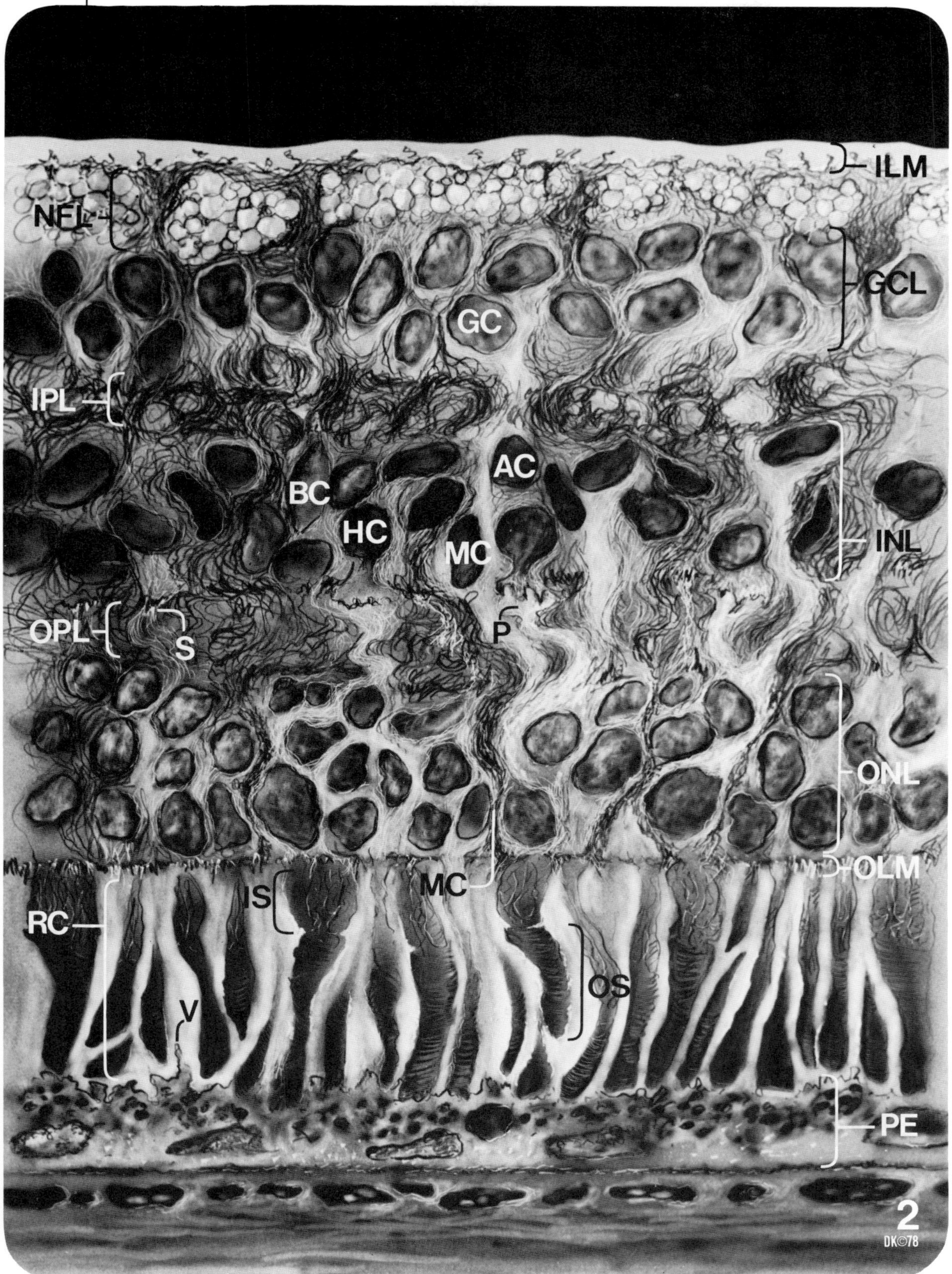

Donald F. Keller

Some controversy exists regarding the nomenclature of the central retina. Therefore, while no definitive classification has been made, we have categorized this region in a manner that we believe to be both clinically and histologically sound. The major regions of the central retina are the macula (MAC), the fovea (FOV), and the foveola (FOVL) 3.

The macula may be clinically defined as that area of the retina characterized by the presence of yellowish pigment. Because of differences in pigmentation, however, this area is poorly defined, and great disparity exists among individuals. Post mortem, it appers as a yellowish area; in the living eye, it is visible only with the red-free light of the ophthalmoscope. The macula measures up to 5 mm in diameter and contains approximately 650,000 cones. Histologically, the macula terminates at the site where the ganglion cells are reduced to a single layer.

The fovea is the central portion of the retina that is completely rod-free. While the limits of the fovea are undefined, it may be said to occupy a space just slightly larger than the capillary-free zone. The fovea measures approximately 500 microns in diameter and contains approximately 34,000 cones.

We have defined the foveola as the area inside the capillary-free zone that measures approximately 250 to 300 microns and is responsible for acute central vision.

An understanding of the structure and organization of the central retina is essential when treating pathology in this area. The macula may be photocoagulated without danger to the patient's central vision. Treatment in the fovea, however, is only safe outside the capillary-free zone. The foveola is never treated, as this will certainly disrupt central vision.

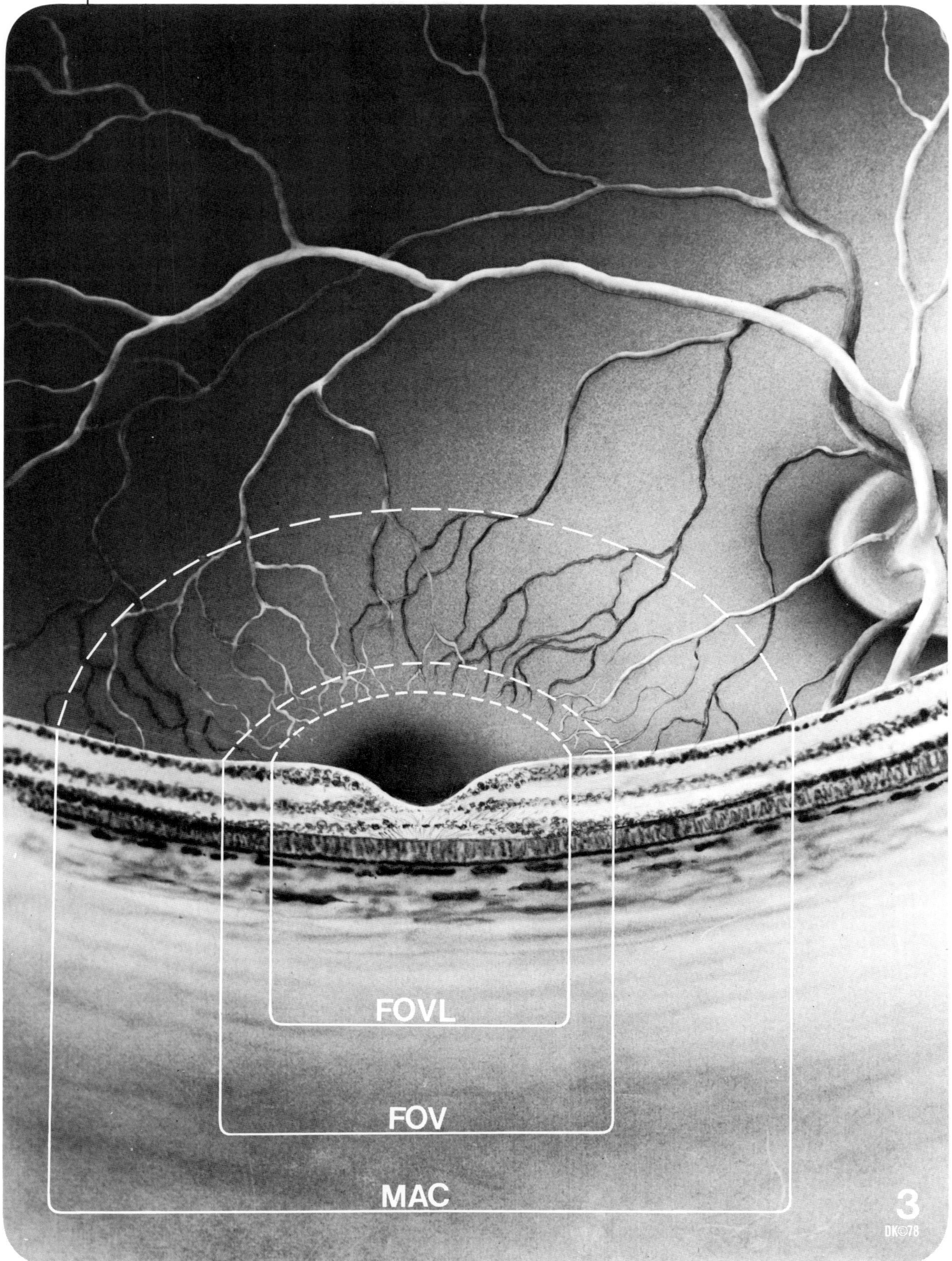

Donald F. Keller

SURGERY OF THE RETINA

Gonin's discovery that a hole in the retina is the cause of retinal detachment provided the basis for modern retinal surgery. Schepen's development of the binocular indirect ophthalmoscope greatly improved the ability to evaluate the peripheral retina and thus the ability to locate the tears. Thanks to the development and general acceptance of the scleral buckling procedure, the prognosis for retinal detachments has progressed from one of inevitable blindness to one that carries a good probability of the patient's maintaining useful vision.

This chapter will describe our management of patients with retinal holes and retinal detachments. These procedures are cryotherapy, used in the treatment of retinal holes; radial silicone-sponge explants, used in retinal holes with localized detachments; scleral buckling procedure with encircling fascia lata, used in cases of routine rhegmatogenous retinal detachments; and scleral buckling procedure with encircling silicone sponge, used in patients who have developed massive vitreous retraction.

CRYORETINOPEXY

Frederick H. Davidorf, M.D.
William H. Havener, M.D.

Early diagnosis and treatment of retinal holes have reduced the incidence of retinal detachments. The incidence of retinal holes in the general population is approximately 5 percent, while the annual incidence of retinal detachments is one in 10,000; therefore, the vast majority of patients with retinal holes never develop retinal detachments. We recommend the treatment of symptomatic holes, horseshoe tears, and tears in patients with a history of retinal detachment. Cryotherapy has simplified the creation of chorioretinal scar and reduced many of the complications inherent with the use of diathermy.

Cryoretinopexy is a rapid, safe procedure. The surgeon wears the indirect ophthalmoscope, holds the hand lens in one hand, and cryoprobe in the other. The tip of the probe is used for localization, and the hole can be frozen immediately when the probe is positioned properly. This eliminates the need for a first assistant and separate localization of the hole and thus shortens the procedure.

An eye may be adequately anesthetized for cryoretinopexy with a subconjunctival injection near the hole. A retrobulbar or lid block is not necessary in most cases. The patient should be able to move the eye during the placement of the cryoprobe. This is especially valuable for the treatment of peripheral holes. If the hole is located too posteriorly for transconjunctival treatment, a 2-cm conjunctival and Tenon's incision is made with a forceps and Westcott scissors. The surgeon separates Tenon's capsule from the underlying sclera by blunt dissection to facilitate passage of the cryoprobe [1].

Before placement of the probe on the eye, the surgeon makes sure that the probe is freezing properly and that the silicone sleeve is not covering the tip. Prior to localization of the hole, the surgeon should be positioned comfortably to activate the foot pedal easily. Most cryoprobes have some type of marker 180 degrees from the freezing tip. The second finger rests on this mark throughout the procedure so that the surgeon can be aware of the location of the tip as it is moved along the scleral surface. As the surgeon looks through the indirect ophthalmoscope, the tip appears as a round indentation that is positioned directly over the retinal hole. When it is in the correct position [2] [3] [4] the surgeon activates the foot pedal. If no freeze occurs

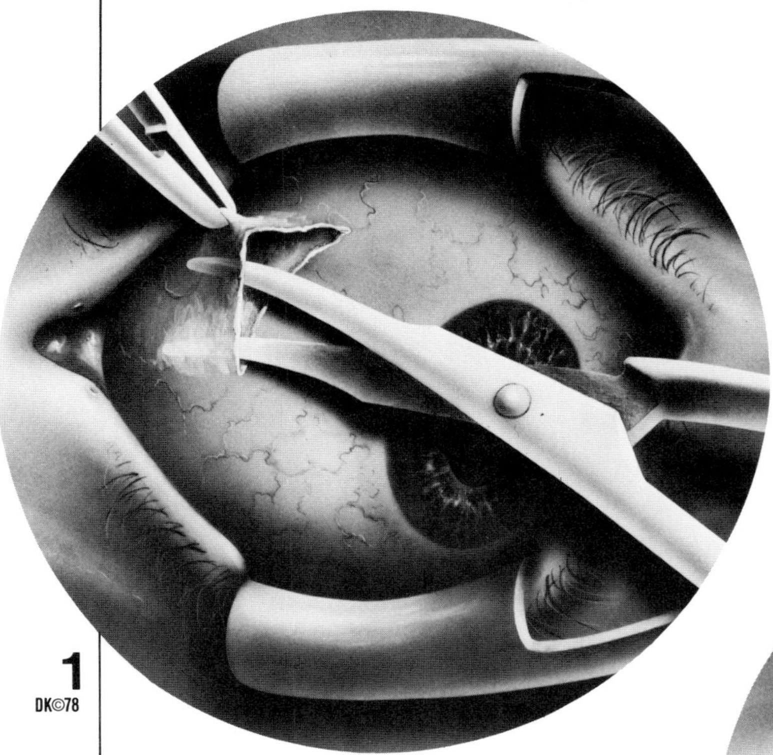

1
DK©78

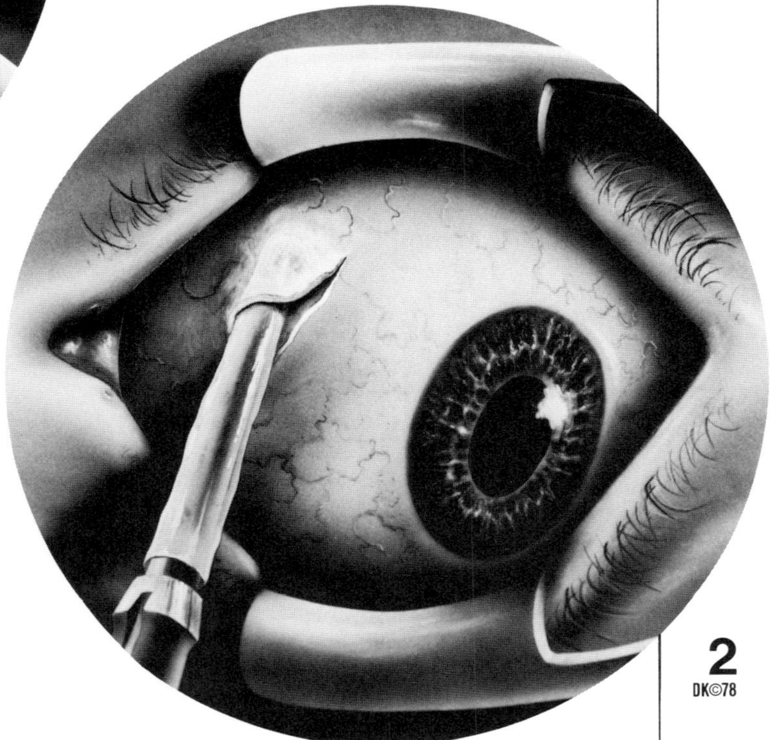

2
DK©78

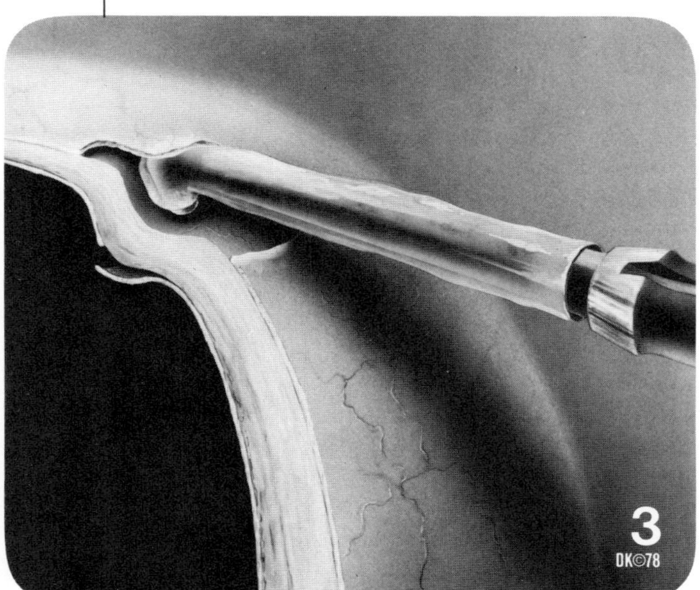

3
DK©78

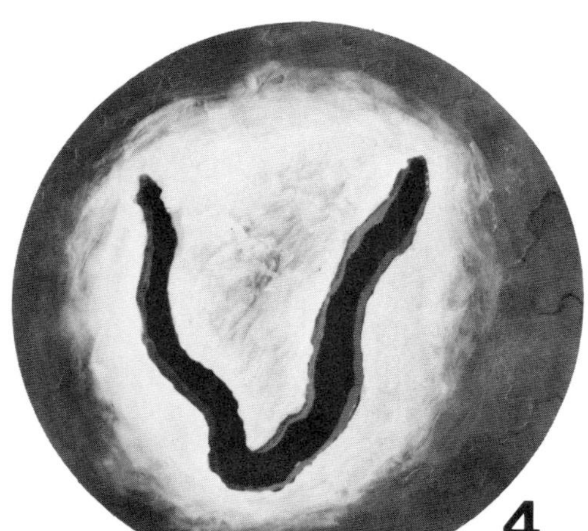

4
DK©78

Donald A. Keller

within five to ten seconds, the surgeon should recheck the position of the probe to make sure that the indentation is not the shaft and that the tip is freezing further posteriorly [5] [6] . A major error in this procedure is to mistake the shaft of the probe for the tip. The edges of the hole must be frozen 360 degrees. When the retina turns white, adequate freezing has occurred. This insures a sufficient chorioretinal scar. The surgeon should avoid excessive freezing, especially in the treatment of large holes, for this may mobilize retinal pigment epithelial cells into the vitreous. This multipotential cell may initiate further vitreous shrinkage and preretinal membrane formation. A small hole may require only a single application of the cryoprobe; a large tear may warrant multiple applications. Some holes with limited retinal detachments may be treated with cryoretinopexy alone. The surgeon should include 2 mm of attached retina in the treatment.

Cryoretinopexy should be a painless procedure since no pain fibers are present in the sclera. If a muscle is frozen, however, considerable discomfort may occur. If a hole is located under the belly of one of the rectus muscles, therefore, we recommend passing the probe between the muscle and sclera. The hole may then be frozen without the use of additional anesthesia.

After the hole is satisfactorily treated, the probe is removed, and the conjunctiva may be closed with bipolar cautery or a single 6-0 catgut suture [7] . The chorioretinal adhesion is secure after two weeks. The patient is ambulatory after surgery but should refrain from strenuous activity for several weeks.

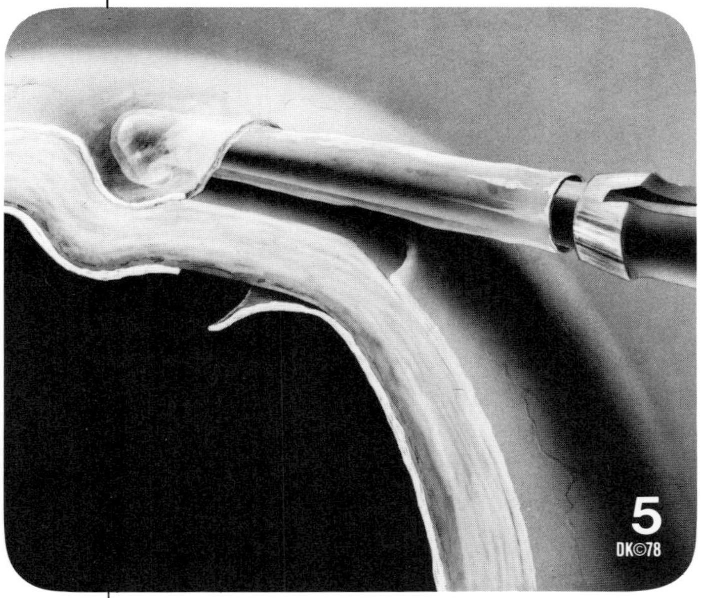

5
DK©78

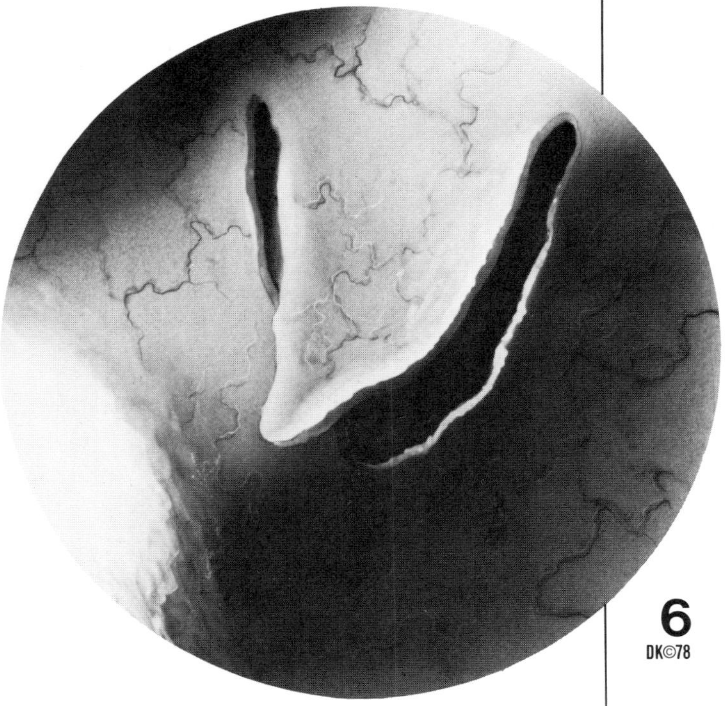

6
DK©78

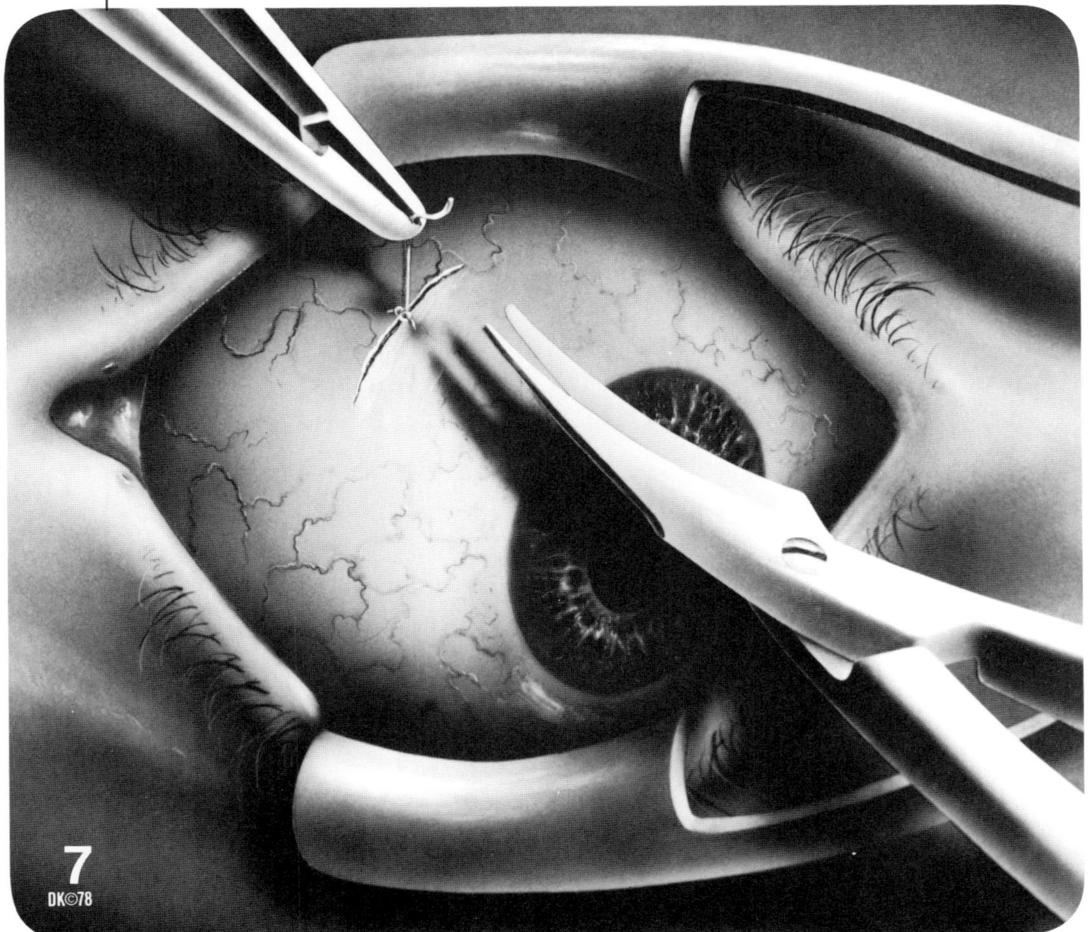

7
DK©78

Donald A. Keller

RADIAL SILICONE-SPONGE EXPLANT

Frederick H. Davidorf, M.D.
William H. Havener, M.D.

A scleral buckling procedure creates an indentation in the sclera and choroid which approximates the retina to the pigment epithelium. The procedure may be accomplished by either the creation of a local indentation or with the use of an element that encircles the globe.

Over a decade ago, Lincoff introduced the concept of suturing an elastic silicone sponge, which is placed under tension, to the sclera. The subsequent expansion of the sponge creates a local indentation that seals the retinal hole without the release of subretinal fluid. We believe that this procedure is particularly effective in patients with localized detachments in which the hole may be approximated or nearly approximated to the RPE with bed rest or scleral depression. This generally is the safest of the scleral buckling procedures since it eliminates the need to drain fluid.

After the introduction of the silicone sponge for retinal surgery, a significant rate of infection occurred. This problem has been largely overcome by impregnating the sponge with an antibiotic solution just prior to its use and irrigating the surgical field with the same solution throughout the procedure.

The procedure may be performed with the patient under either local or general anesthesia. Adequate exposure of the surgical field and accurate localization of the hole are essential to successful scleral buckling procedures. Inadequate exposure results in unnecessary trauma to tissues and generally compromises the procedure. A generous conjunctival incision is made in the region of the retinal hole. If the hole is located between the rectus muscles, 4-0 black silk traction sutures, passed through the edge of the muscle insertion, facilitate the exposure [1]. Should a hole lie under a muscle, the muscle is tenotomized, and a 4-0 black silk suture is passed through the muscle stump to provide traction. The localization of a retinal hole is frequently a difficult and time-consuming maneuver. Forceps localization, the most rapid and reliable method to identify the location of the hole, can be accomplished without the aid of an assistant. A 0.3-mm Castroviejo forceps is used to grasp the sclera in the approximate area of the hole [2]. The surgeon rotates the globe and observes the indentation while wearing the indirect ophthalmoscope. The tips of the forceps appear as a round indentation [3]. The surgeon must take care not to mistake the shaft of the forceps for the tip. As the fundus is viewed, the globe should be indented with the tips of the forceps. The observer identifies the tips as a rounded indentation which disappears as the pressure is released [4].

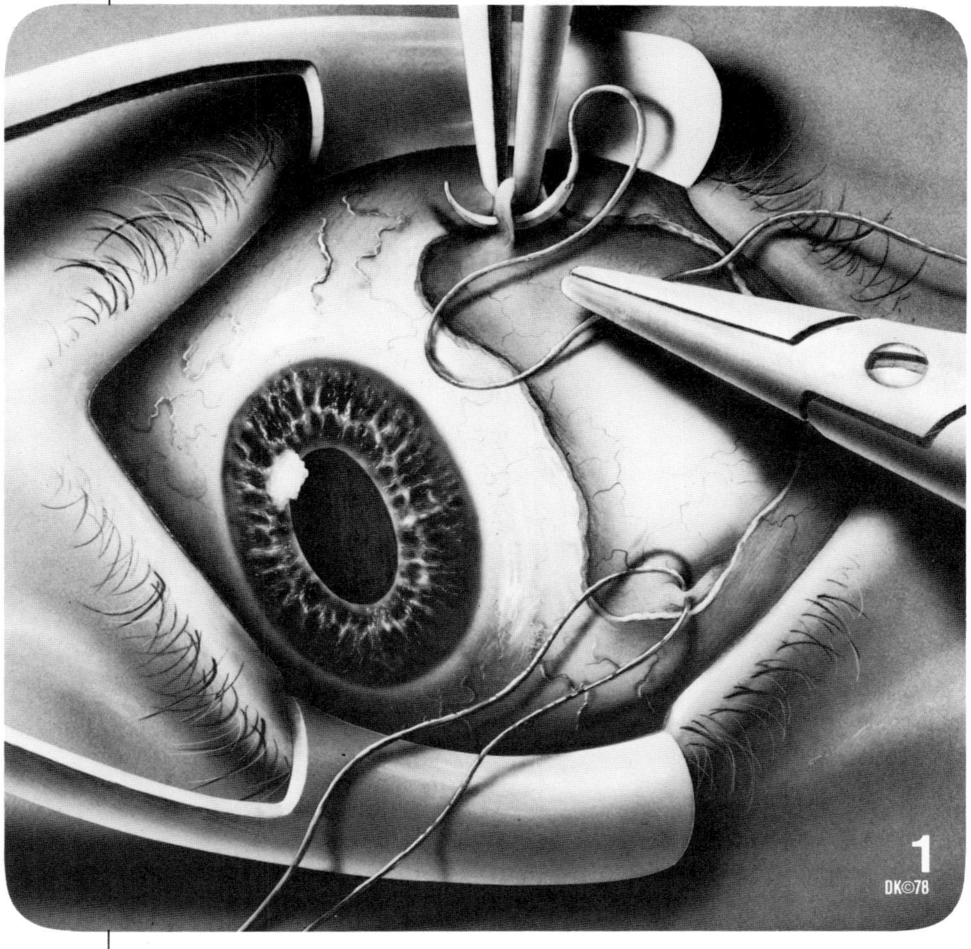

1
DK©78

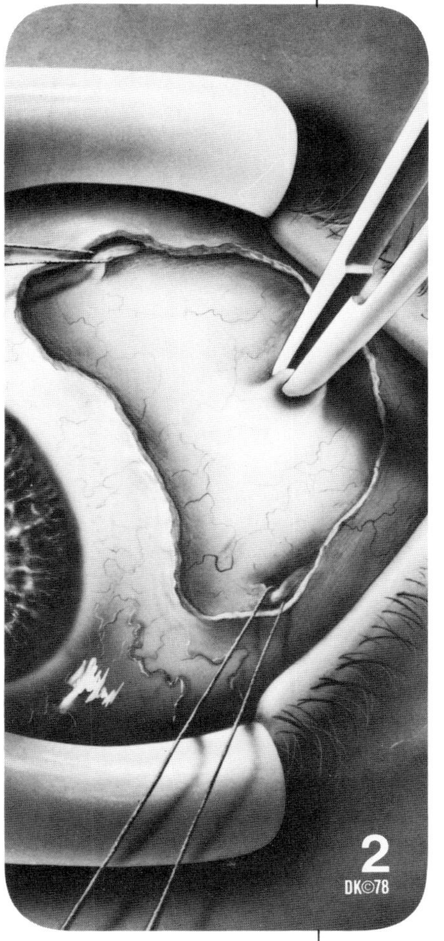

2
DK©78

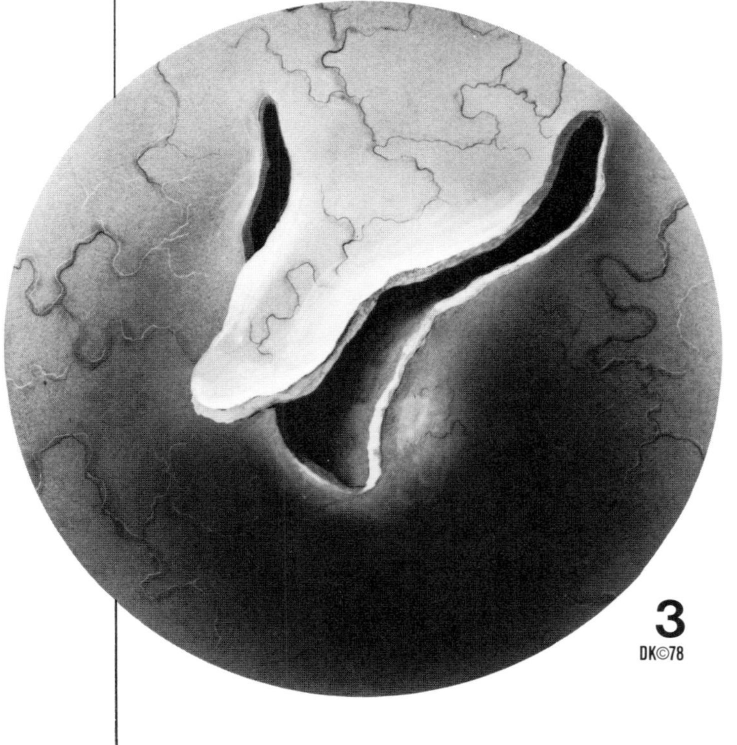

3
DK©78

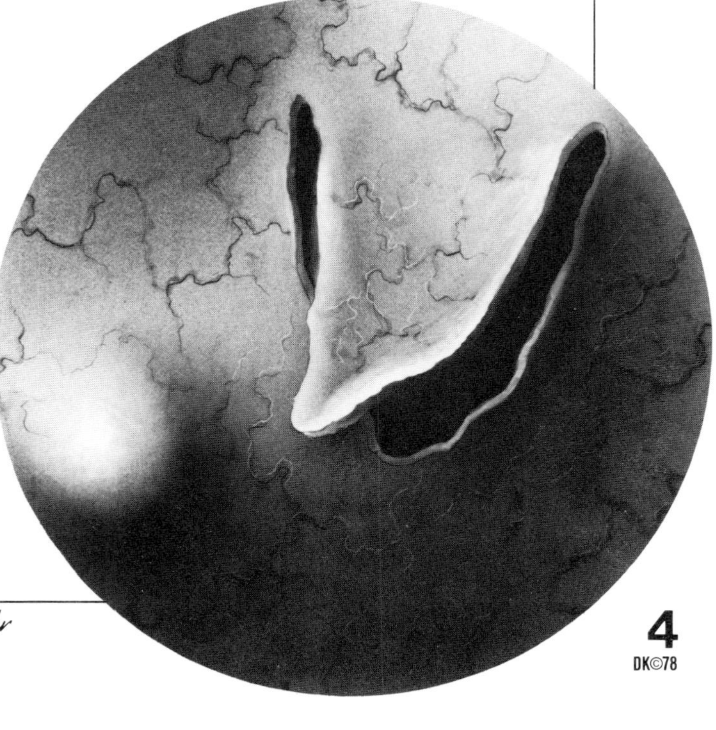

4
DK©78

To localize the hole, the surgeon uses two 0.3-mm Castroviejo forceps. One forceps is used to localize the hole and rotate the globe, while the other fixates the globe as the localizing forceps is positioned [5]. During the localization of the hole, the surgeon observes whether the detachment can be flattened as the sclera is indented. This determines if a local buckle is sufficient to repair the retinal detachment. If the hole cannot be flattened or nearly flattened, the surgeon may want to switch to a scleral buckling procedure with an encircling element.

After the hole has been localized, a marking pencil marks the location of the hole on the scleral surface [6]. The cryoprobe is placed on the scleral mark, and as the tip freezes to the sclera, the globe is rotated [7]. The region of the hole is observed with the indirect ophthalmoscope. Formation of an ice ball at the retinal hole confirms accurate localization. The hole is frozen until the retina turns white so that at least a 2-mm margin is treated around its periphery [8].

To treat relatively small holes, a sponge sutured to the sclera, overlying the localizing mark, will adequately flatten the hole. With larger holes, however, the placement and orientation of the sponge are more difficult. The orientation is best determined by the use of a cotton-tipped applicator applied to the scleral surface, while the indentation is viewed with the indirect ophthalmoscope [9]. The exact

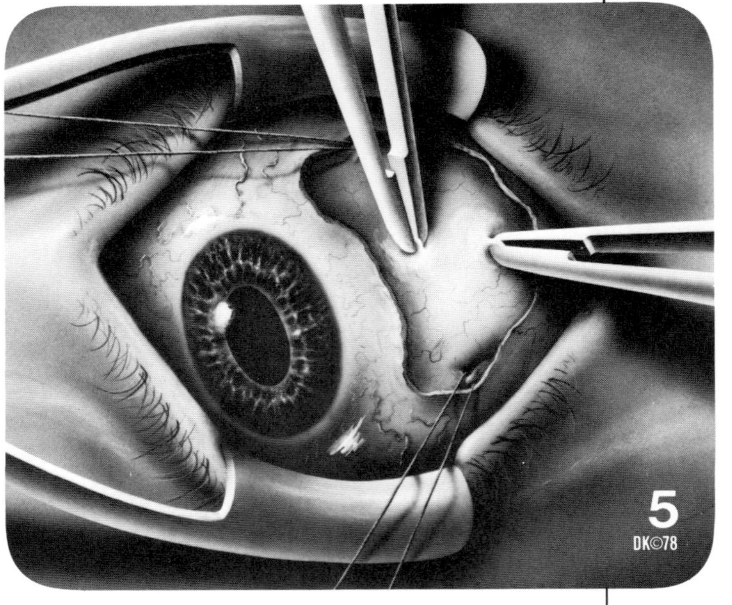

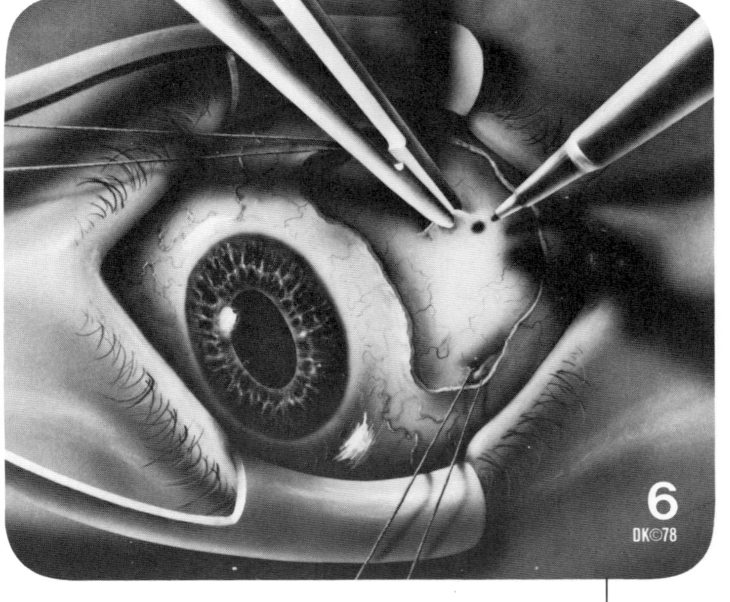

Donald A. Kilby

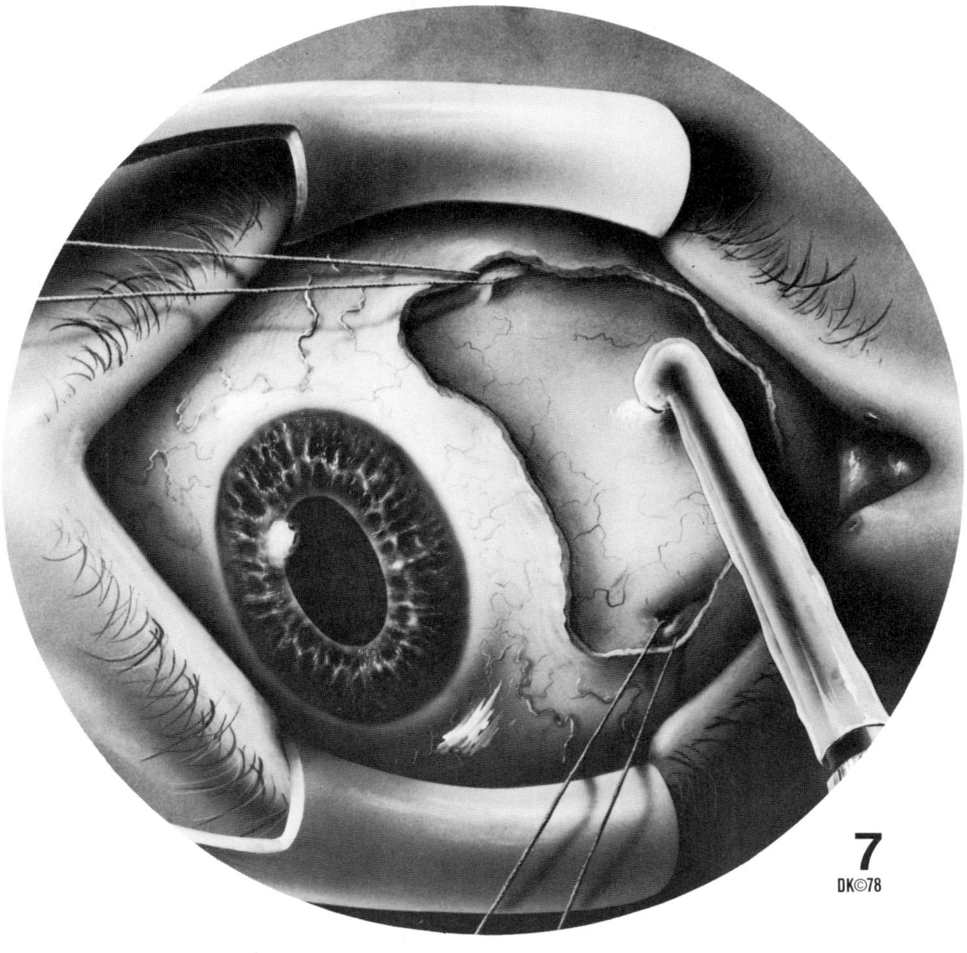

7
DK©78

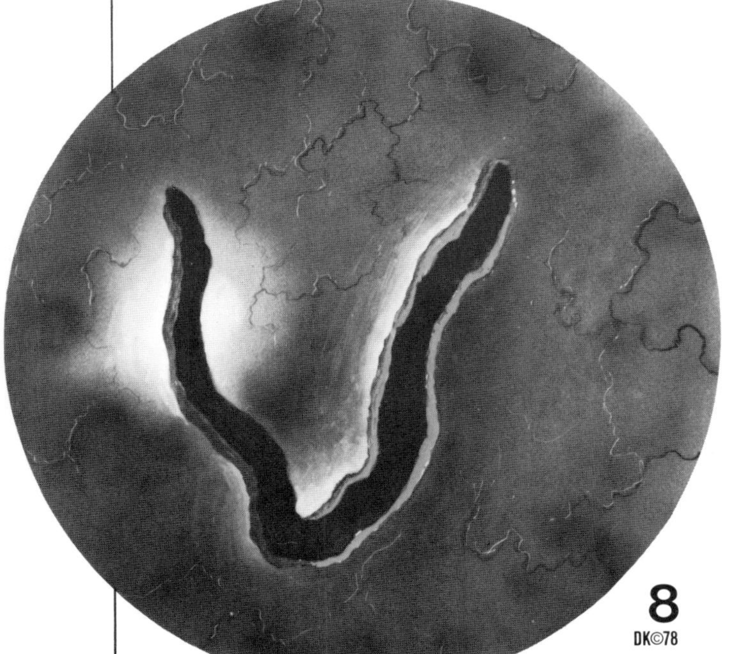

8
DK©78

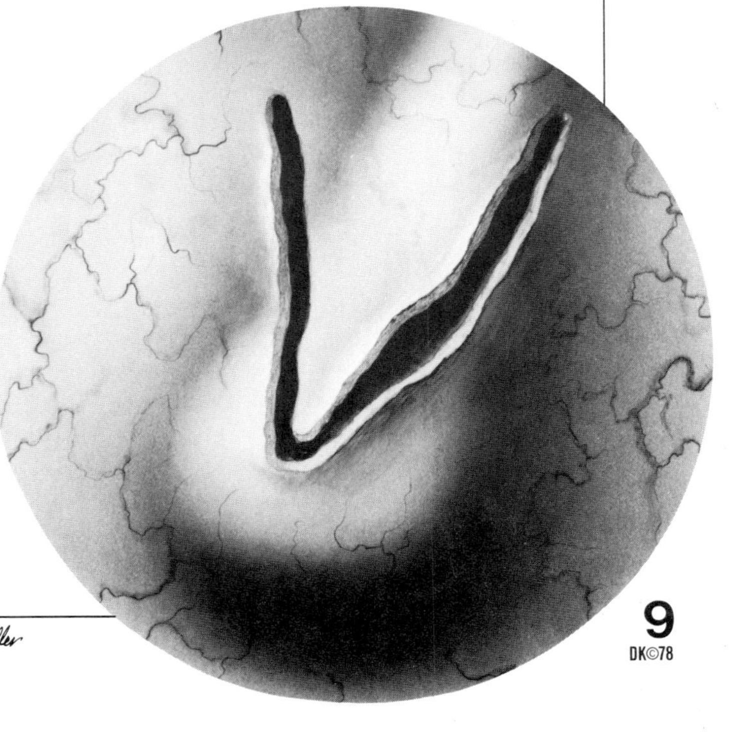

9
DK©78

Donald A. Keller

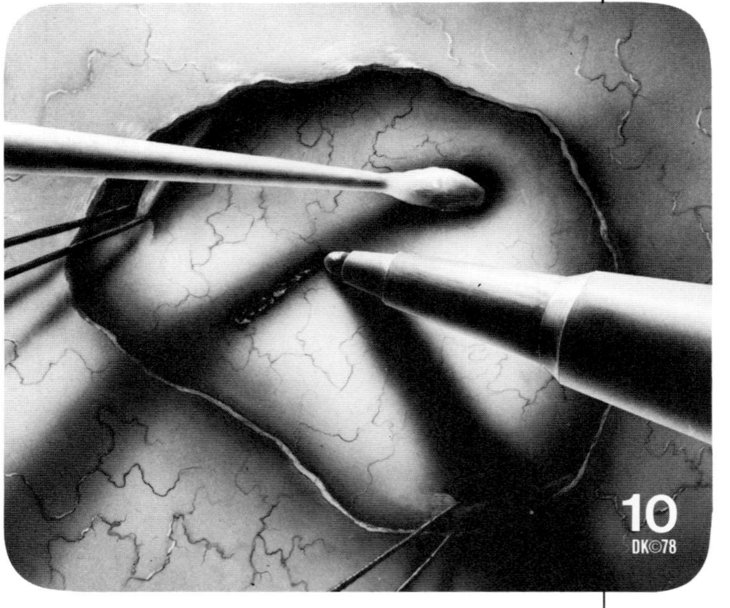

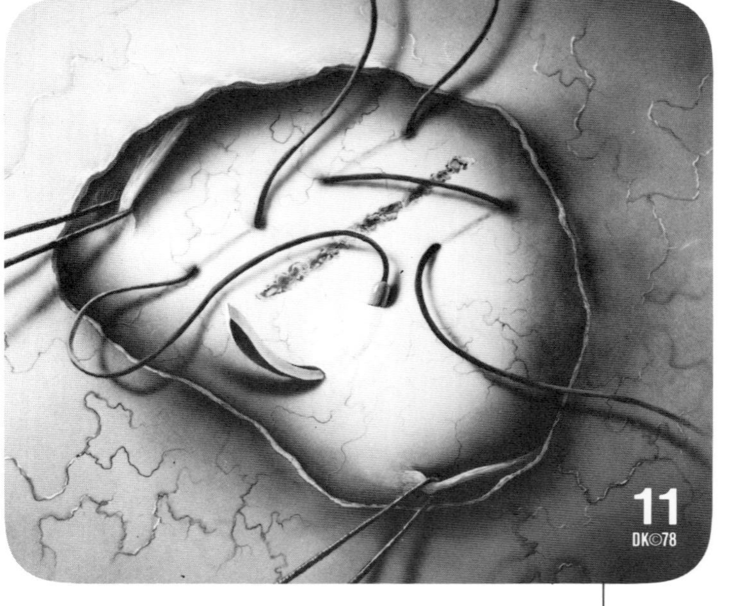

radial orientation of the sponge is marked on the sclera [10]. Two variables affect the creation of an indentation when a silicone sponge is used: the distance between the sutures and the amount of tension on the sponge. The greater the distance and tension, the greater will be the indentation. We recommend suturing a 5-mm sponge to the sclera with a radial orientation. This eliminates one problem inherent with circumferential indentation; that is, a large horseshoe tear will frequently fish-mouth. If correctly positioned, a radial indentation created by the sponge will flatten the tear. We recommend the use of a 4-0 synthetic suture (Mersilene) with a spatula needle to secure the sponge to the sclera. This gauge suture is strong enough to create tension without breaking and large enough not to cut through the sclera when the suture is tied. We also recommend the use of long scleral bites parallel to and placed 5 mm on either side of the scleral mark [11]. As the needle courses through the superficial scleral fibers, the tip should always be visible to reduce the possibility of perforating the globe. The scleral bite should be approximately 5 mm long to provide a firm scleral attachment to anchor the sponge.

After the sutures are placed, the surgeon passes the sponge beneath the loops of the suture [12], and the assistant grasps both ends of the silicone with toothless forceps or hemostats. The sponge is placed on stretch along the line previously marked on the sclera. The assistant must pull in a tangential fashion directed toward the globe. If tension is directed away from the globe, the sutures may rip out of the sclera as they are tied. With the sponge on stretch, a triple-loop surgeon's knot is firmly tied. A second tie locks the suture, and the assistant can release the tension on the sponge [13]. The third tie com-

Donald J. Keller

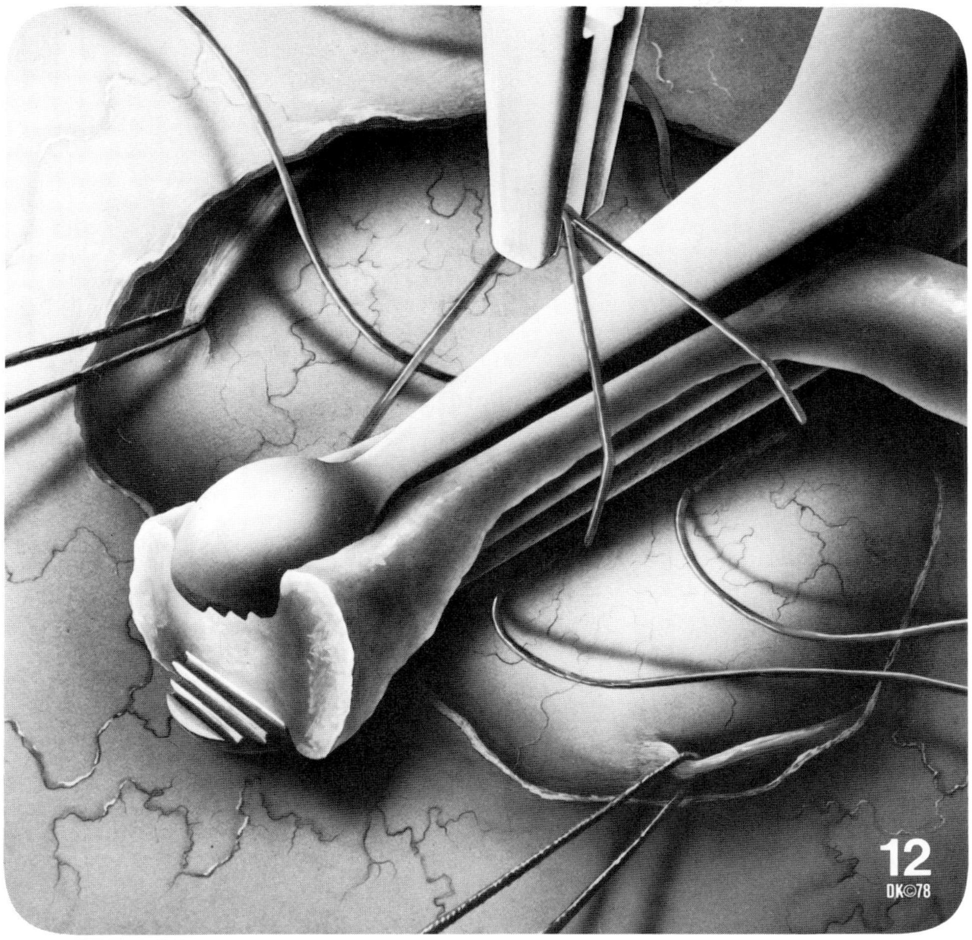

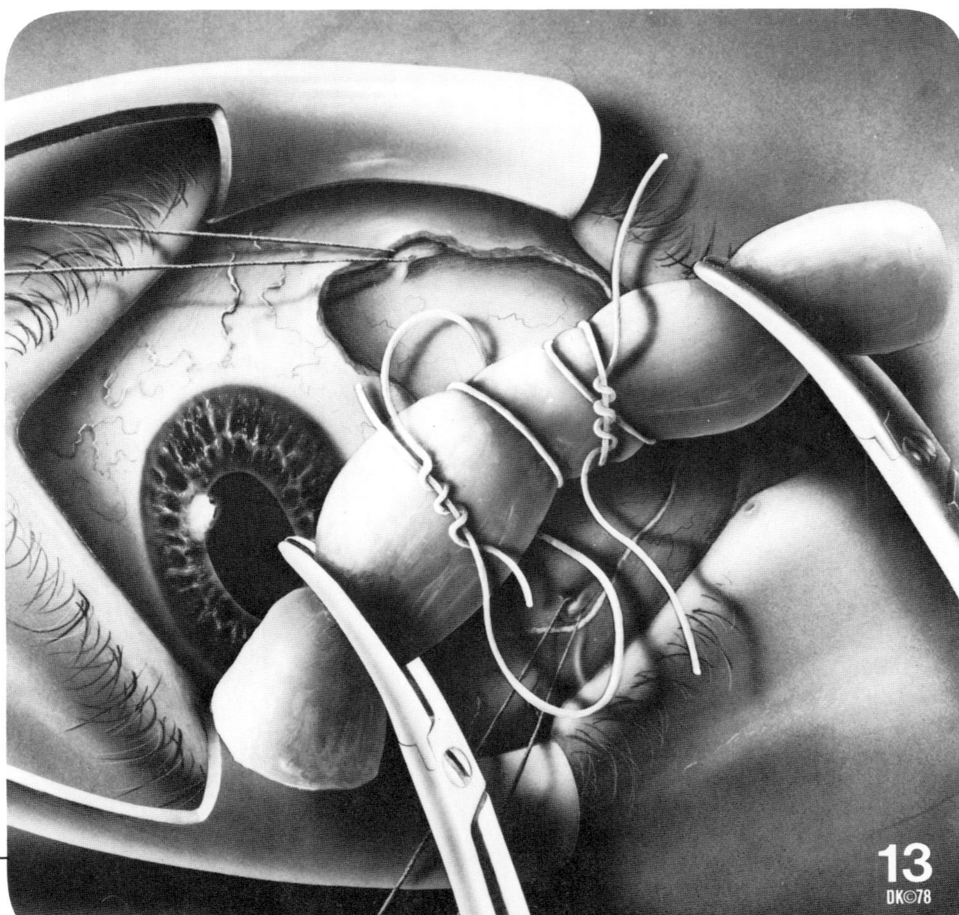

Donald A. Killer

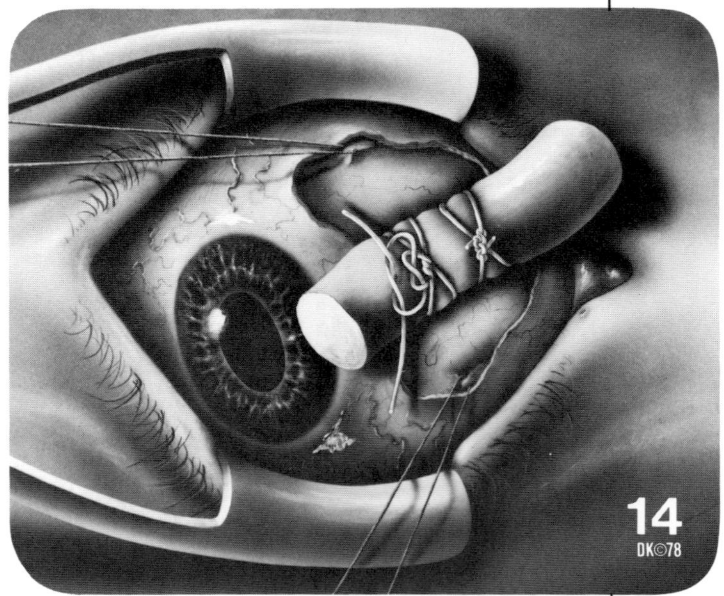

pletes the knot. The explant is firmly secured with two additional knots, and the redundant ends of the sponge are cut [14] [15] . If the initial localization was accurate, fundus examination at this time reveals a radial indentation that approximates the hole to the retinal pigment epithelium [16] .

Additional sutures may be placed to create a longer indentation if necessary. If a large hole is present, a broader buckle is needed, and two or even three radial sponges may be placed side by side. Tenotomized muscles are replaced, and the conjunctiva and Tenon's capsule are meticulously closed to cover the sponge [17] . Any gap in the wound that exposes the sponge will eventually result in infection and extrusion of the sponge. We recommend the use of atropine sulfate 1 percent once a day and antibiotic solution four times a day in the immediate postoperative period. The patient is fully ambulatory the day after surgery but should refrain from vigorous activity until after the first postoperative visit in two weeks.

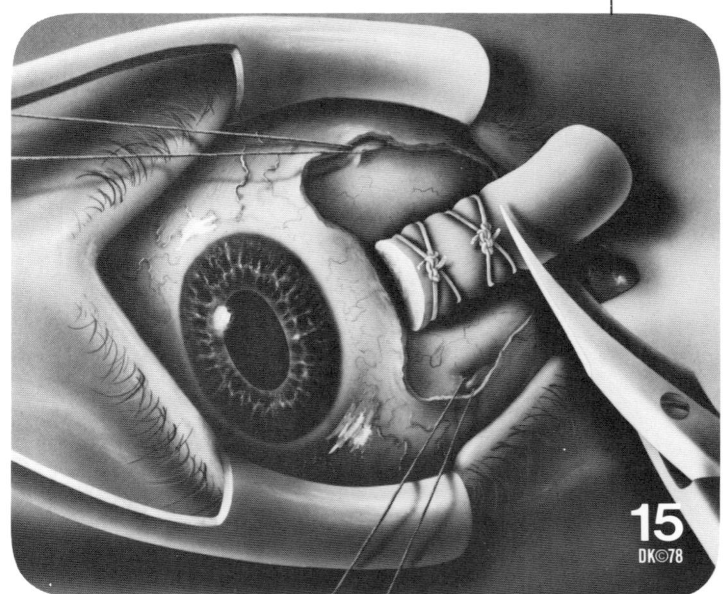

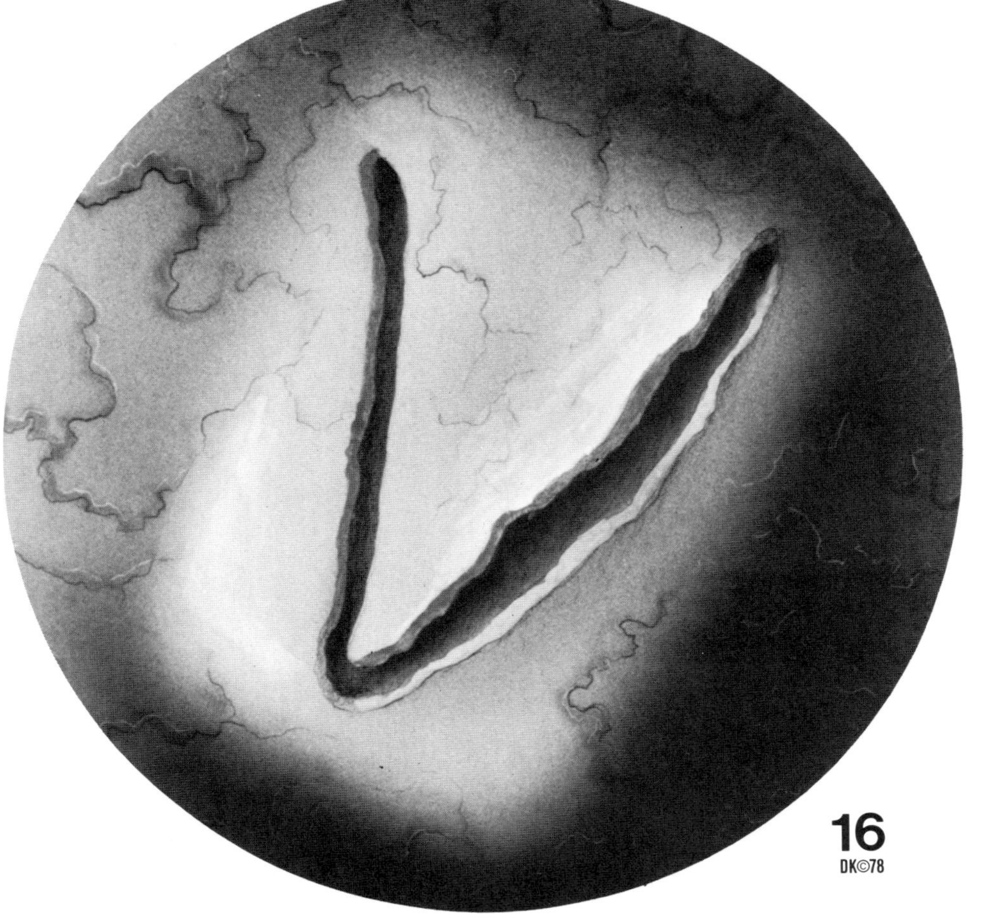

16
DK©78

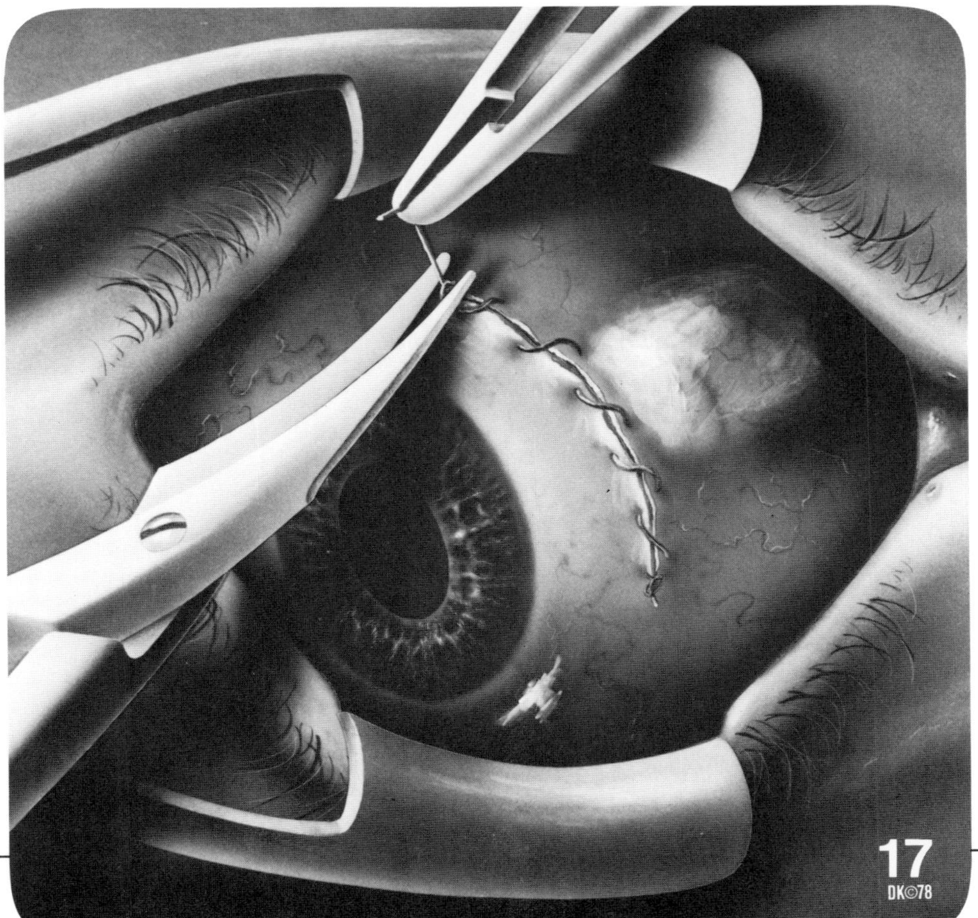

17
DK©78

PREPARATION OF FASCIA LATA STRIPS

Frederick H. Davidorf, M.D.
William H. Havener, M.D.

Human fascia lata has been used in surgery since McArthur used strips of the external oblique aponeurosis for sutures to repair inguinal hernias in 1901. The ophthalmic surgeon has found many uses for human fascia: suspension procedures for ptosis repair, treatment of scleromalacia perforans, and repair of ectropion and entropion.

Homologous fascia lata, the conjoint aponeurosis of the gluteus maximus muscle (GM) and the tensor fascia lata muscle, TFL [1], is the primary encircling element used for repair of retinal detachments at our institution. It is ideal because of the exceptional strength of its long parallel fibers. Although it surrounds the entire thigh, only the lateral fibers are suitable since they are fairly dense and run parallel to one another. We have found that preparation of fascial strips from cadavers has eliminated the need to use the patient's own fascia. Obtaining the fascia from cadavers is a relatively simple procedure, and elaborate equipment is not required. Fifty strips can be obtained from one cadaver. The fascia strips are frozen in antibiotic solution and have been stored up to six months with no loss of strength. Neither infection nor host rejection has been encountered in over 7,000 scleral buckling procedures with use of homograft fascia lata.

Depending on state law, the formal consent for autopsy is usually sufficient for removal of fascia. We recommend its removal from the body as soon as possible, and no longer than 24 hours after the donor's death. We have avoided the use of material from donors who have died of infectious diseases or who have a history that suggests the possibility of hepatitis. The age of the donor is not a consideration, except that infants and children are usually not suitable donors because the fascial strips are not of sufficient length.

The method of stripping fascia is extremely important if the surgeon is to obtain strips that are strong and will not tear during surgery. Therefore, it is important to identify the parallel fibers and to prepare the strips by tearing, rather than cutting, the fascia into linear bundles.

The donor site, extending from the greater trochanter to the knee on the lateral side of the thigh, is prepared as for sterile surgery. The initial skin incision is made on the lateral aspect of the thigh [2]. Starting the incision about 8 cm distal to the greater trochanter in the region of the greatest fat accumulation decreases the possibility of damaging the fascia lata. The incision is extended to 8 cm above the patella. The amount of subcutaneous fat varies, but eventually a glistening white layer is seen as the incision is deepened. When the fascial plane is reached, the initial longitudinal skin incision is extended posteriorly at a right angle from its upper end, creating an L-shaped opening [3].

Due to the loose areolar tissue that surrounds it, the dissection of the surface of the fascia lata is relatively easy. While the surgeon uses a Kelly clamp or hemostat to hold the lateral skin flap stationary, blunt dissection with the fingers divides the fat from the fascia lata [4]. Occasionally, a scalpel is needed to sever some of the lateral femoral

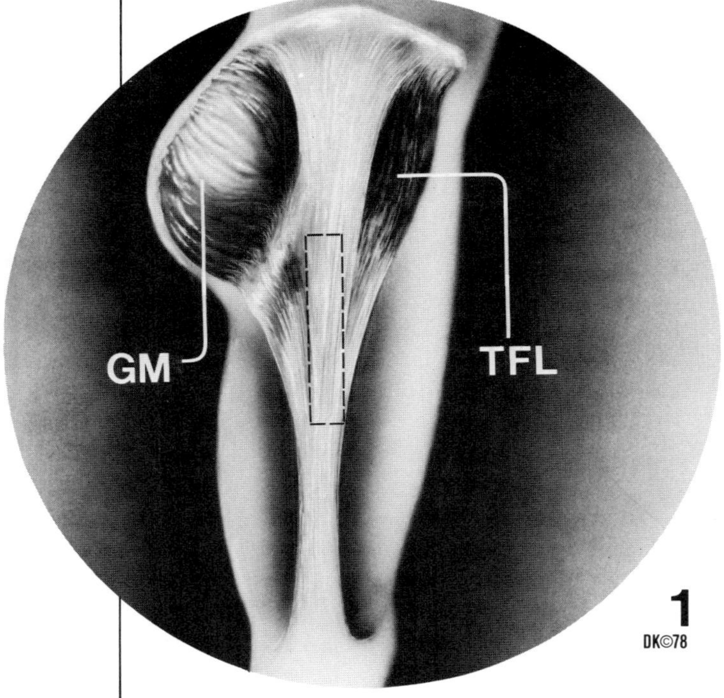
GM
TFL
1
DK©78

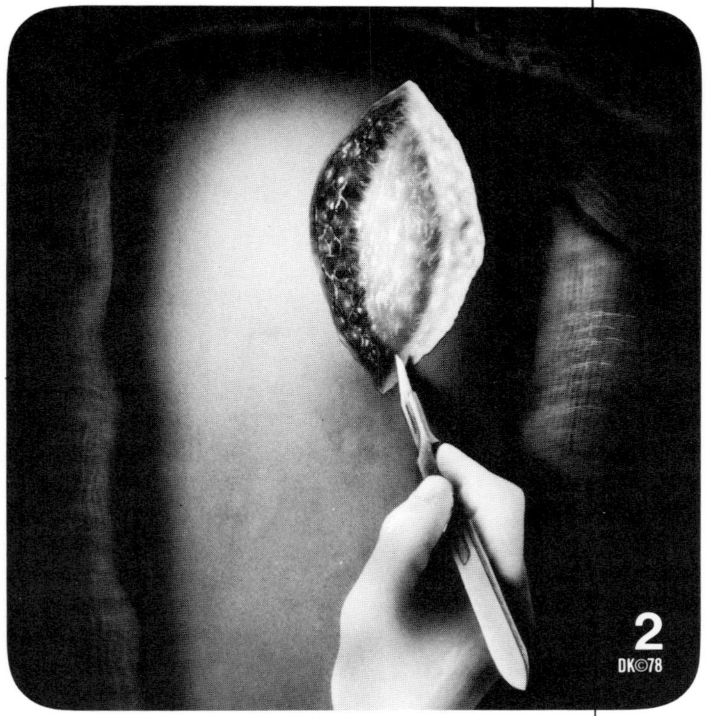
2
DK©78

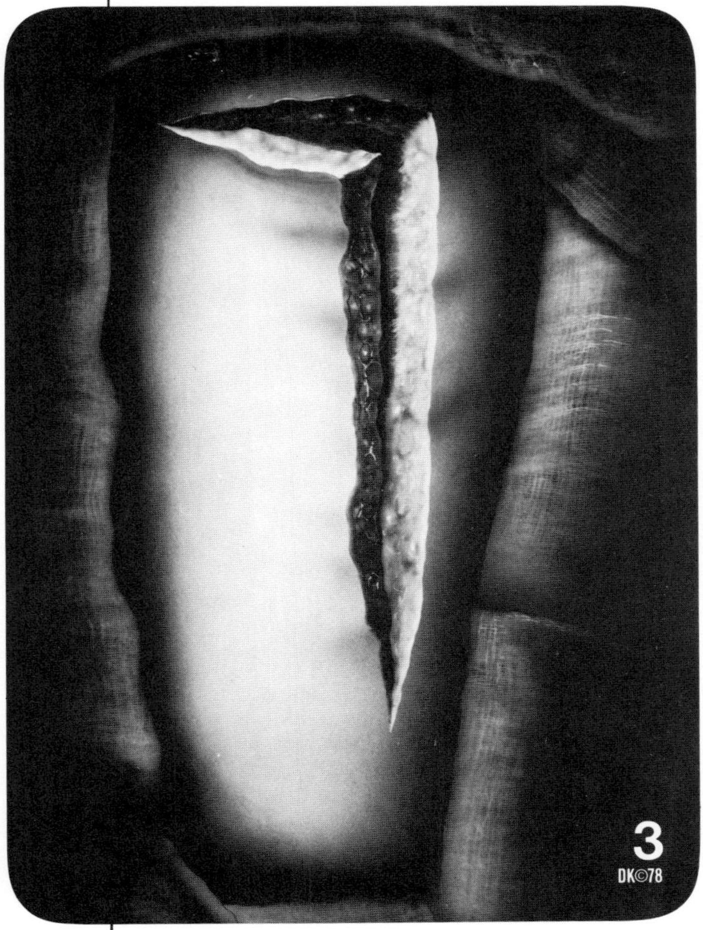
3
DK©78

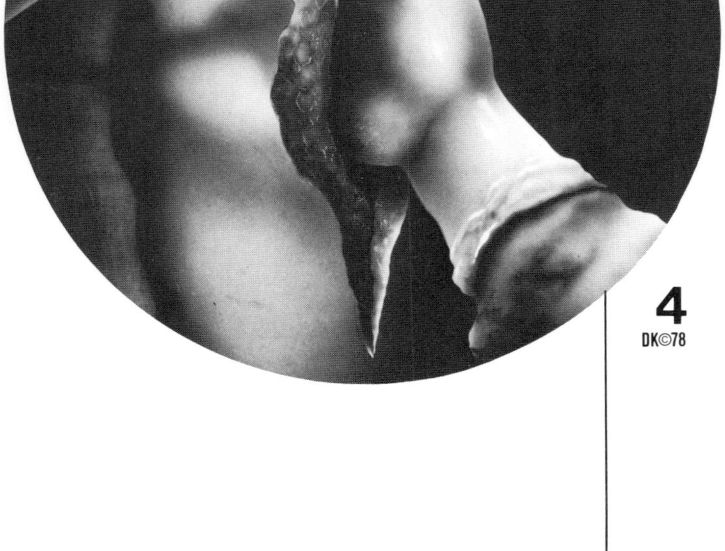
4
DK©78

cutaneous nerves that pierce the fascia. The scalpel, held perpendicular to the fascia fibers, also helps to remove some of the adhering loose areolar tissue and fat [5]. By a combination of blunt and sharp dissection, the skin and underlying fat are separated from the fascia as far as possible in all directions.

With the same dissecting technique, the surgeon exposes the anterior portion of the fascia. Usually this anterior skin flap is only 2 to 5 cm wide since the fascia lata fibers in this area become much thinner and poorly defined and hence are unsuitable for donor tissue. After the outer surface of the fascia has been generously exposed, several dry sponges are rubbed vigorously over the exposed surface of the fascia lata to remove most of the remaining fat [6].

At the junction of the thin, obliquely oriented, anterior fibers and the longitudinal, lateral fibers, an incision is made extending from the proximal to the distal end of the exposed fascia [7]. The surgeon can easily slip a 4″ x 4″ dry sponge behind the fascia lata and free the entire deep surface of the fascia by blunt dissection [8]. To remove the fascia from the thigh, the surgeon extends the superior end of the fascial incision about 8 cm posteriorly. With blunt large Mayo

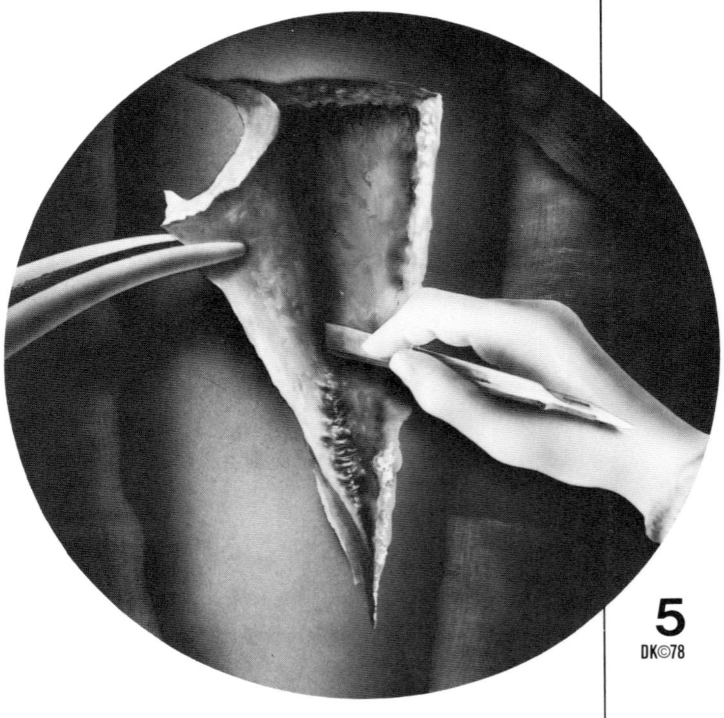

5
DK©78

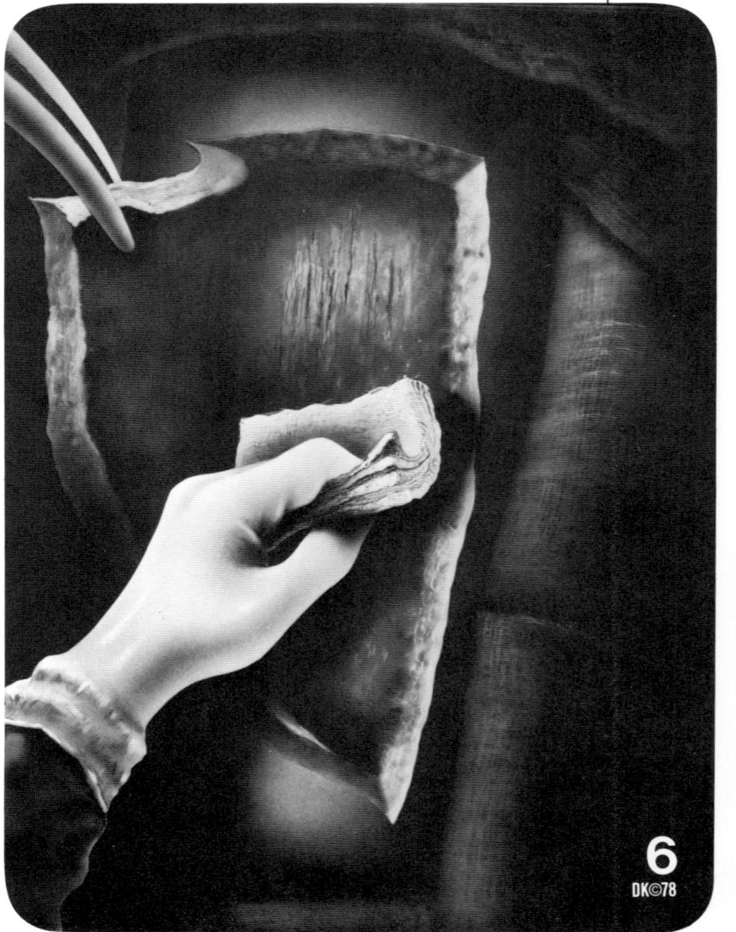

Donald F. Keller

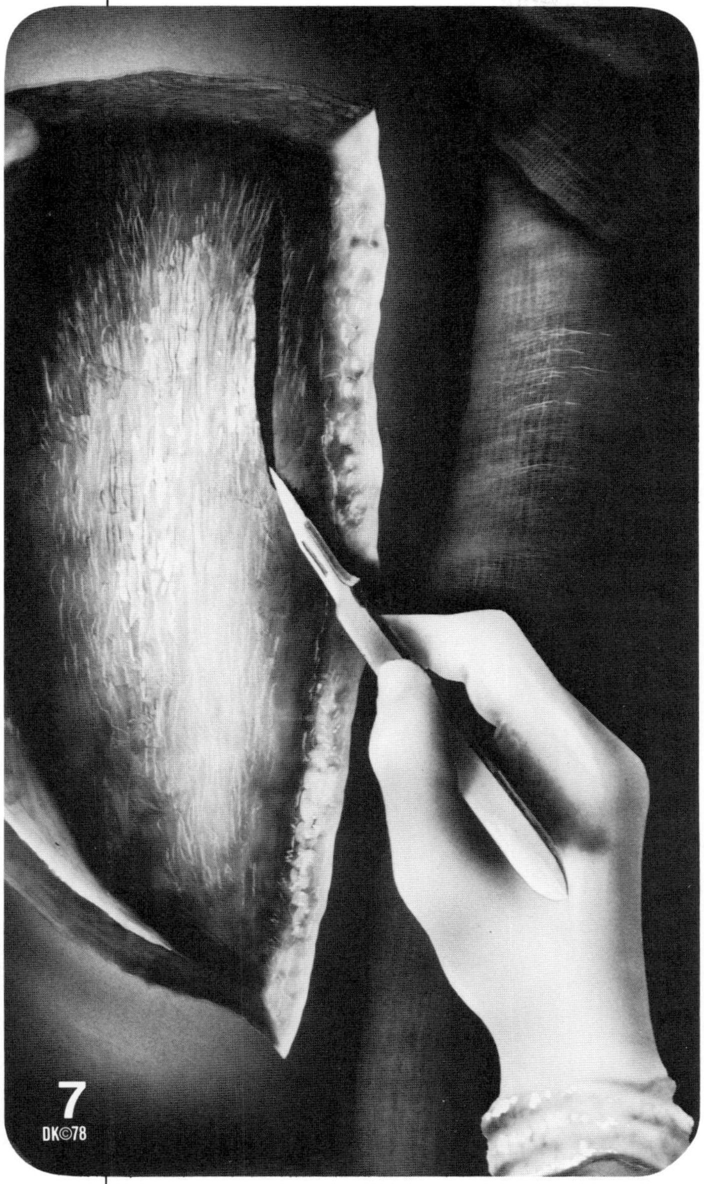

7
DK©78

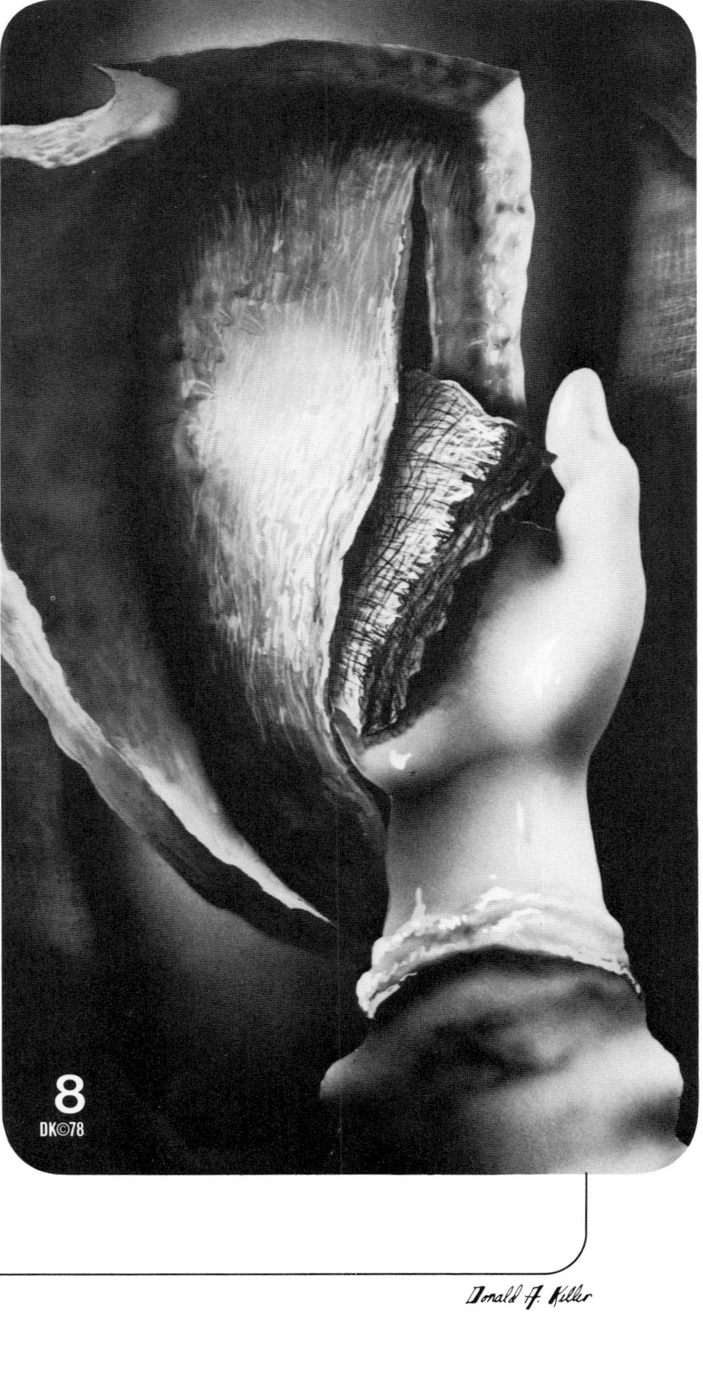

8
DK©78

Donald A. Kilhr

scissors, the superior end of the fascia is cut just distal to the end of the tensor fascia lata muscle [9]. With the aid of traction from clamps, the posterior fascial border is cut. Finally, the inferior margin is incised to remove the fascia lata from the thigh [10].

The dissected piece of fascia should be roughly rectangular in shape. The most common error in obtaining fascia is to take the material from the anterior thigh (thin, nonlinear tissue) or to excise a diamond-shaped or oval piece (which provides only a small amount of long-fibered fascia).

The fascia lata is placed in a sterile container and immersed in the antibiotic solution of the surgeon's choice. We use Neosporin solution, a mixture of polymyxin B sulfate, neomycin sulfate, and gramicidin. Subsequent cultures of this preparation have never resulted in bacterial growth.

The process is repeated on the second thigh. The skin incisions are closed with any appropriate suture. Both pieces of fascia can be placed in the same container and antibiotic solution. The fascia is frozen and can be stored for many months without deterioration.

The strips of fascia can be prepared in a sterile environment at a later date. After thawing, the fascia is spread, and the loose fat is rubbed off with a dry sponge [11]. A hemostat may be needed at one end to hold the fascia in place. A No. 22 Bard-Parker blade may be used to scrape off the fat by holding the scalpel perpendicular to the piece of fascia at 90 degrees to the axis of the long fibers. Care must be exercised not to cut the fascia. The oblique fibers on the undersurface can also be removed by traction with a hemostat or forceps.

Once the fascia has been cleaned on both sides, it can be divided into strips. Several methods of creating thin, uniform strips have been described, most of which involve cutting the fascia. However, it is difficult to cut between two bundles of fibers without cutting diagonally which destroys the continuity of the longitudinal fibers. The problem can easily be avoided by tearing the fascia [12]. With one hemostat placed parallel to the edge at the end of the broad fascia lata band, a second large hemostat is placed as close to the first as possible. The hemostats are pulled in opposite directions forming a thin, uniform strip of fascia about 3 mm wide. Rubbing the thin strip with a dry cotton sponge removes all remaining fat as well as any loose areolar tissue. The ideal fascial strip is about 3 mm wide and 12 to 16 cm long.

The strip of fascia is placed in a sterile test tube. Ten drops of antibiotic solution placed in the test tube rinses the fascia to the bottom of the tube. A piece of plastic drape, about 10 cm square, is placed over the top of the test tube, and a stopper is pushed into the mouth of the tube outside of the plastic drape. A rubber band is wrapped around the plastic to hold it securely to the tube. In this manner the fascia remains sterile when poured from the tube, since the end of the tube remains covered during storage.

The fascia lata from one thigh usually makes about 20 to 25 strips. The test tubes are placed into a basket that has been labeled with the donor's name, date and time of death, date and time of collection of the fascia lata, and the cause of death. The basket is placed in the freezer. The fascia is removed from the freezer just prior to use in surgery, is permitted to thaw, and is shaken directly from the tube onto the instrument table.

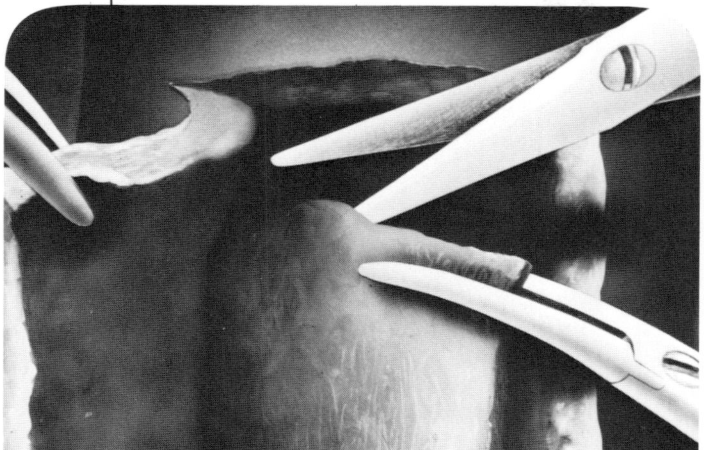

9
DK©78

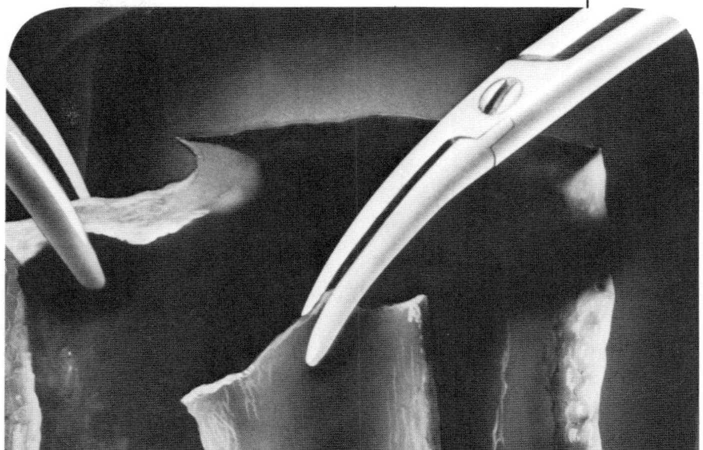

10
DK©78

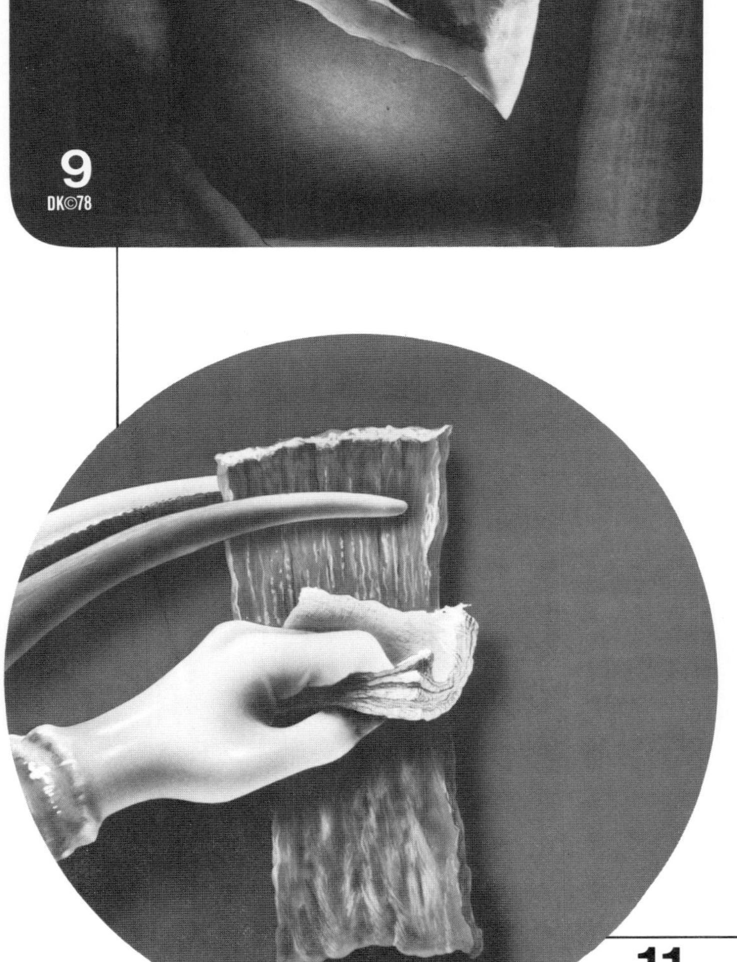

11
DK©78

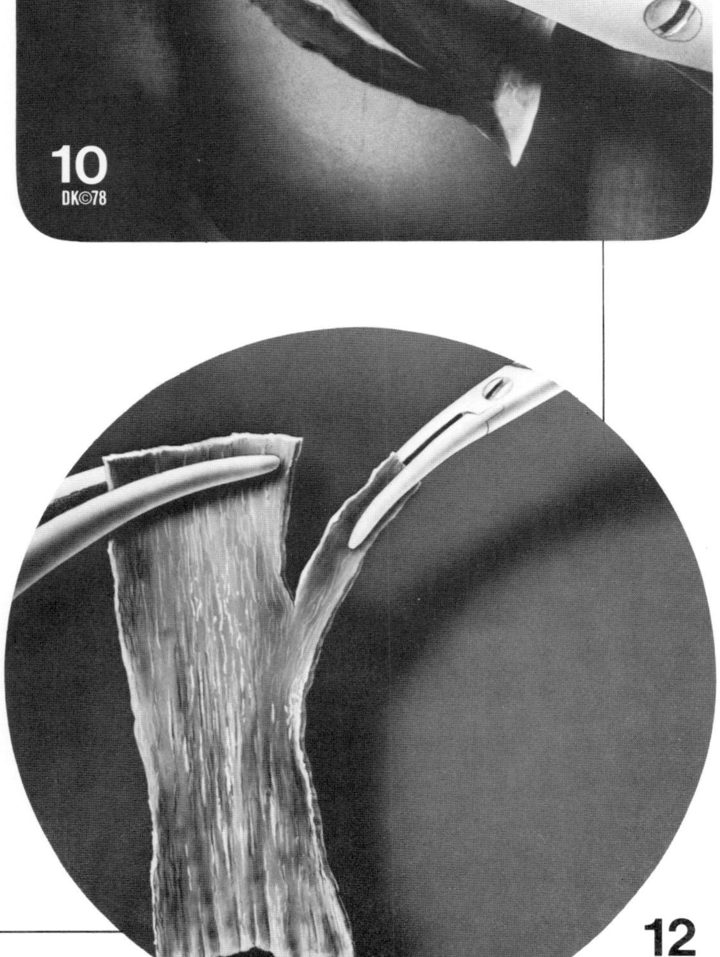

12
DK©78

Donald A. Keller

ENCIRCLING FASCIA LATA

Frederick H. Davidorf, M.D.
William H. Havener, M.D.

We have used homologous fascia lata in retinal surgery at our institution since 1961. Since that time, we have performed over 7,000 scleral buckling procedures using an encircling fascia lata strip and have not encountered complications, such as erosion and infection, that have occurred as a result of silicone and other synthetic encircling elements. Because of the ease with which fascia can be manipulated during surgery and the lack of postoperative complications, we feel that it approaches the ideal material for use in scleral buckling procedures.

Most of the operations are performed with the patient under general anesthesia. However, a medical problem that precludes the use of a general anesthetic may warrant the use of retrobulbar anesthesia.

Conjunctival incisions are made in the two quadrants away from the retinal hole. With a fine-toothed Bishop-Harmon forceps, the conjunctiva is grasped 3 to 4 mm from the cul-de-sac. The conjunctiva is elevated, and a 1- to 2-cm incision is made through the conjunctiva and Tenon's capsule with a Westcott scissors. Sclera is exposed with blunt dissection made by the Westcott scissors [1] . The fixation sutures are placed just anterior to the equator. Adequate scleral stabilization is essential for the placement of the 4-0 fixation sutures (Mersilene) and is best accomplished with the use of two 0.3-mm Castroviejo forceps. Superficial scleral fibers are grasped initially at the site of the conjunctival incision, and the globe is rotated for better exposure. A second forceps grasps sclera several millimeters posteriorly, just anterior to the equator. The surgeon then grasps the sclera with a forceps in the nondominant hand, which frees the dominant hand for passage of the needle through superficial scleral lamella [2] . If the conjunctiva interferes with exposure, it may be retracted with the hub of the fixation needle as it is passed through the sclera.

After placement of the fixation sutures, the conjunctiva and Tenon's capsule are opened overlying the muscle in the region of the hole [3] . A muscle hook is passed beneath the rectus muscle to expose its insertion [4] . As the tendon is elevated with the muscle hook, cautery is applied to the insertion along the entire length of the hook. This avoids inadvertent damage to the underlying sclera. The

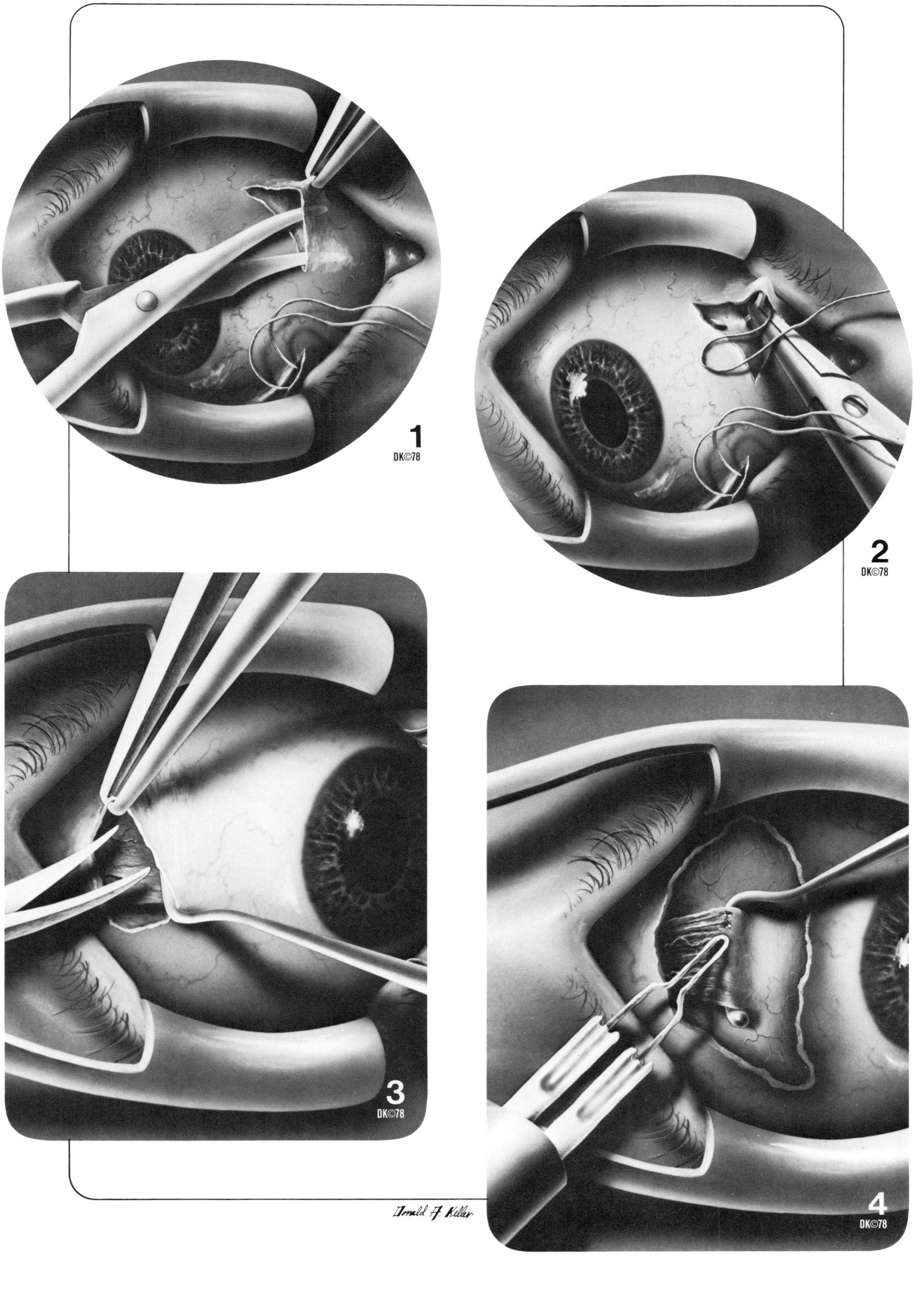
1
DK©78
2
DK©78
3
DK©78
4
DK©78

muscle is tenotomized with a Westcott scissors; less than 1 mm of tendon is left attached to the sclera [5]. It is not necessary to tag the rectus muscle prior to disinsertion. It is easily retrieved at the end of the procedure by everting the conjunctival surface with one forceps while a second forceps grasps and elevates the muscle sheath. This exposes the cut end of the muscle. A 4-0 black silk suture is passed through the stump of the tendon and should incorporate the superficial scleral fibers. One pass through each end of the stump is sufficient to secure the suture, which is used for traction throughout the procedure.

The success of the scleral buckling procedure depends on accurate localization treatment of all holes [6] [7]. Forceps localization (see Radial Silicone Sponge Explant section) is used to identify the position of the retinal hole.

After the hole has been localized and marked, cryoretinopexy is applied to the retinal hole under direct visualization. When the retina around the hole turns white, cryoapplication is adequate. In bullous detachments, where a considerable amount of subretinal fluid is present, it is frequently difficult to determine where the hole will rest after the fluid is drained. In these cases, we frequently freeze the retinal hole after the subretinal tap. This reduces the amount of cryotherapy necessary to create an adequate adhesion.

The fascia is passed under the rectus muscle and secured to the sclera with the use of the previously placed fixation sutures. To insure that the fascia passes beneath the muscles, initially a muscle hook is passed beneath the rectus muscle, and the fascia is then directed along the same pathway underneath the muscle hook [8]. To accomplish this, the Castroviejo forceps grasps the end of the fascia and passes it between muscle and sclera and then through the conjunctival opening. An alternative method for the passage of fascia uses a second muscle hook and may be necessary when directing fascia under horizontal rectus muscles [9].

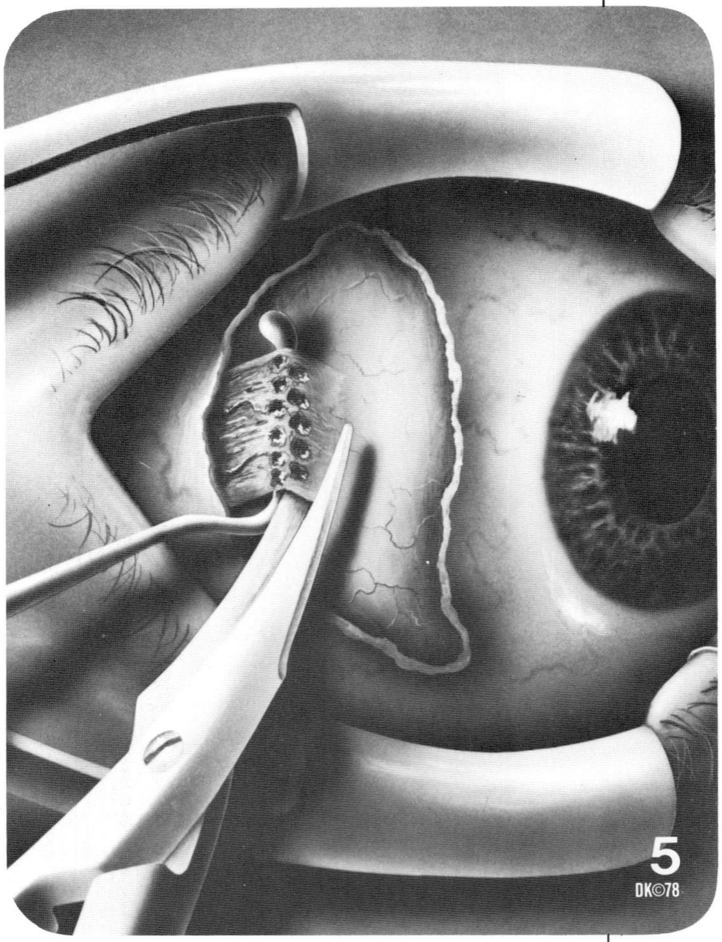

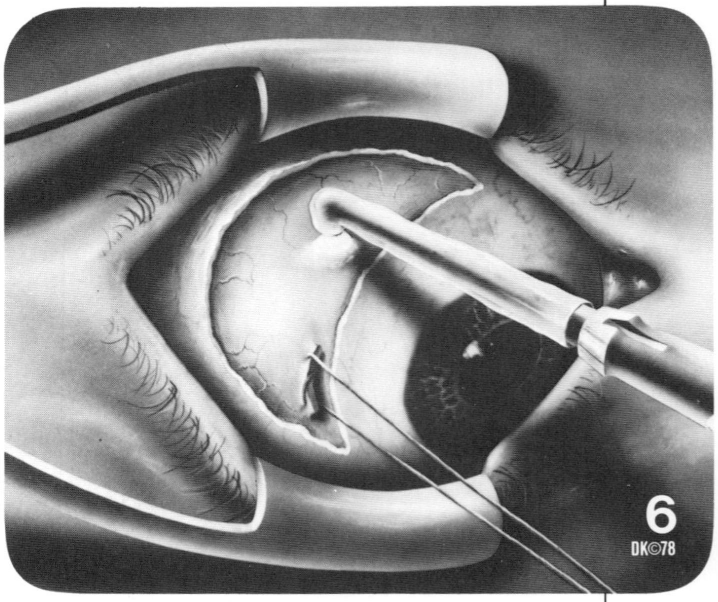

Donald A Keller

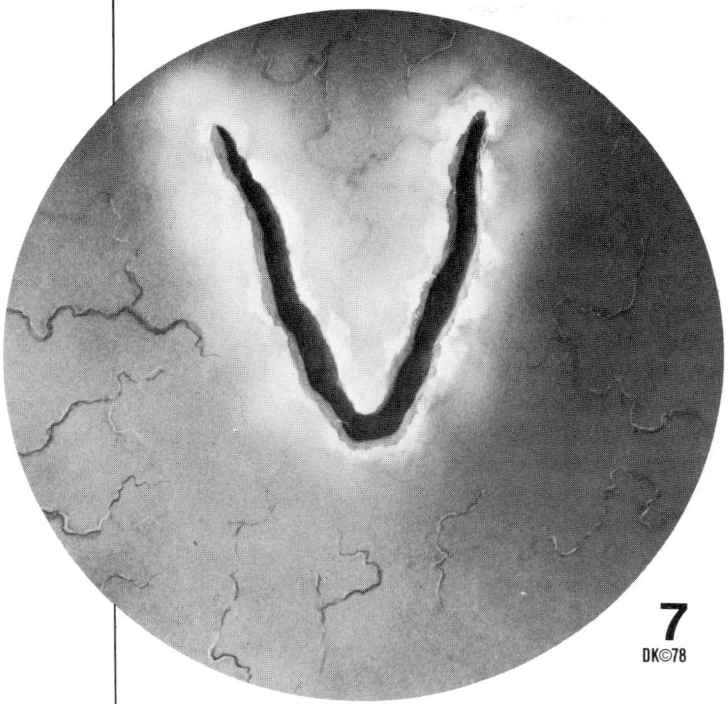

7
DK©78

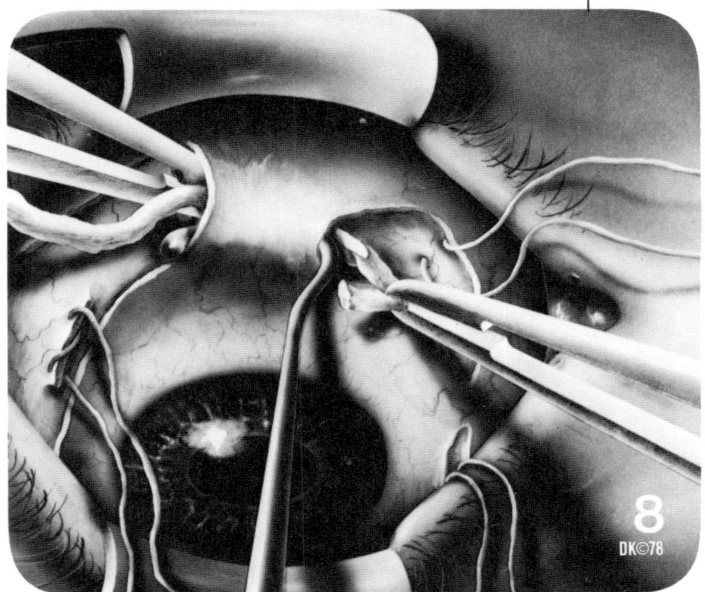

8
DK©78

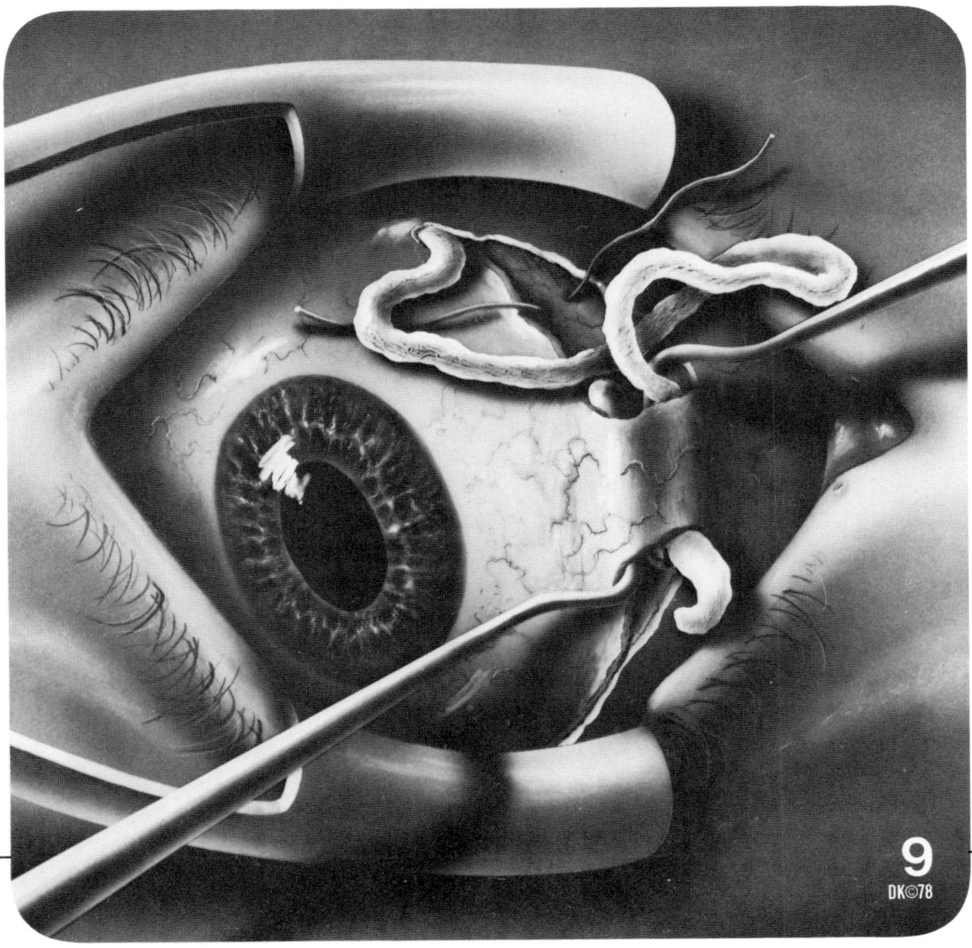

9
DK©78

The exposed end of the fascia is grasped and advanced with a forceps. As the fascia is advanced, 5 to 10 cm is left on each side of the retinal hole to be used for subsequent tying. The Mersilene suture secures the fascia to the sclera. When the suture is tied, the pull should be tangential to the globe **10** . If the surgeon lifts when tying the fixation suture, the suture may tear from the sclera.

After the initial muscle hook is passed beneath the tendon of the muscle, the end of the fascia is placed at the edge of the muscle, and a second muscle hook with a rounded tip may be used to engage the fascia and guide it beneath the muscle and through the conjunctival opening. The fascia is passed under the remaining rectus muscles, and the fixation sutures are tied and cut.

The selection of the proper drainage site requires a great deal of experience and judgment. Although a number of acceptable drainage sites exist, we believe that the ideal one is located just posterior to the retinal hole, since this insures flattening of the hole and minimizes fish-mouthing of the tear. However, this site may have to be altered to avoid two potential problems sometimes encountered. To avoid hemorrhage, the surgeon should observe the exposed choroid prior to the tap for evidence of visible choroidal vessels. If the choroid has a deep-red color, a large choroidal vessel is present and should be avoided. Another site must be chosen.

The surgeon also may wish to choose a different tap site when draining fluid in a patient with a retinal detachment that contains shifting subretinal fluid. Since this usually results in the immediate incarceration of the retina at the tap site, with little or no drainage, the surgeon risks the creation of an iatrogenic retinal hole, which compounds the problem and complicates the procedure. In these patients, the surgeon should turn the head and rotate the globe to create a dependent tap site. This usually allows access to the subretinal fluid and thus avoids retinal incarceration.

To drain the subretinal fluid, a No. 15 Bard-Parker blade is used to make a sclerotomy in the region of the hole to expose the choroid **11**. A 4-0 Mersilene suture is passed through the edges of the sclerotomy. This suture is looped out of the incision and is used to close the tap site after the subretinal fluid has been released. Before the choroid is perforated, the fascia is knotted over a second 4-0 Mersilene suture **12** . Two hemostats are attached to the ends of the fascia. The edge of the scler-

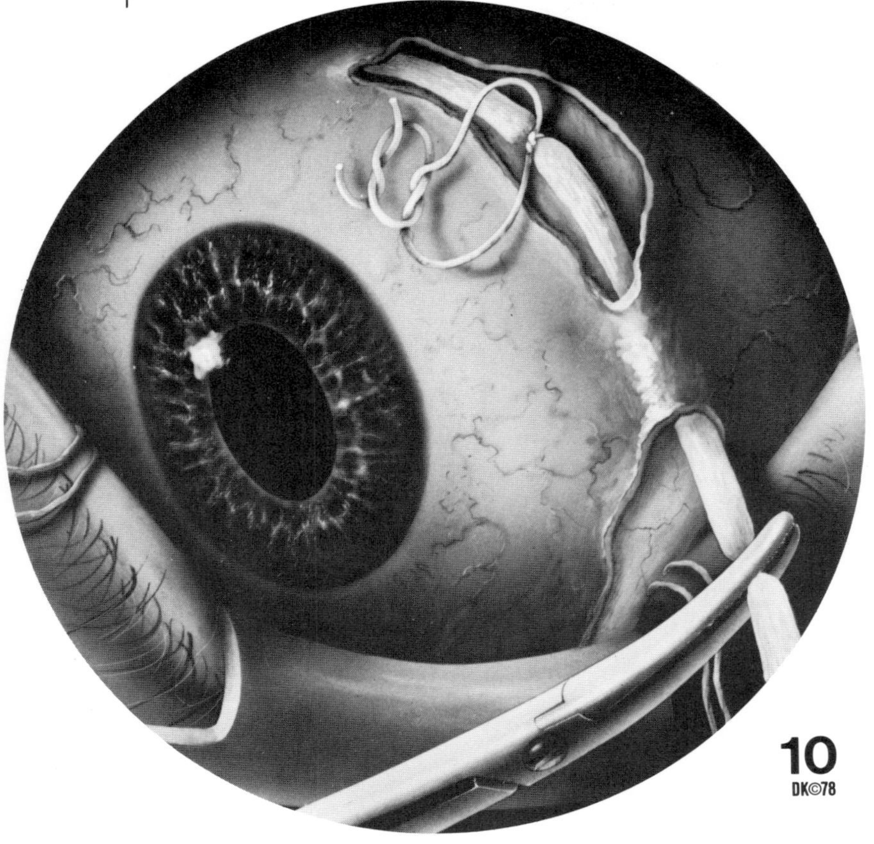

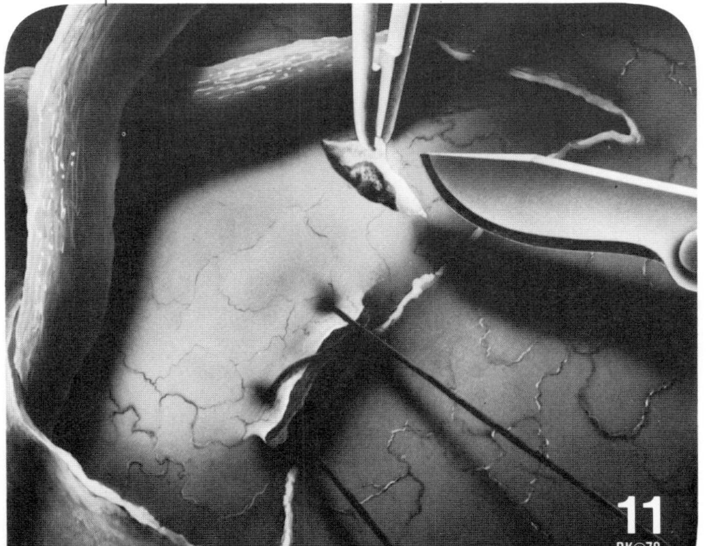

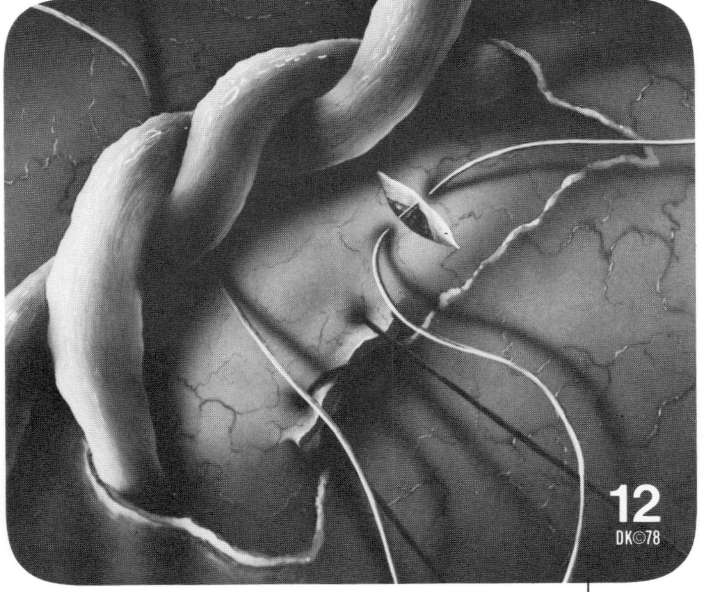

Donald A. Killer

otomy is grasped with a 0.3-mm Castroviejo forceps, and the choroid is perforated with a fine spatula needle [13] . This releases the subretinal fluid.

To monitor the flow of subretinal fluid, the globe is rotated with a cotton-tipped applicator applied to the sclera in the region of the tap, while the surgeon observes the fundus with the indirect ophthalmoscope [14] . The retina exhibits a flapping motion as the fluid escapes from the subretinal space. Direct observation of the fundus during drainage has several advantages. It provides a dependent tap site, and with the use of the cotton-tipped applicator, the site can be manipulated to facilitate removal of the fluid. Also, the surgeon knows when the subretinal space has been evacuated. Finally, complications, such as retinal incarceration and choroidal or subretinal hemorrhage, are promptly recognized. The cotton-tipped applicator also helps maintain pressure. Once the subretinal fluid has been evacuated completely, the sclerotomy site is closed by tying the previously placed suture.

Since the ends of the fascia cannot be tied together, the Mersilene suture secures the fascia with three passes through the fascial knot [15] [16] [17] . The surgeon continues to tuck fascia with additional bites until the desired intraocular pressure is reached. Because fascia shows no tendency to erode into the eye, it may be secured tightly, creating a high buckle, without fear of subsequent erosion. Once the knot is secured and the redundant ends of the fascia are cut, the retina is examined with the indirect ophthalmoscope to insure that the hole is well approximated to the pigment epithelium.

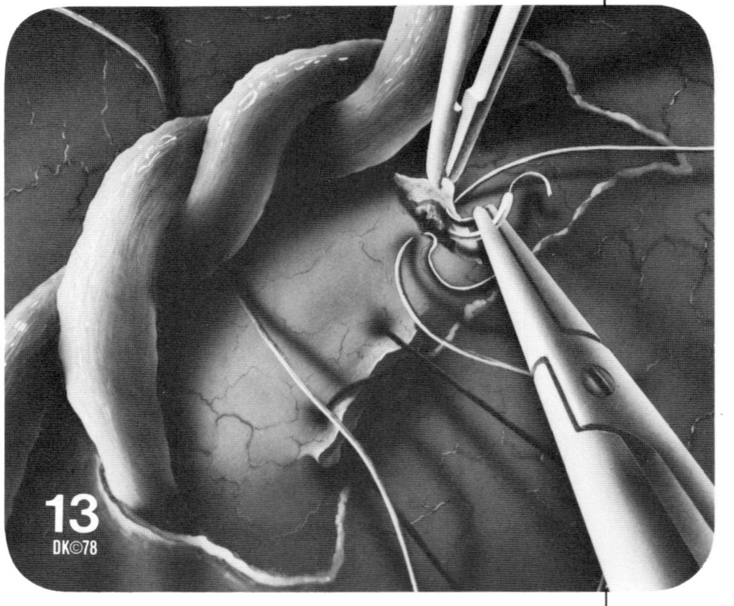

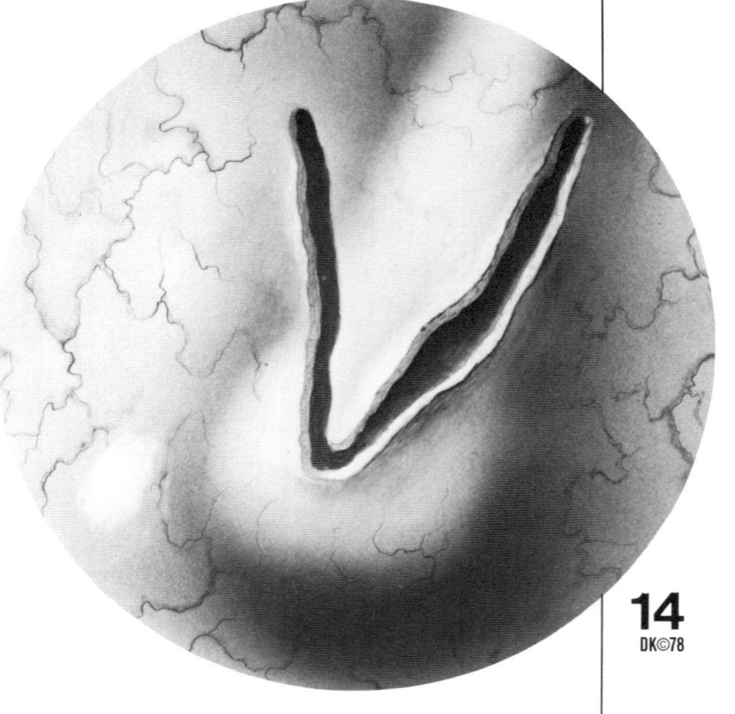

14
DK©78

Donald H. Keller

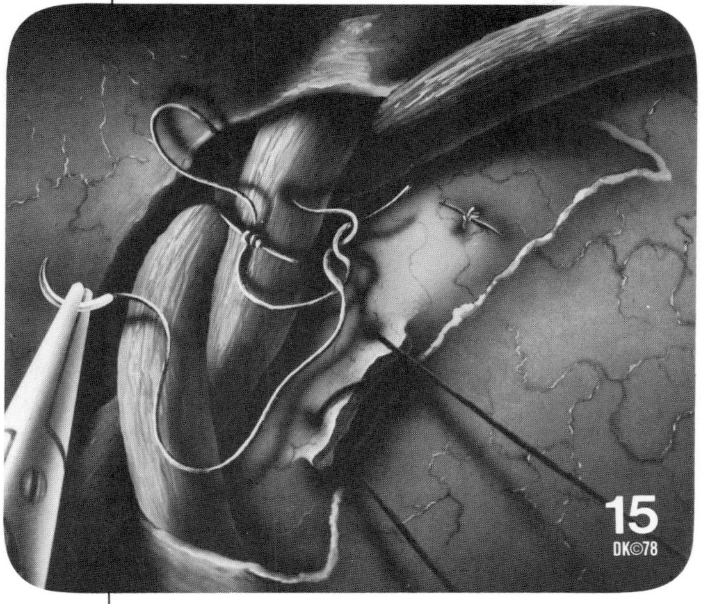

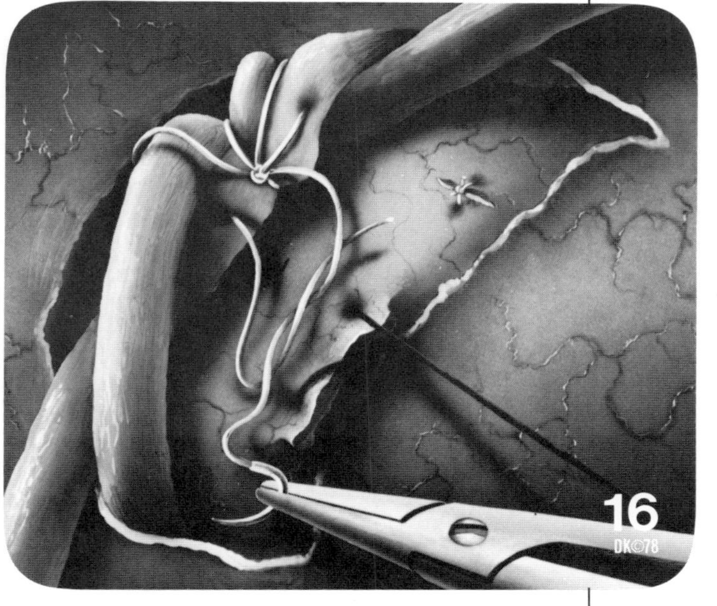

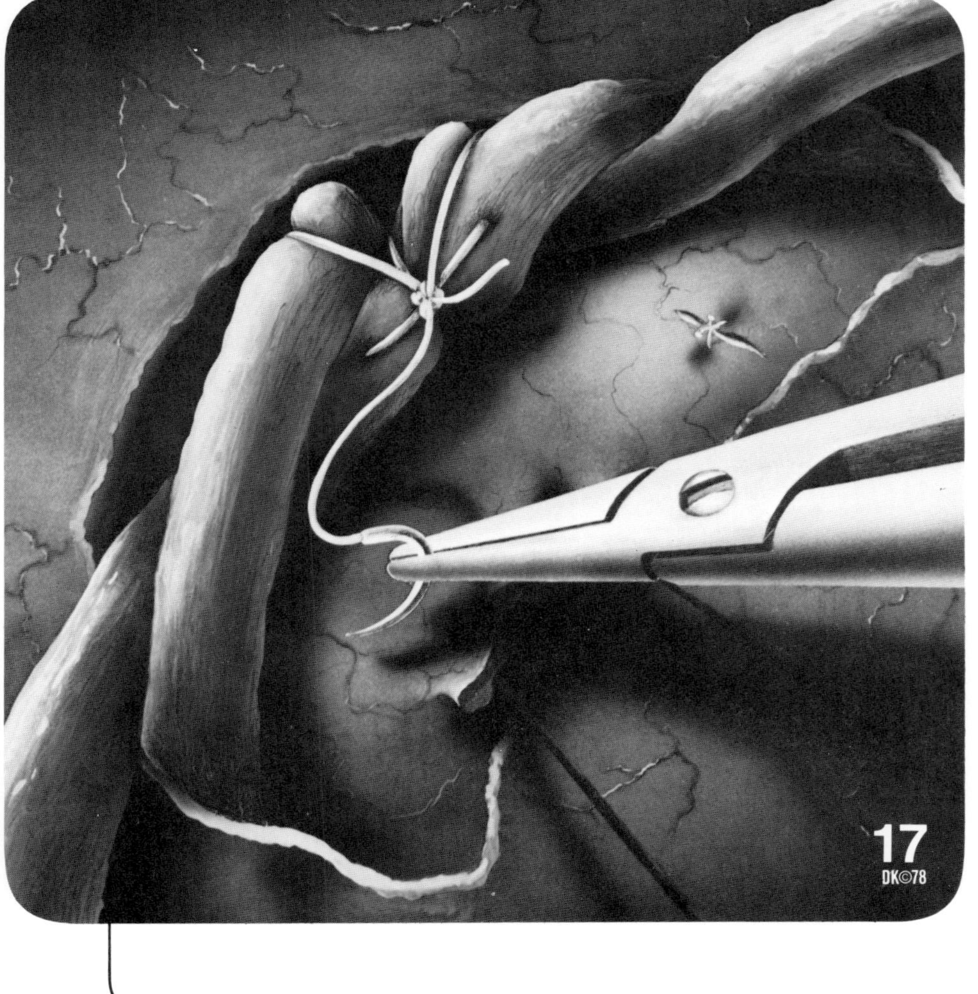

Donald F. Keller

If additional subretinal fluid is present, a second subretinal tap can be made at another site. The position of the buckle can be altered if the surgeon moves the fascia either anteriorly or posteriorly. Ideally, the hole will lie flat on the anterior edge of the buckle with no subretinal fluid 18 .

Once the encircling fascial strip is correctly positioned, the Mersilene suture, which anchors the encircling element to the globe, is passed through the sclera 19 . The redundant ends of the fascia are now cut. If a retinal hole fish-mouths, a subretinal tap will flatten it by incarcerating the posterior edge of the tear.

Alternatively, one sutures a 5-mm radial silicone sponge to the overlying sclera beneath the encircling fascial strip. The radial silicone sponge is sutured to the globe with the same suturing technique described in the radial explant procedure. This usually provides a sufficient buckle to flatten a fish-mouthed tear 20 . When a radial sponge is used in conjunction with an encircling fascial strip, two Mersilene sutures are used to secure the fascia to the sclera on either side of the sponge.

After the retina is satisfactorily reattached, the sutures are permanently tied and cut. The previously tenotomized muscle is replaced with the use of 5-0 catgut suture, and the conjunctival and Tenon's capsule incisions are closed with a 6-0 catgut suture 21 .

The patient is fully ambulatory the day after surgery and may be discharged from the hospital. One drop of atropine sulfate administered once a day is used for a two-week period. No antibiotics are necessary.

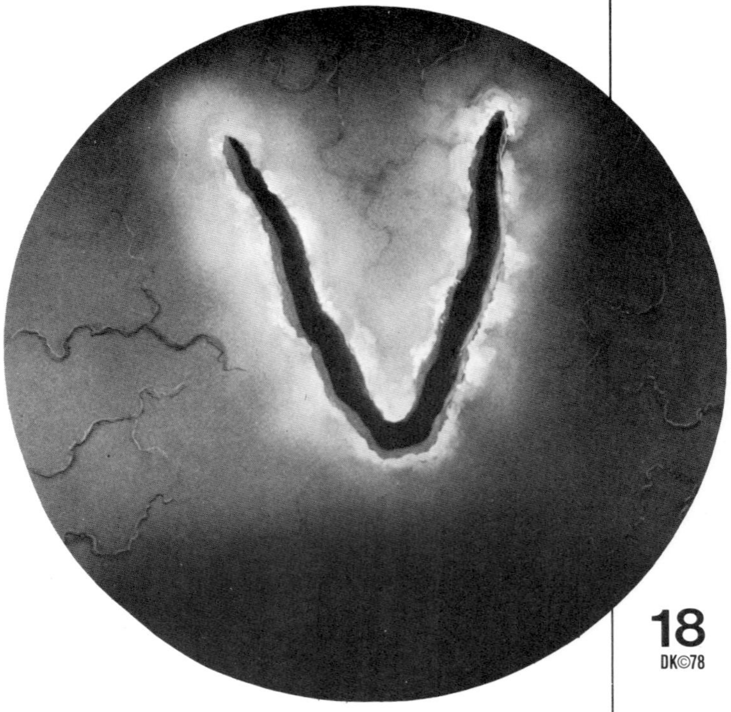

18
DK©78

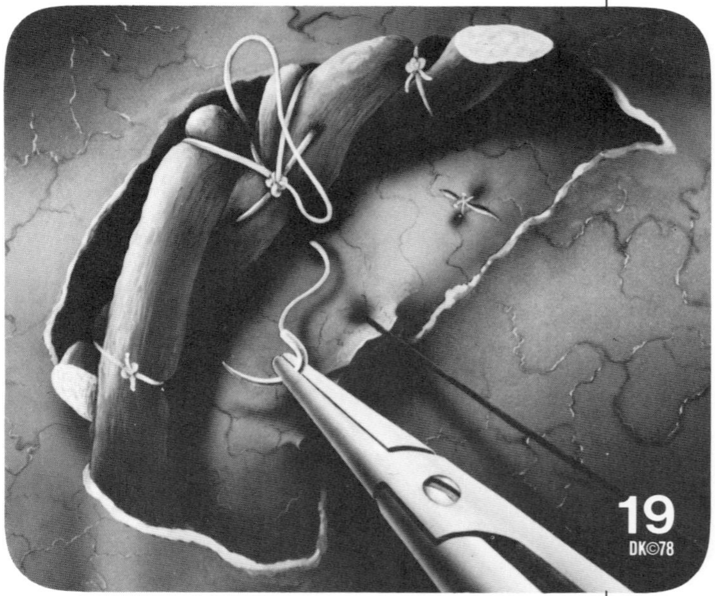

19
DK©78

Donald A. Keller

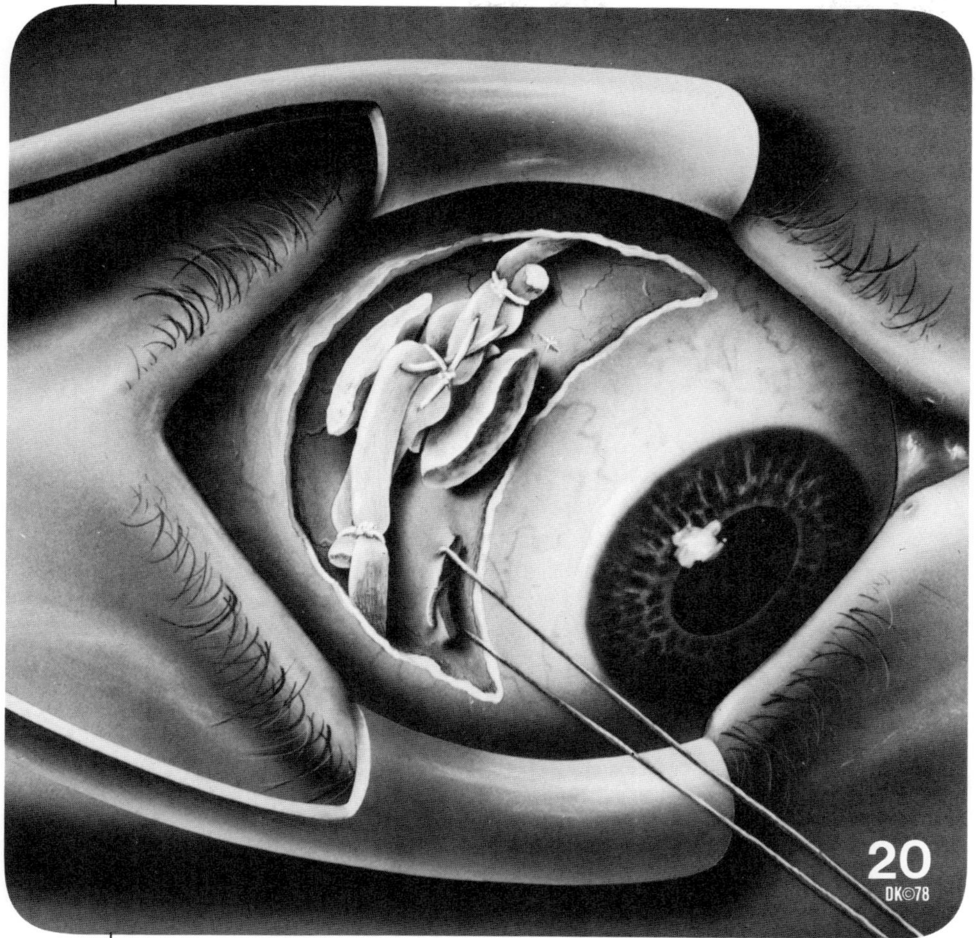

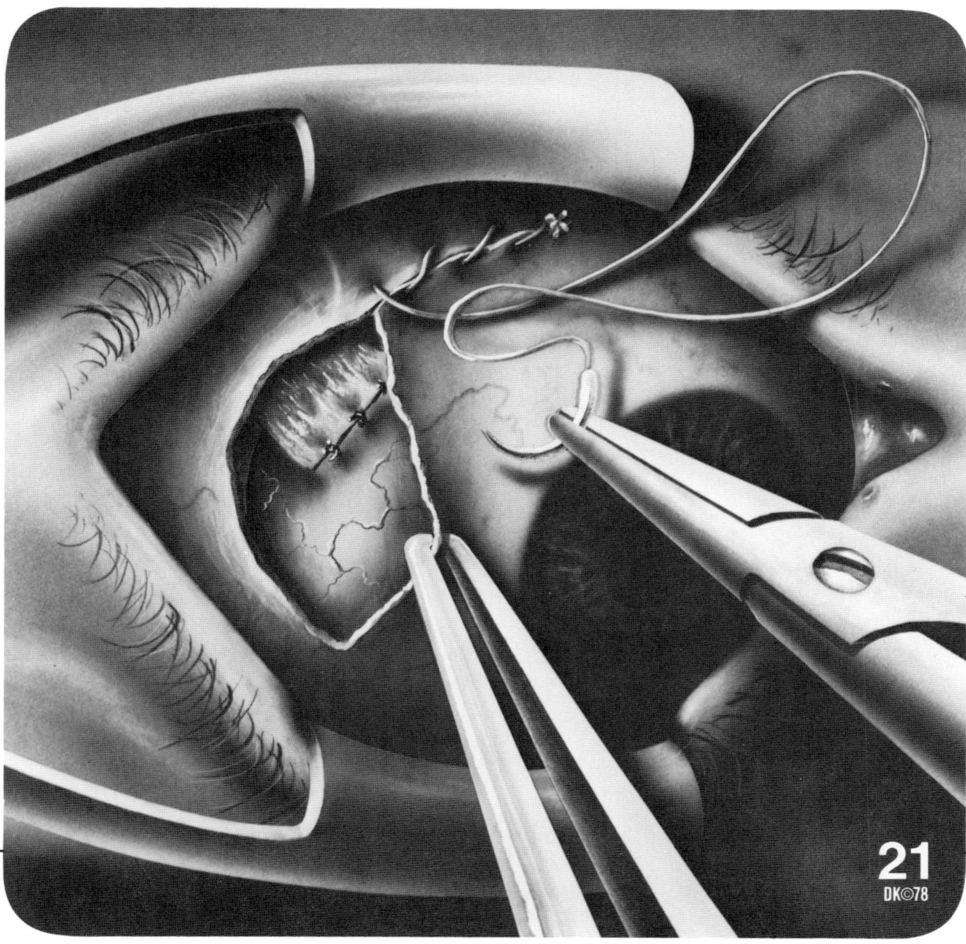

Donald A. Kelker

ENCIRCLING SILICONE SPONGE

Frederick H. Davidorf, M.D.
William H. Havener, M.D.

Although prognosis for patients undergoing scleral buckling procedures for rhegmatogenous retinal detachments has dramatically improved during the last two decades, the development of massive preretinal fibrosis or massive vitreous retraction (MVR) remains the most common cause for operative failure. These patients develop characteristic fixed and immobile retinal folds, a hazy vitreous with many pigment cells present, and a morning-glory appearance to the retina. Attempts to repair these detachments by performing a vitrectomy combined with membrane stripping have been uniformly disappointing.

Since 1970, we have used an encircling silicone sponge for treatment of patients with MVR. While anatomic reattachment is possible in a considerable number of these patients who were previously considered inoperable, the visual results are frequently poor. The degree of cellular infiltrate in the vitreous and the amount of preretinal fibrosis in the macular area are major factors that affect the ultimate vision. Finger-counting or 20/400 postoperative vision is not uncommon in patients who have MVR. Therefore, this operation should be reserved only for those patients in whom this level of vision would constitute improvement. The reaction of eyes to this procedure is surprisingly greater than to a circling band of fascia lata. Redness and swelling may be quite marked; pain may be intense and can last from four to six weeks.

This procedure is designed to evacuate all of the subretinal fluid which usually represents most of the liquid vitreous. The encircling silicone sponge exerts continued external pressure on the globe after surgery that flattens the retinal holes in spite of the multiple surface irregularities due to the preretinal membrane.

The basic steps in implanting an encircling silicone sponge are identical to those used in the encircling fascia procedure. First, the sponge is secured to the sclera. All holes must be localized and treated with cryotherapy. Finally, the subretinal fluid is evacuated.

Since a great deal of subretinal fluid is usually drained, the quadrant fixation sutures should be located in the equatorial region. If they are placed too far anteriorly, the resulting constriction of the globe will cause a distortion of the anterior segment and create a cosmetically unacceptable eye. On the other hand, if fixation sutures are placed too far posteriorly, the buckle may interfere with the venous drainage by compromising the vortex veins. This will result in a severely inflamed eye secondary to venous stasis.

The conjunctival incisions are made several centimeters anterior to the cul-de-sac. Since many of these patients have had previous surgery, the surgeon frequently encounters a significant amount of scar tissue before reaching the scleral plane. The sclera is grasped with a 0.3-mm Castroviejo forceps to stabilize the globe for placement of the 4-0 Mersilene fixation sutures in the same manner as shown in the scleral buckling procedure. We also recommend tenotomizing the muscle in the region of the retinal hole. The location of all holes is identified with forceps localization and marked on the scleral surface. Following cryotherapy, the sponge is passed around the globe beneath the extraocular muscles. A 3-mm silicone sponge, previously impregnated with antibiotic solution (Neosporin), is grasped with either a capsule forceps or fine hemostat [1]. It is then passed underneath the muscle, which is elevated with a muscle hook, and out the conjunctival opening. The end of the sponge is grasped with a Castroviejo forceps and advanced to leave a sufficient length for subsequent tying. The Mersilene fixation sutures are tied to secure the sponge firmly to the globe. The sponge is passed under the remainder of the muscles and anchored to the globe with the second fixation suture. Two additional fixation sutures are placed in the sclera on either side of the tenotomized muscle [2]. The placement is selected so that the hole will lie on the anterior surface of the buckle after the subretinal fluid is released, and the sponge is secured.

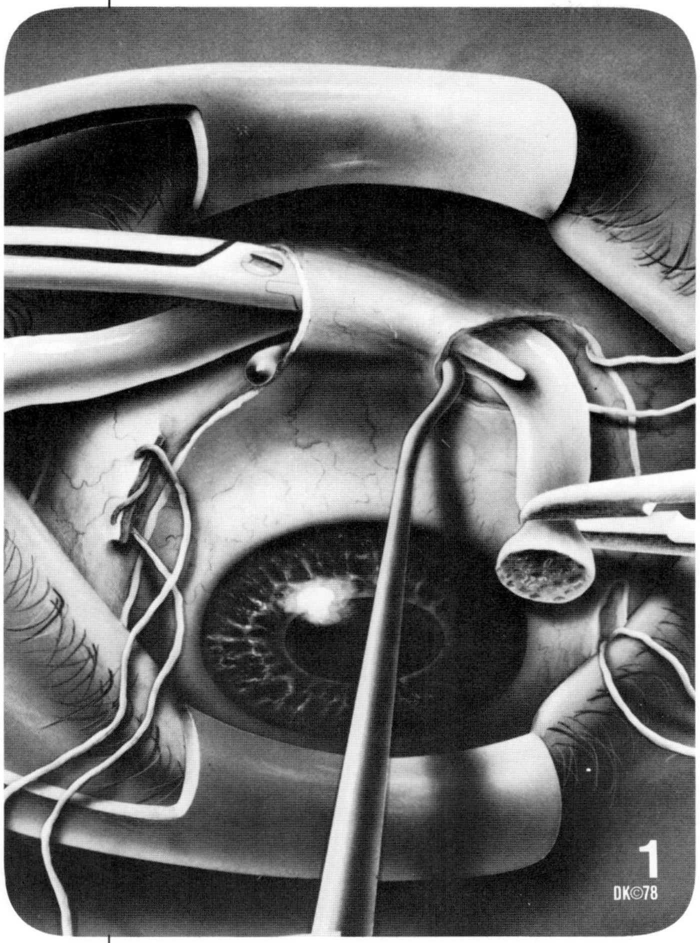

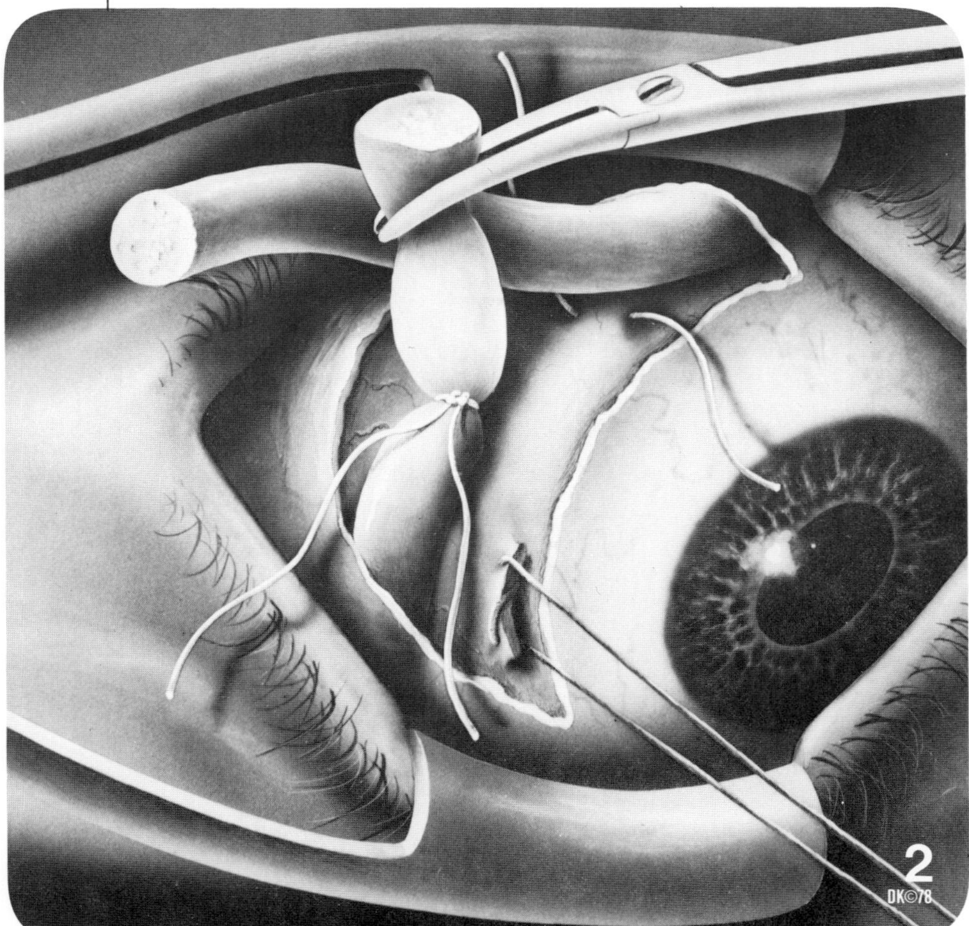

Donald A. Keller

A sclerotomy is performed in a manner similar to that used in the routine scleral buckling procedure. The edges of the sponge are grasped with a hemostat rather than a toothed forceps to prevent tearing the sponge when it is placed on stretch. An additional Mersilene suture is placed under the sponge between the two fixation sutures, and the subretinal tap is performed. The hemostats are used to keep the sponge on stretch and to maintain the intraocular pressure throughout the drainage. After all of the fluid is evacuated, the tap site is closed with a previously placed 4-0 Mersilene suture. When the desired amount of pressure (20 to 30 mm Hg) is exerted on the globe, the Mersilene suture is tied with a surgeon's knot.

The remaining two anchoring sutures are then tied over both arms of the sponge [3]. The surgeon must observe the optic nerve before the sutures are permanently tied to be sure that there is perfusion of the retina, for it is possible to occlude the central retinal artery if the intraocular pressure is too high. When all of the fluid is drained and the hole is flat on the buckle, the sutures are permanently tied, and the ends of the sponge are trimmed. The muscle is replaced, and the conjunctiva and Tenon's capsule are closed in a manner similar to the other scleral buckling procedures. No part of the encircling element should be exposed since any defect in the conjunctival covering of sponge will inevitably result in infection and require its removal.

Postoperatively, we recommend the use of atropine sulfate drops once a day and antibiotic solution four times a day until the eye is white and quiet. The patient is fully ambulatory the day after surgery and may be discharged at that time.

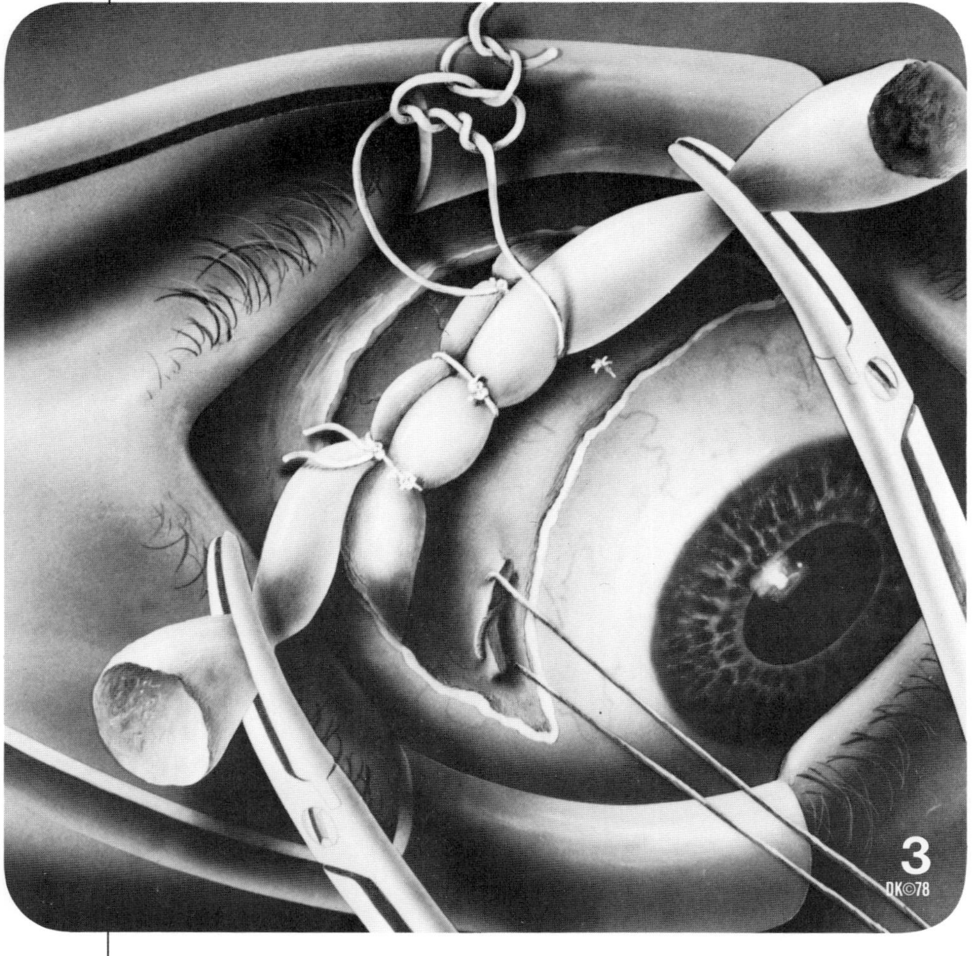

Donald F. Killer

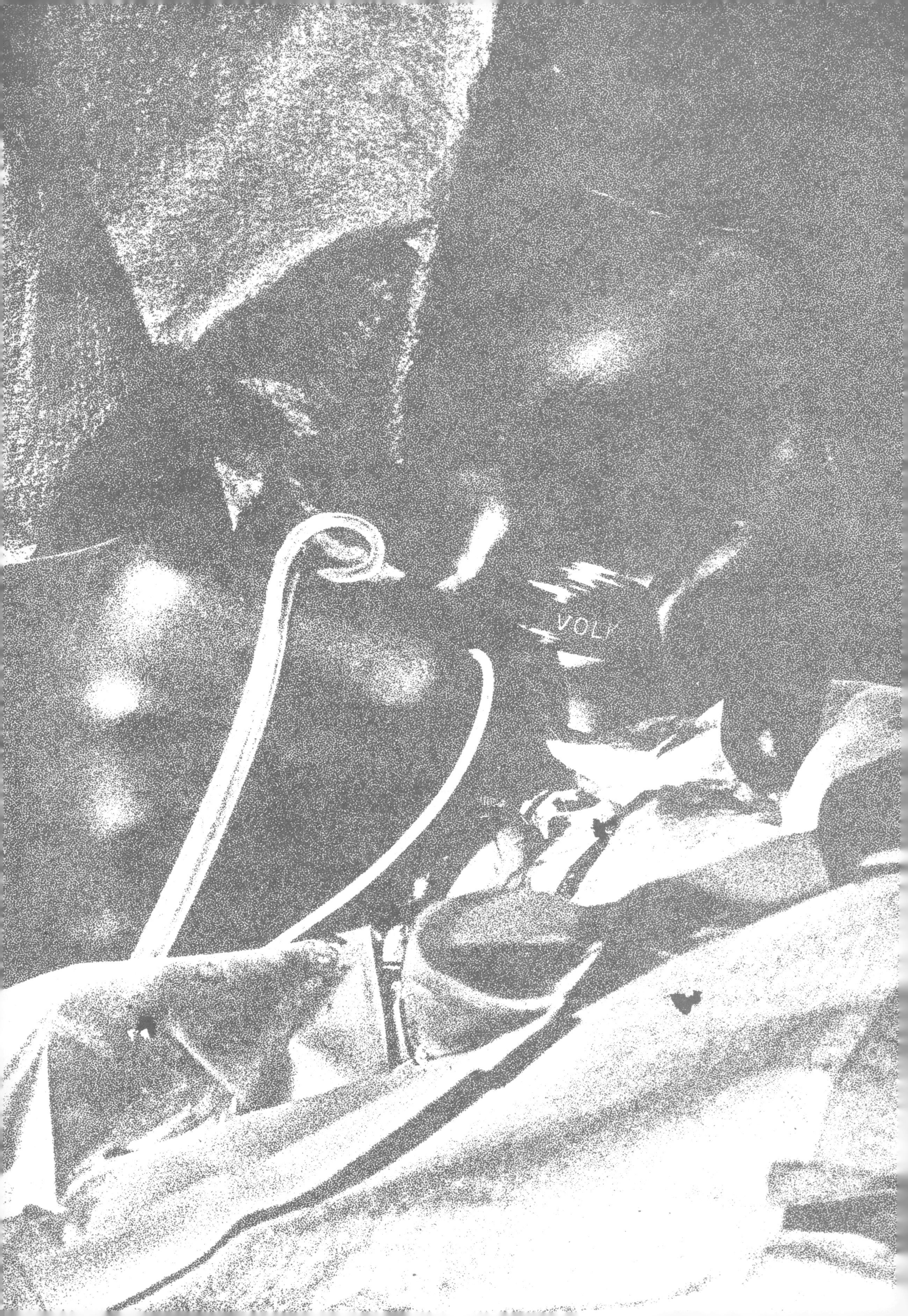

5
VITREOUS
SURGERY

ANATOMY OF THE VITREOUS

Frederick H. Davidorf, M.D.

The vitreous body occupies four fifths of the volume of the globe; its volume is 4 ml, and it weighs 4 gm. The liquid portion of the vitreous accounts for 99 percent of its volume. The viscosity of the vitreous differs markedly from individual to individual. The vitreous humor is similar in composition to aqueous humor, except for the presence in vitreous of collagen and hyaluronic acid. The outer surface of the vitreous is quite irregular because it conforms to the contours of the ciliary body and the retina. Vitreous fibrils, VF [1] [2], are arranged randomly throughout the main body of the vitreous and form an irregular mesh. At the vitreous base, VB [1] [2], in the region of the pars plana and ora serrata, the fibrils are parallel to the basement membrane.

Cloquet's canal, CC [1], is a vestigial structure that extends from the optic nerve anteriorly to the lens. It represents the area once occupied by the hyaloid vessels, which atrophy before birth.

The vitreous surgeon must be familiar with the anatomy of the ciliary body, peripheral retina, ora serrata, and the vitreous base. The entire ciliary body has a width of 5.9 mm nasally and 6.7 mm temporally from the limbus and extends posteriorly to the ora serrata. The ciliary body consists of two basic parts: the pars plicata, PPLI [1] (corona ciliaris), which occupies about 2.0 mm, and the pars plana, PPLA [1] (orbiculus ciliaris), which is 3.5 to 4.0 mm wide.

The pars plana is the posterior aspect of the ciliary body. It is 3.5 to 4.0 mm wide and extends from the ciliary processes, or pars plicata, to the ora serrata. Since the vasculature of the pars plana is relative, tenuous incisions through this area rarely evoke hemorrhage.

The neurosensory portion, NSP [2], of the retina ends at the ora serrata but continues forward on the inner aspect of the ciliary body as a single layer of nonpigmented cells. The pigment epithelium (PE) layer continues, but the cells contain larger melanin granules and are more densely pigmented than the adjacent pigment epithelial cells posterior to the ora serrata. The choroid (CHOR) in the pars plana is similar to the peripheral choroid; however, an accumulation of collagen (COL) separates the choroid from the two epithelial layers. The peripheral retina ends with many finger-like processes that are separated by scalloped bays composing the ora serrata.

The vitreous base is the area of adhesion between the vitreous cortex, the retina, and pars plana. It is 2 to 3 mm wide and forms a circular band straddling the ora serrata and occupying approximately the posterior half of the pars plana.

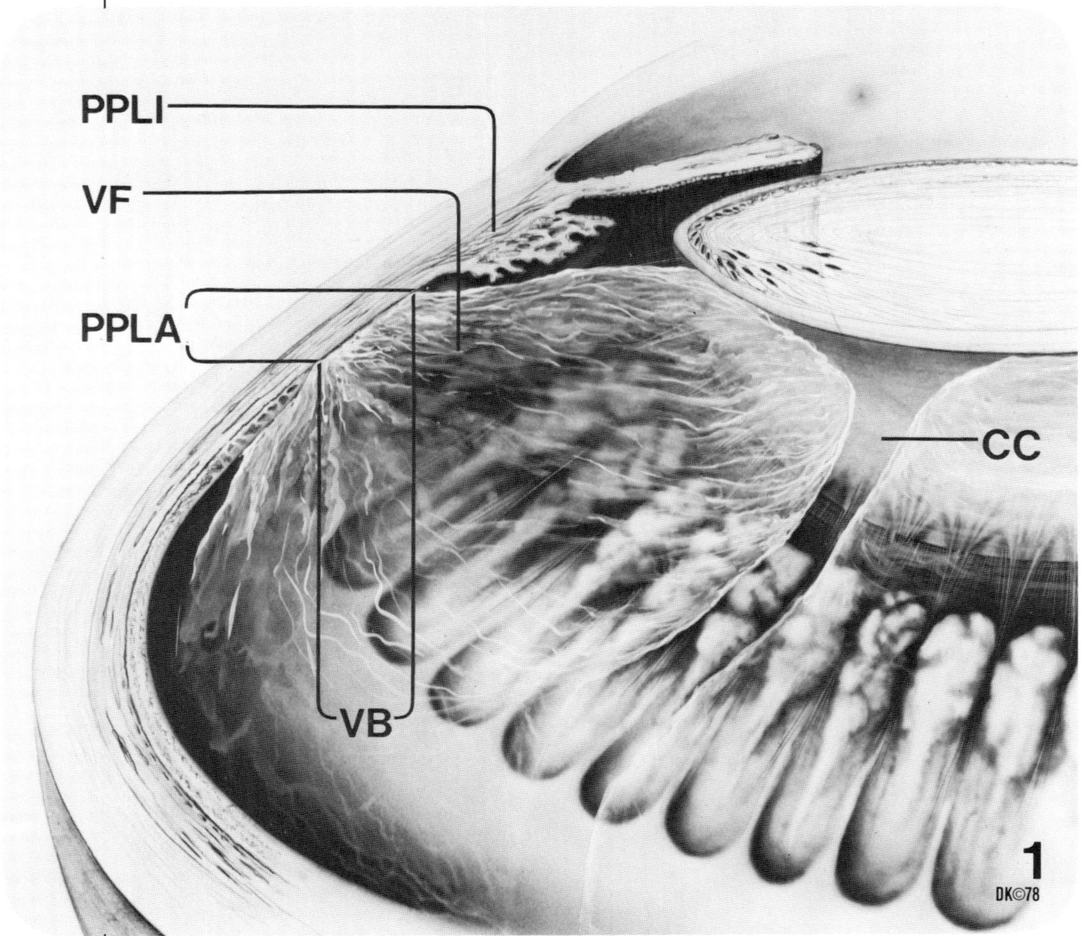

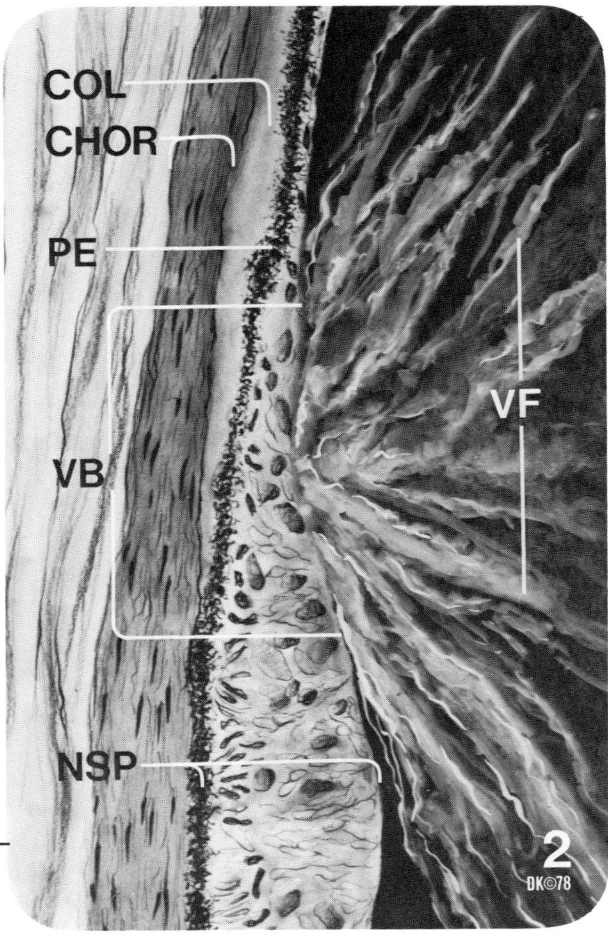

Donald A. Keller

Normally the vitreous fibrils break down with age. This is referred to as syneresis or liquefaction of the vitreous gel. As the cortex becomes syneretic, a point is reached when the vitreous collapses, resulting in a separation of the posterior vitreous from the retina [3] . The vitreous nearly always remains firmly attached at its base; only under unusual cases of ocular trauma does a detachment of the vitreous base occur. The presence of blood or inflammatory cells within the vitreous enhances the syneretic process. In the patient who has a dense vitreous hemorrhage that fails to reabsorb, a separation of the posterior vitreous face occurs. Red blood cells become entrapped between the anterior and posterior vitreous face, causing a dense opaque membrane composed of vitreous remnants and blood breakdown products. In some instances, attachments may exist between the posterior vitreous face and the retina and/or disk. These connections are usually located at neovascular areas that have proliferated into the vitreous.

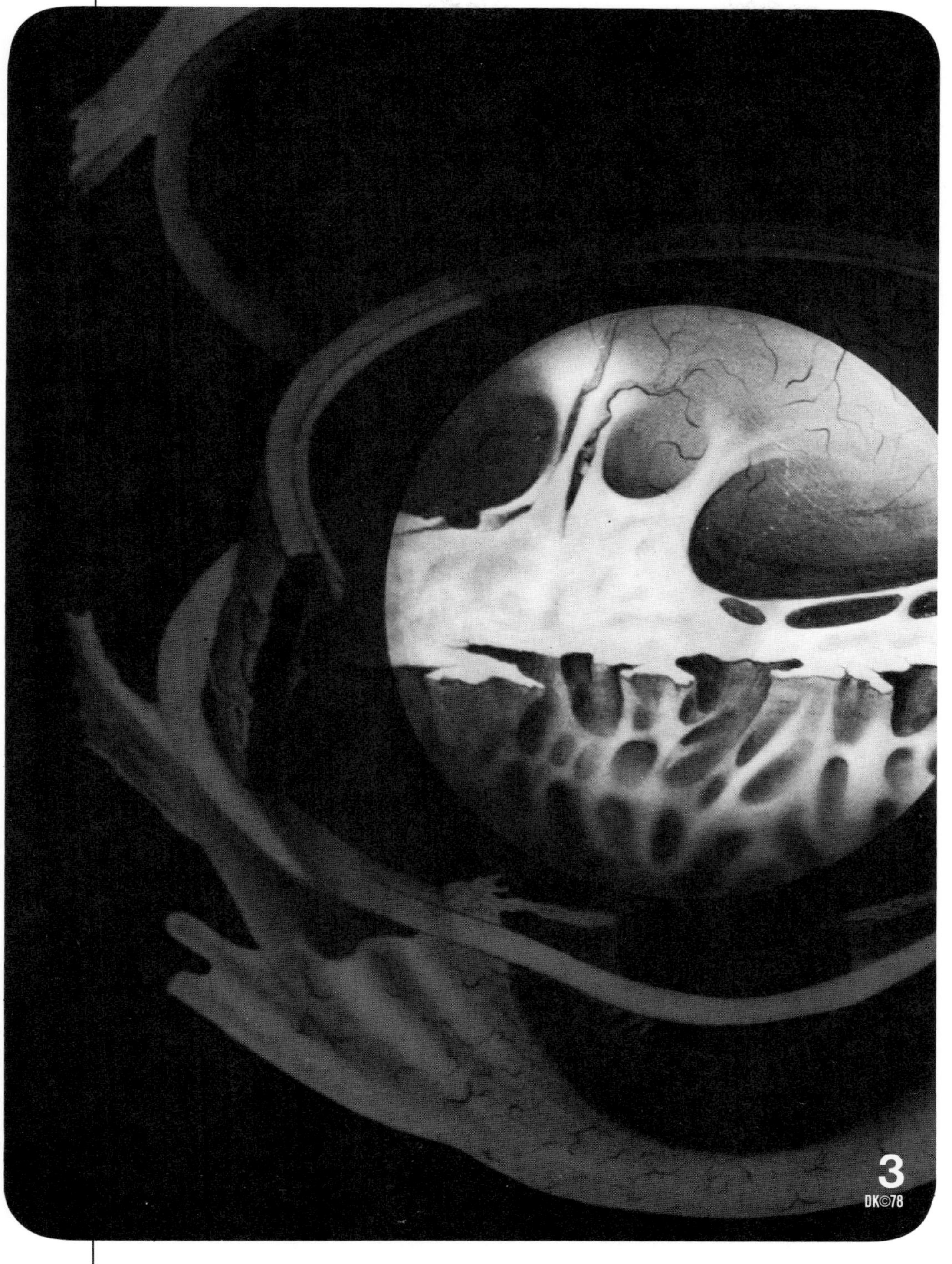

Donald A. Keller

PARS PLANA VITRECTOMY

Frederick H. Davidorf, M.D.

The advent of pars plana vitrectomy has brought help to many patients who were previously considered hopelessly blind because of vitreous opacities. This surgery is a new and rapidly expanding field; no discussion of it could possibly cover all of the latest advancements in instrumentation and technique. It is the primary purpose of this chapter, therefore, to outline standard techniques for pars plana vitreous removal.

Classically, the vitreous was considered a sacred structure to be manipulated as little as possible. The removal of the anterior vitreous during cataract surgery when vitreous loss occurs has become an accepted procedure. Surgical approaches to the deeper vitreous, however, were previously directed toward correcting secondary retinal pathology and included the cutting of vitreous bands and vitreous replacement. Until recently, little consideration had been given to removal of vitreous opacities. It now has been established that the eye can tolerate the total vitreous removal and continue to function normally.

The most common candidate for vitrectomy is the diabetic patient with an unresolved hemorrhage. While many diabetics develop irreparable proliferative retinopathy and secondary retinal detachment, others have only minimal retinal proliferative changes but develop dense vitreous hemorrhages which do not resolve even after months and years. This latter group is ideally suited for pars plana vitrectomy [1]. Patients with unresolved vitreous hemorrhages due to other causes, such as trauma, are also surgical candidates.

Several generalizations can be made concerning vitrectomy. Careful patient selection is necessary for successful results. A quiet eye is much easier to operate on and has much fewer postoperative complications than an eye that is actively hemorrhaging. Intraoperatively, hemorrhage is a major complication which increases operating time and interferes significantly with the surgeon's view. The problem of intraocular hemorrhage can be dramatically reduced if one selects patients who have no active hemorrhage for at least six months prior to surgery.

Preoperative ultrasonography is essential to outline retinal topography. Sites of vitreoretinal adhesion as well as proliferative stalks and even local traction detachments must be noted. During the initial part of the operation, the surgeon avoids these problem areas, since cutting into a proliferative stalk might create significant hemorrhage or traumatize the retina and cause an iatrogenic retinal hole. As the vitreous cavity is cleared, the sites of vitreoretinal traction can be seen and manipulated more safely.

A great number of vitrectomy instruments are available. There are similarities among the instruments, each with its own advantages and disadvantages. They vary in diameter from 0.9 mm to 1.7 mm, and all instruments consist of a cutting blade/suctioning mechanism, an infusion system to maintain the intraocular pressure during surgery, and a method of internal illumination.

There are two types of cutting movements: rotating [2] or up-and-down [3]. Some cutters rotate continuously, while others oscillate. The up-and-down cutters offer greater safety for surrounding tissue because they avoid the problem of "wrapping" tissue, which can occur with the rotation instruments. The instruments can be either electrically, hydraulically, or airdriven. A major drawback of the electrically powered instruments is the risk of an electrical shock. Most systems have an automatic suction mechanism which is controlled by the surgeon. This is a marked improvement over the older systems which utilized manual suction.

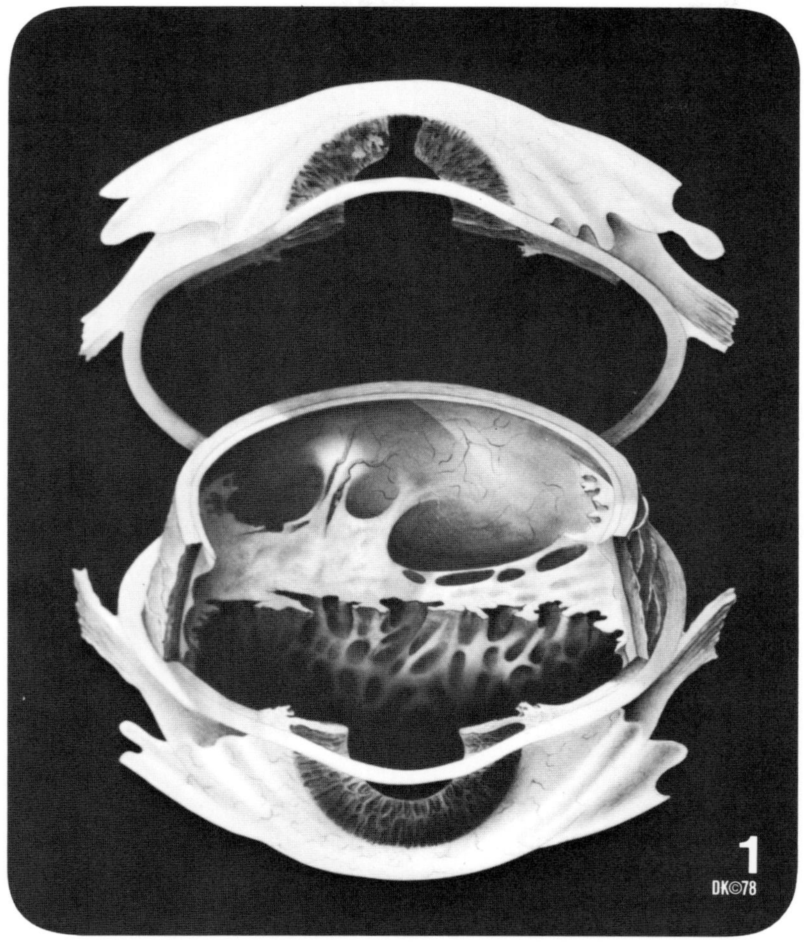

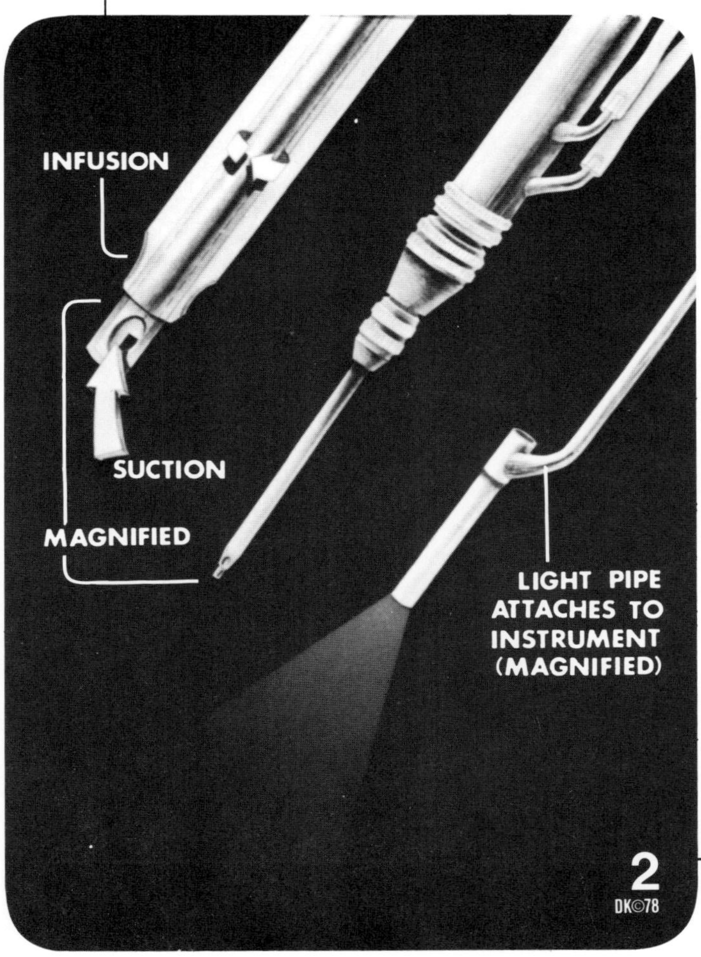

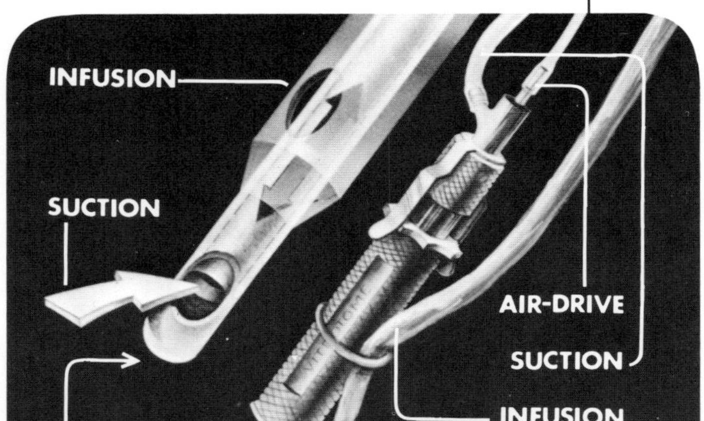

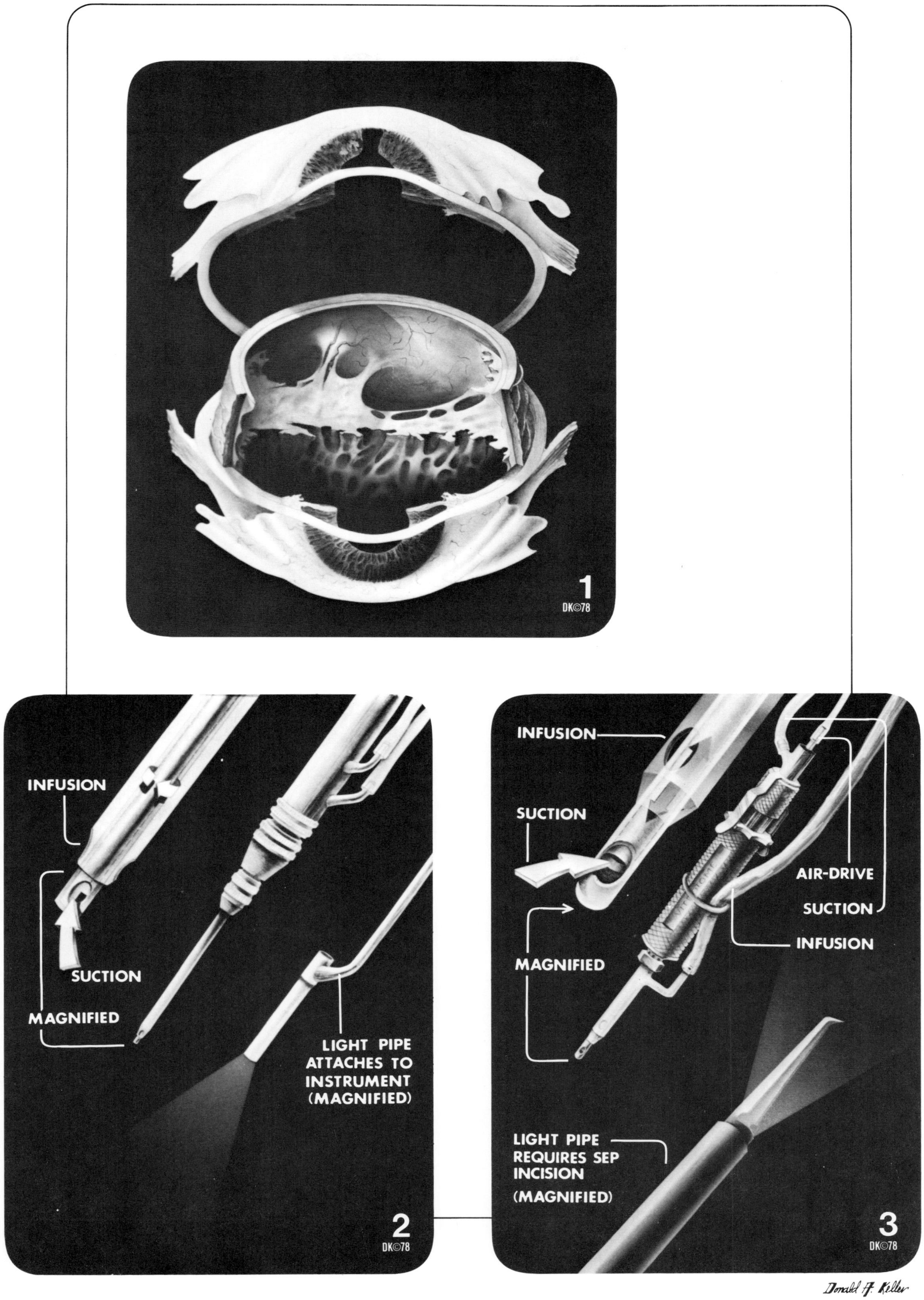

Donald A. Keller

Some manufacturers separate the cutting/suctioning elements from the infusion mechanism. These systems require two incisions in the pars plana to accommodate both instruments. The major advantage of this method is that less infusion fluid is required, reducing the eddy currents within the eye. However, there is a distinct disadvantage of needing two incisions instead of one.

Internal illumination is most often provided by a light pipe directly attached to the vitrectomy instrument. Some light pipes are used separately and are introduced into the eye through a second incision. They may be equipped with hooks and needles to feed the vitreous material into the cutter.

The operating microscope used in pars plana vitrectomy should have an incorporated X-Y mechanism. This allows the surgeon to change the surgical field throughout the operation. The focusing mechanism of the microscope should be controlled with a foot pedal to free the surgeon's hands for the procedure.

If the combined cataract extraction-vitrectomy procedure is performed in two stages rather than one, ocular morbidity and secondary complications such as corneal edema, uveitis, and secondary glaucoma can be reduced. Previous cataract surgery with a large sector iridectomy facilitates visualization of the posterior pole during vitreous removal and shortens the operating time.

A serious postoperative complication, especially in the diabetic patient, is that of secondary glaucoma with rubeosis iridis. Therefore, the surgeon must carefully examine the iris prior to surgery. Preoperatively, if very fine vessels are seen at the pupillary margin or confined to a portion of the angle, the chances of developing secondary glaucoma are greatly increased.

Of vital importance is a properly functioning vitrectomy instrument. It should be checked grossly after assembly, and in order to evaluate the cutting/suctioning mechanism, it must be examined again under the operating microscope prior to surgery. During the procedure excess fluid frequently flows out of the field. To collect this, the patient should be draped in such a manner that a trough is created between the head and the arm rest.

Initially, a superotemporal limbal incision is made in the conjunctiva to expose the sclera overlying the pars plana [4]. An incision posterior to the pars plicata is unlikely to cause a hemorrhage. The large, long posterior ciliary artery and nerve, which enter at the 3-o'clock and 9-o'clock meridian, should be avoided. Transilluminators are available which can be placed on the cornea to identify the ciliary body for localization of the sclerotomy site. The incision should be made 5.0 mm from the limbus in the phakic eye and 4.5 mm in the aphakic eye. If a lensectomy is planned, a more anterior incision 4.0 mm from the limbus can be employed. A single traction suture of 6-0 Mersilene placed in the sclera 3 mm from the limbus is sufficient to manipulate the globe during the procedure.

The incision site is marked on the sclera with a hand cautery [5]. The sclerotomy is made with a disposable No. 51 Beaver blade to accommodate the cutting/suctioning instrument. Generally a 3-mm opening is sufficient for most vitrectomy instruments. The sclera is grasped with fixation forceps at the site of the traction suture, and the globe is rotated inferonasally. The knife is directed centrally until it is visible through the microscope [6]. This insures that a tract has

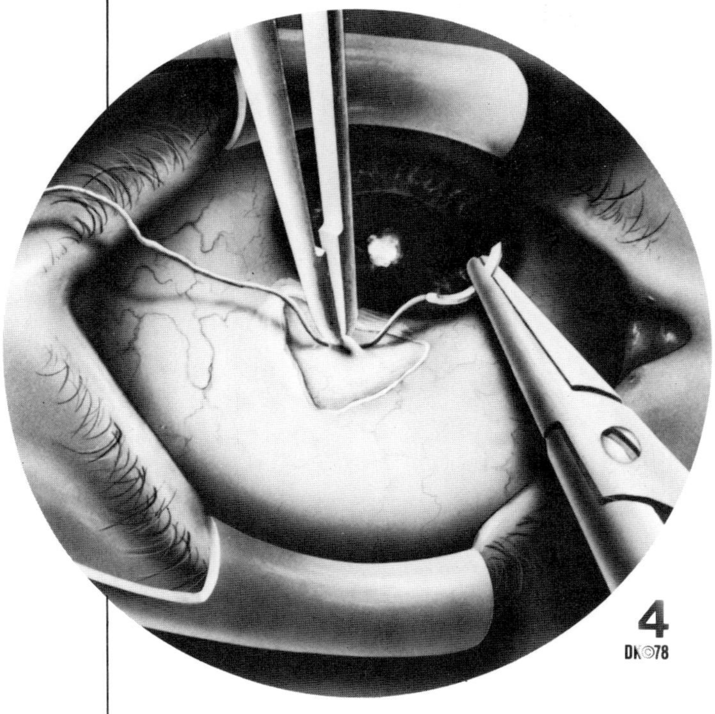

4
DK©78

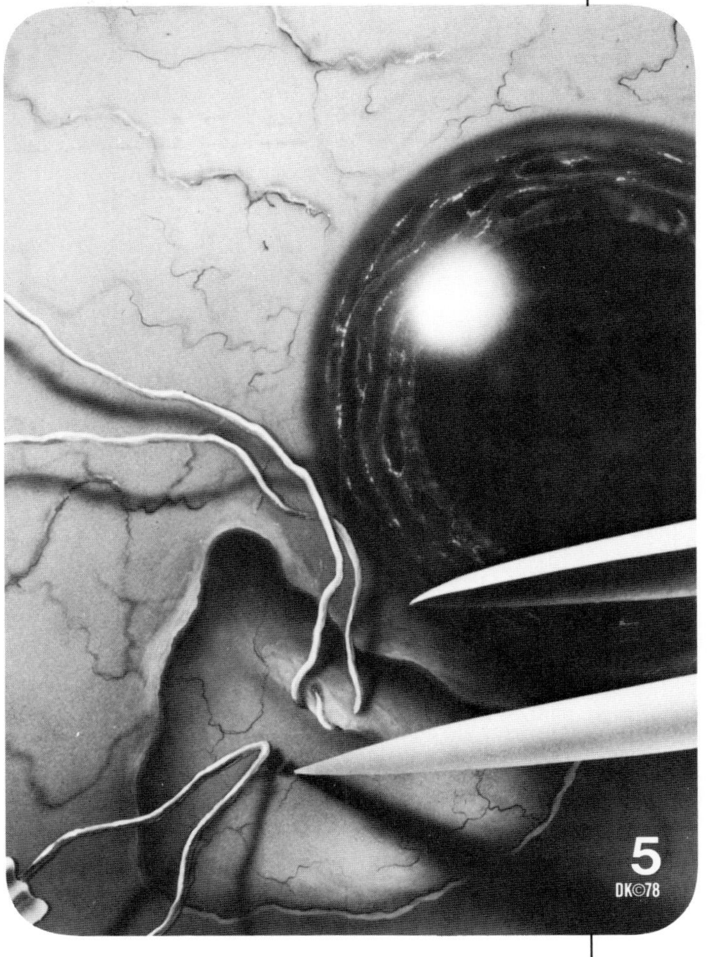

5
DK©78

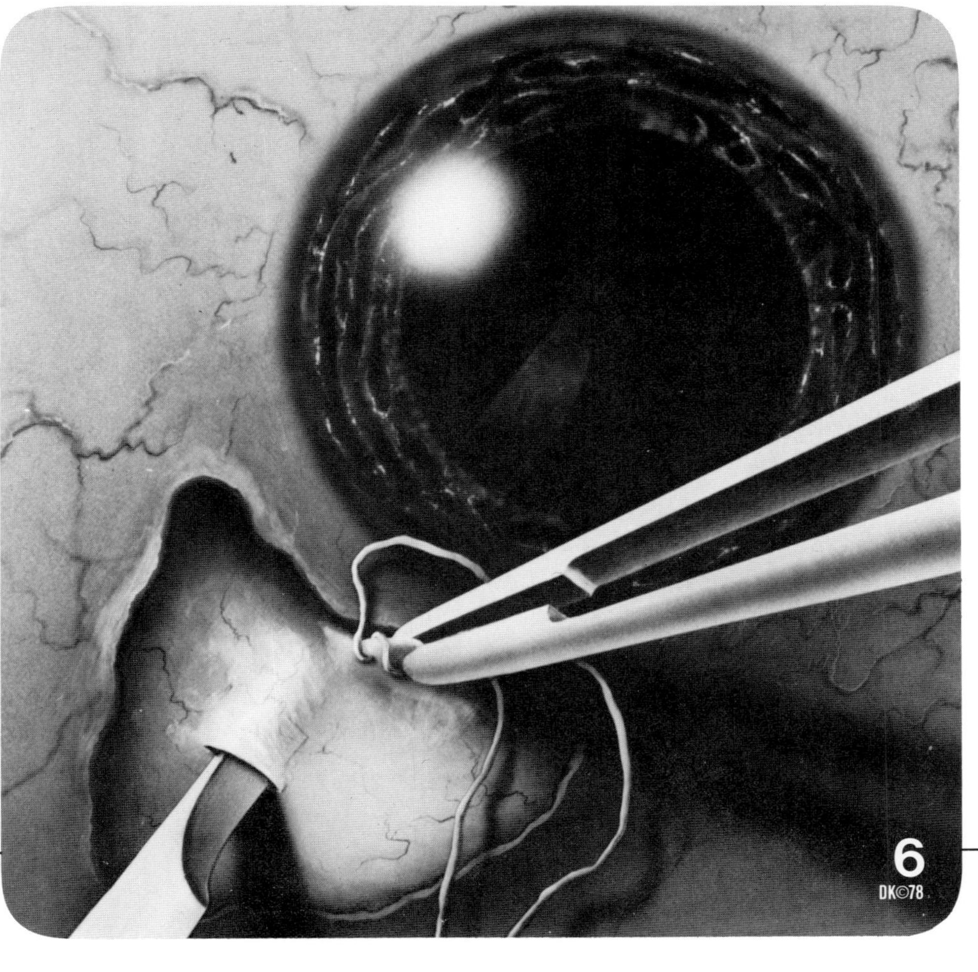

6
DK©78

Donald A. Killer

been made through the vitreous base [7]. When the knife is withdrawn, a significant loss of fluid may occur. Frequently, however, the flow is stopped by internal plugging of the incision site with formed vitreous. At this point, a double-armed 6-0 Mersilene suture is placed through the incision and looped out of the wound so that it may be closed at the end of the procedure.

As the vitrectomy instrument is inserted into the eye, it must be monitored visually with the operating microscope. Low power permits visualization of both the incision and central axis of the globe [8].

The intraocular pressure can be altered by changing the height of the infusion bottle. During the procedure it may be necessary to raise the intraocular pressure if excessive bleeding occurs.

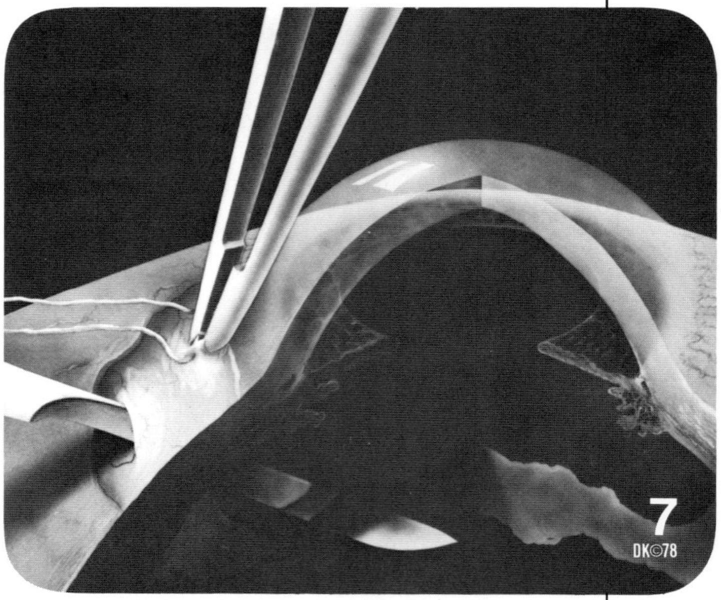

The tip is centered in the field and the anterior vitreous is removed first [9]. As the vitreous is eliminated, the instrument is gradually directed posteriorly. Since much of the cutting of the vitreous needs to be done under high-power magnification, the ability to focus in the deeper vitreous is essential.

Understandably, as one progresses posteriorly, less light is available. Internal illumination is achieved with a fiberoptic light pipe. Two types are available. The first fits over the cutting tip and is introduced through the same incision; the other is inserted through a second incision in the nasal pars plana, providing for more versatile posterior illumination. Light pipes are available with hooked ends, which are particularly useful in membrane stripping. The hook allows the surgeon to lift the membrane as it is cut with the vitrectomy instrument [10].

Donald F. Keller

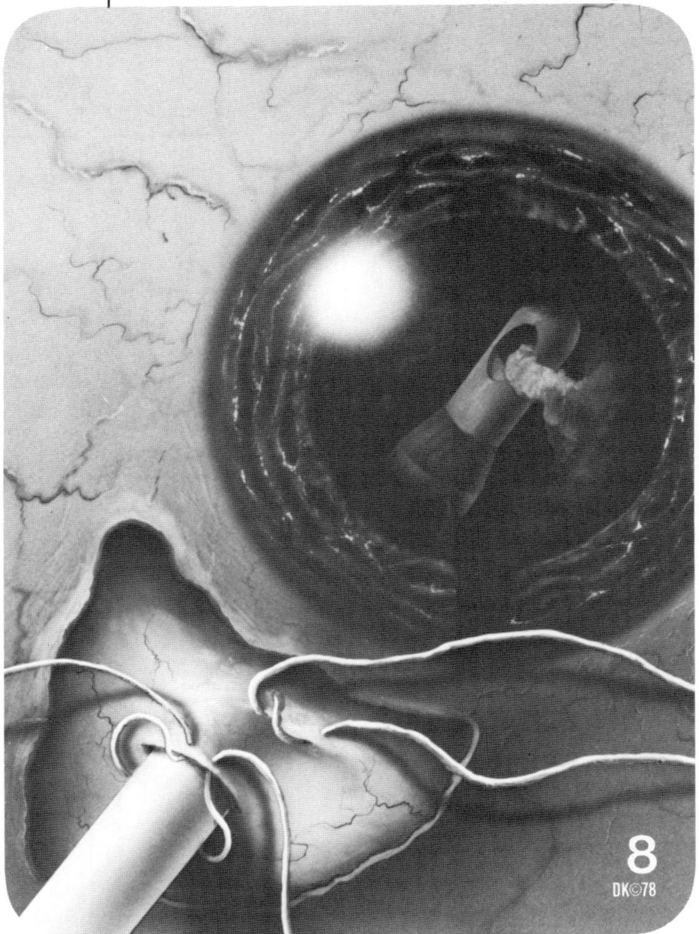

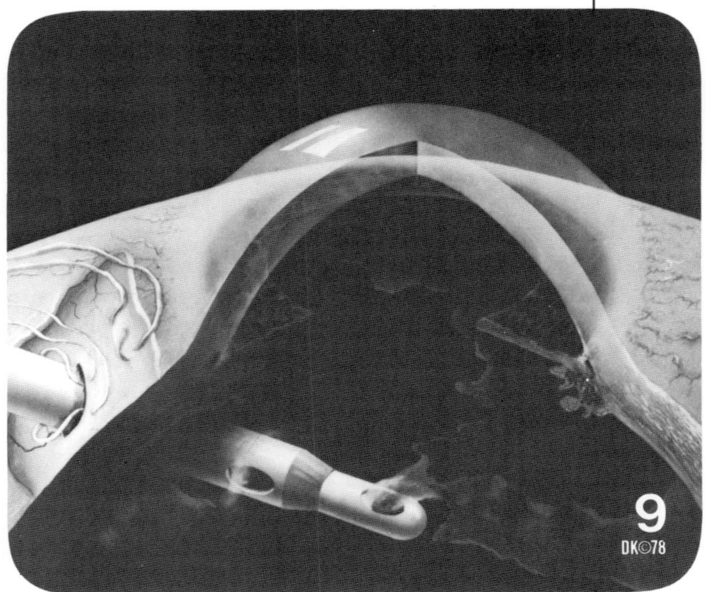

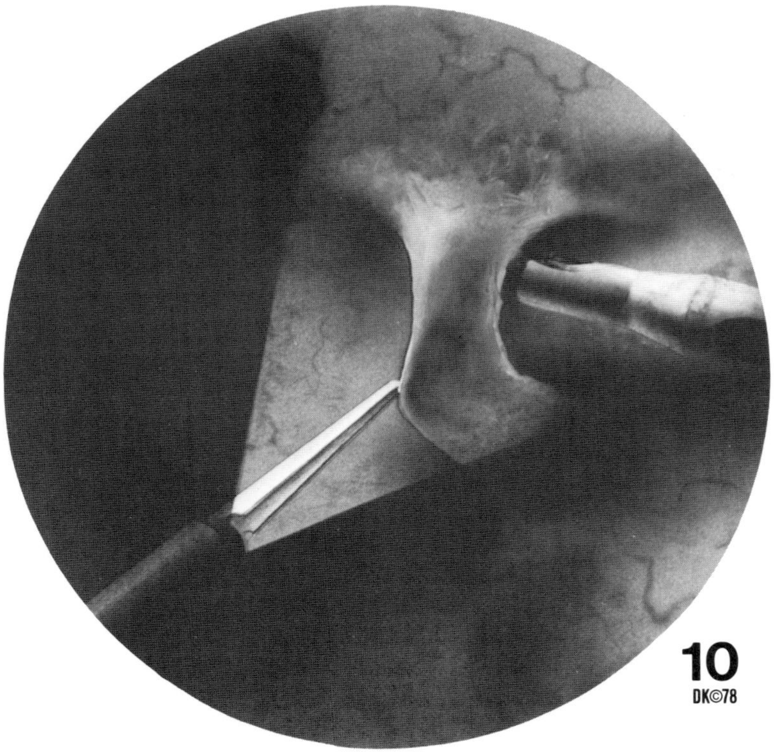

Donald F. Keller

It is possible in most situations to achieve adequate visualization of the deeper vitreous by still another method, the use of the indirect ophthalmoscope in place of the operating microscope [11] . The microscope is pivoted away from the patient, and the vitrectomy instrument is held in one hand while the hand lens of the indirect ophthalmoscope is held in the other. This provides a much larger surgical field, frequently easier identification of the retina, and better visualization of the peripheral vitreous is possible which facilitates its removal. In some instances, a partially opaque lens must be removed to create adequate visualization for vitrectomy. With the use of the indirect ophthalmoscope, it is possible to remove the vitreous in some patients with relatively dense lens opacities, thereby eliminating the need for a lensectomy. If a manual suction method is employed when the indirect ophthalmoscope is used, the first assistant can monitor the procedure through the teaching mirror on the ophthalmoscope.

During the removal of the posterior vitreous, the surgeon may find that his view has become obscured by fresh bleeding. Since the surgeon must be able to visualize the tip of the vitrectomy instrument before the vitreous can be safely cut, the instrument must be brought anteriorly until the tip can be seen. The cloudy fluid is removed predominately by infusion and suction, with the cutting mechanism turned off. The instrument is moved posteriorly until the source of the bleeding can be identified. Active bleeding can be controlled by raising the intraocular pressure. This is done by raising the height of the infusion bottle. If bleeding continues, cautery is accomplished using bipolar coagulation. The positive pole is attached to the vitrectomy instrument, while the negative pole is attached to a small needle knife inserted into the pars plana. To cauterize the source of bleeding, the tissue is placed between the two instruments, and the diathermy current is activated.

After the posterior vitreous is removed and the bleeding points are cauterized, the peripheral vitreous is excised. The safest and most rapid method for peripheral vitreous removal is with the use of the indirect ophthalmoscope. Because of the attachments of the vitreous base to the peripheral retina, a small skirt of vitreous should remain. After the peripheral vitreous is excised, the operating microscope is repositioned, and the instruments are withdrawn. The preplaced suture is tied, which closes the incision. If the eye is hypotonous, balanced salt solution is injected with a 25-gauge needle on a 2-ml syringe to normalize the intraocular pressure [12] . A single gut suture at the limbus is used to close the conjunctiva [13] . The patient is fully ambulatory after surgery. Atropine sulfate 1 percent and an antibiotic steroid drop are used once a day for two weeks.

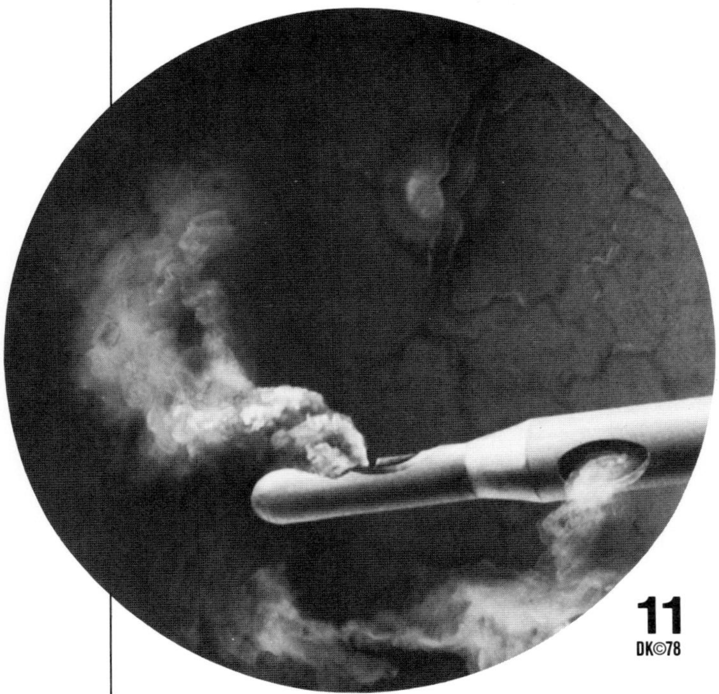

11
DK©78

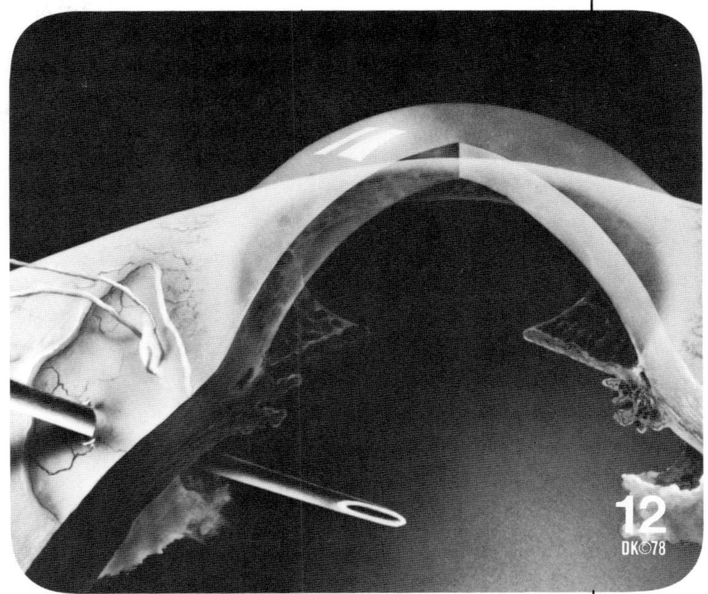

12
DK©78

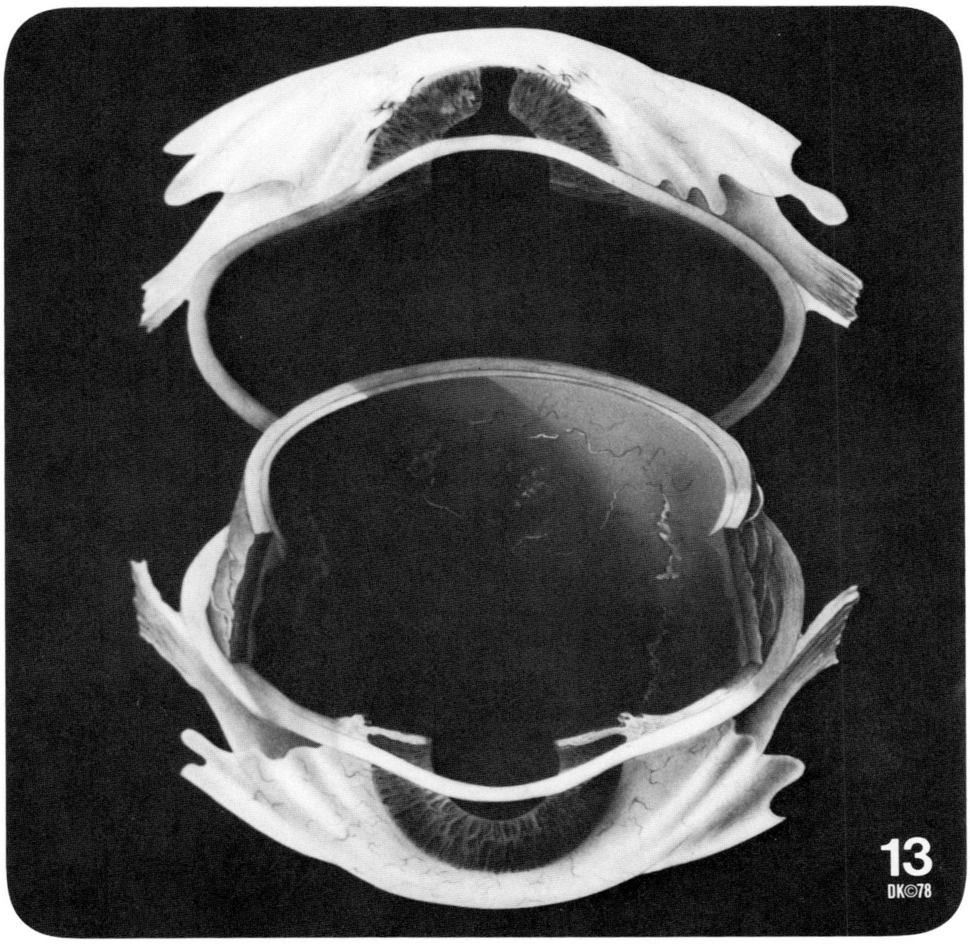

13
DK©78

Donald A Keller

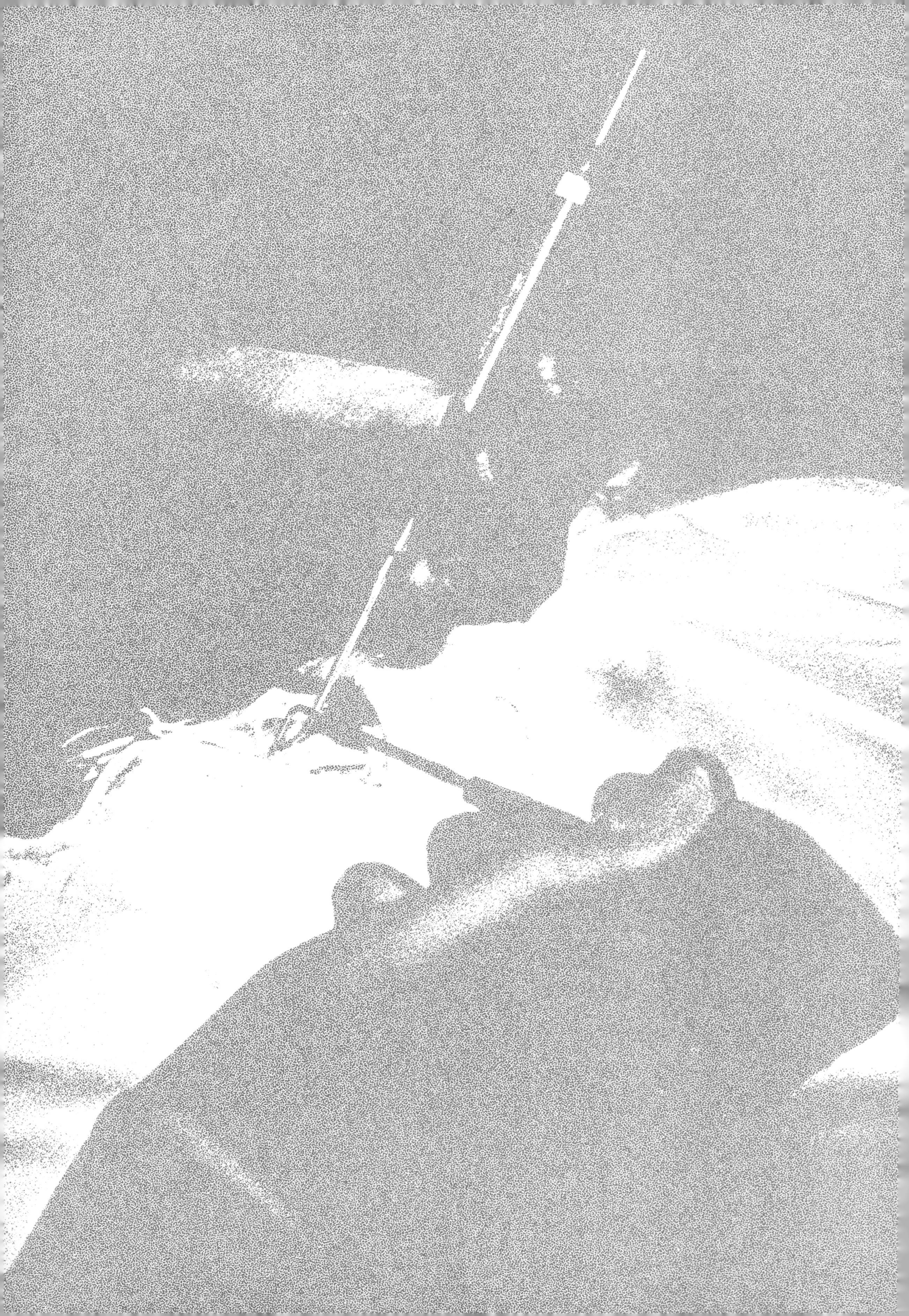

6
EXTRAOCULAR MUSCLE
SURGERY

ANATOMY OF THE EXTRAOCULAR MUSCLES

Gary L. Rogers, M.D.
James A. Savage, M.D.
Richard E. Simmons, M.D.

The six extraocular muscles are the superior oblique (SO) and inferior oblique (IO) muscles and the four rectus muscles: superior (SR), inferior (IR), medial (MR), and lateral, LR [1] [4] .

The superior oblique muscle is the longest and thinnest of the extraocular muscles. It originates close to the annulus of Zinn, AZ [2] [5] , superior and medial to the optic foramen, between the origins of the superior and medial rectus muscles. The tendon is 30 mm long and begins 30 mm from the origin; therefore, the total length measures 60 mm. It courses directly forward, parallel to the nasal wall of the orbit, for a length of 40 mm, to the trochlea, TRO [2] , a fibrocartilage considered to be a specialized part of the sheath of the superior oblique muscle. The trochlea is located 5 mm posterior to the junction of the medial and superior orbital rim.

The tendon passes through the trochlea and inserts on the globe posterior to the equator beneath the lateral border of the superior rectus muscle [4] . Several millimeters before its insertion, it becomes quite broad and thin and has an average width of 11 mm. The bow-shaped insertion of the superior oblique muscle is the most variable of all the extraocular muscles; its concavity faces the trochlea. The course of the tendon from the trochlea to the globe forms an angle of 54 degrees with the optic axis.

The superior oblique muscle is innervated by the fourth cranial nerve, which enters the muscle on the superior surface of its medial side, approximately 12 mm from its origin. Its blood supply is derived from the superior muscular branch, SMB [2] , of the ophthalmic artery (OA). Because of its location and angle of insertion, the superior oblique muscle intorts the globe (incycloduction) when the eye is in the primary position of gaze. Secondarily, it acts as an abductor and depressor.

The inferior oblique muscle, the shortest of the extraocular muscles, varies in length from 35 to 38 mm. At its midpoint, the muscle is 8 to 10 mm wide. The inferior oblique muscle arises from the periosteum of the superior extension of the maxillary bone located several

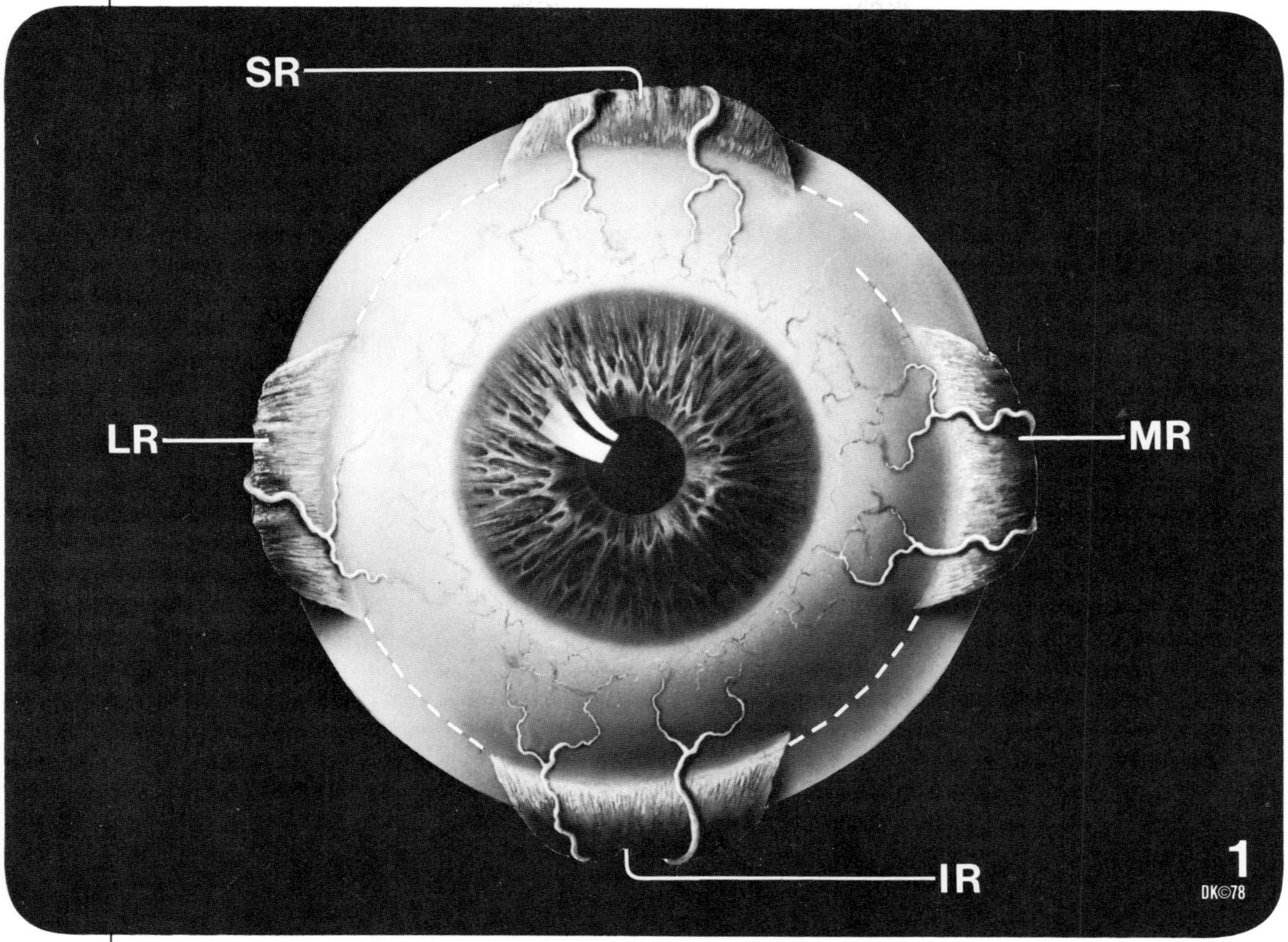

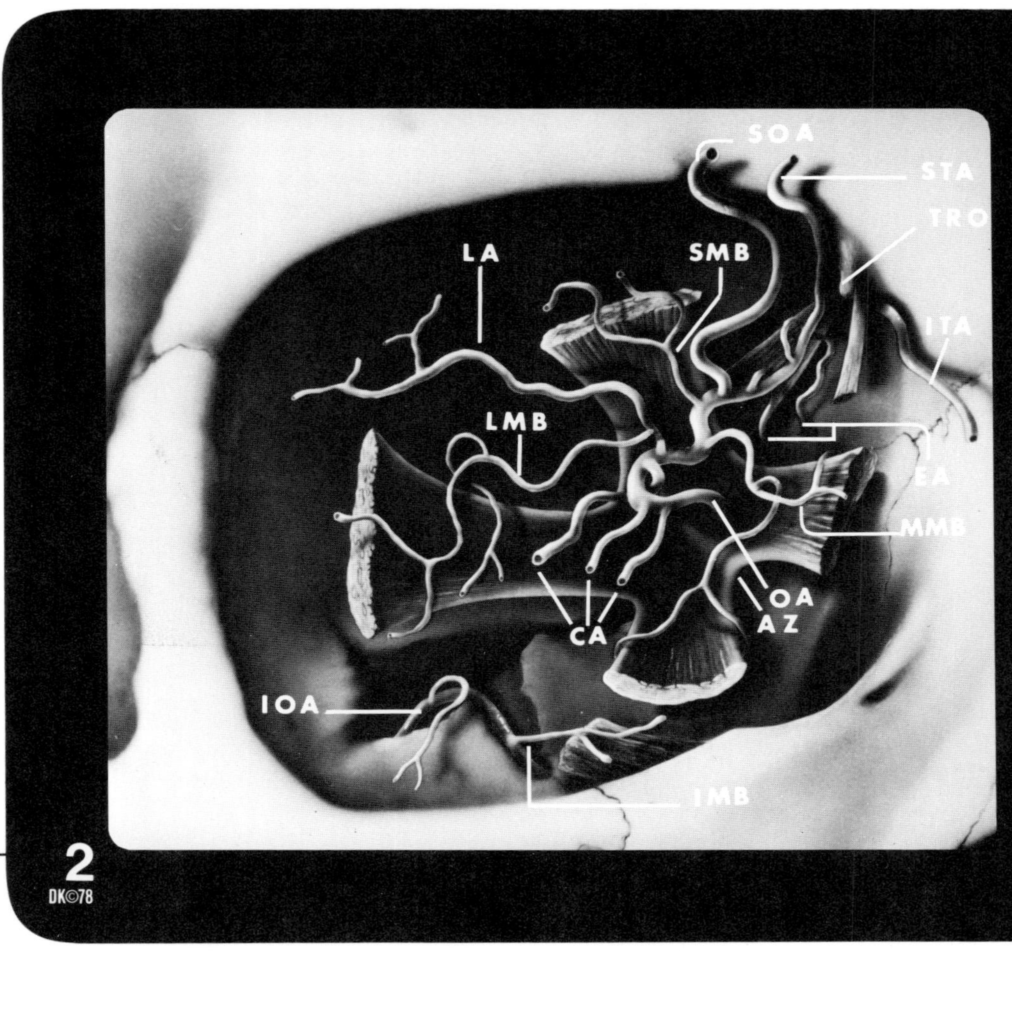

LA
lacrimal artery

LMB
lateral muscular branch

IOA
infraorbital artery

IMB
inferior muscular branch

CA
ciliary arteries

OA
ophthalmic artery

MMB
medial muscular branch

EA
ethmoidal arteries

ITA
infratrochlear artery

TRO
trochlea

STA
supratrochlear artery

SOA
supraorbital artery

Donald F. Keller

millimeters behind the inferior orbital rim, just lateral to the opening of the nasolacrimal duct. The muscle passes posterior, temporal, and slightly superior beneath the inferior rectus muscle. As the inferior oblique muscle and the inferior rectus muscle cross, their fascial coverings fuse to form Lockwood's ligament, LL [3] . A broad arc of scleral contact is maintained as the muscle curves around the globe beneath the lower border of the inferior rectus muscle to its insertion posterior and temporal to the optic nerve in the region of the macula [4]. The muscle is attached to the globe by a short tendon, usually less than 1 mm in length. The line of insertion is oblique and curved; its convexity faces superiorly. The width of insertion varies from 8 to 10 mm; the average width is 9.5 mm. The inferior oblique muscle forms a 51-degree angle with the optic axis.

The nerve and blood supply enter the belly of the inferior oblique muscle just temporal to the lateral border of the inferior rectus muscle, approximately 12 mm posterior to its insertion. The muscle is innervated by the inferior division of the third cranial nerve, and the blood supply is derived from the muscular branches of the infraorbital artery, IOA [2], and inferior muscular branch (IMB) of the ophthalmic artery. Because of its anterior origin and posterior insertion, when the eye is in the primary position, the muscle extorts the globe (excycloduction). Secondarily, it acts as an abductor and elevator.

The four rectus muscles originate in the posterior orbit around the optic foramen (OF) in the annulus of Zinn, AZ [5] . All are 40 mm long, and their nerve supplies enter 26 mm from the insertion. The rectus muscles pass anteriorly to the orbit to insert on the globe where they create an ellipse depicted by the spiral of Tillaux [1] . Except for the lateral rectus muscle, the blood supply of the three muscles originates from the muscular branches of the ophthalmic artery. In addition to these common characteristics, each rectus muscle exhibits some other properties.

As the superior rectus muscle passes anteriorly from the annulus of Zinn, it courses beneath the levator muscle, LV [5] , to insert

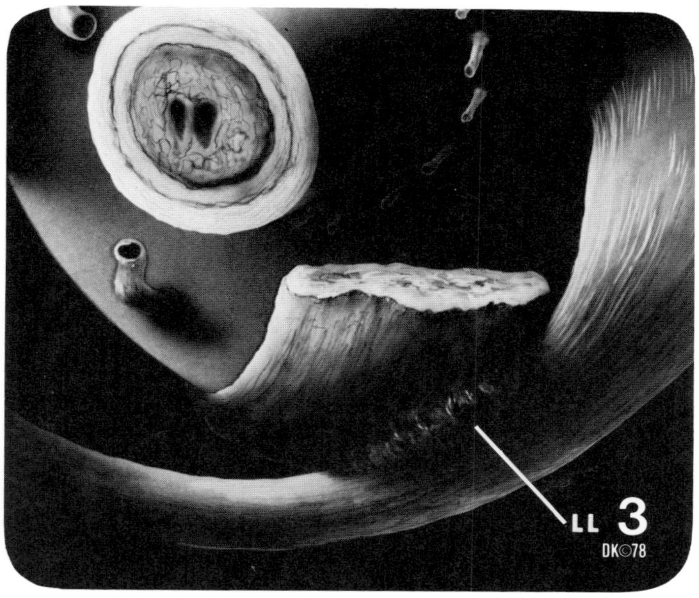

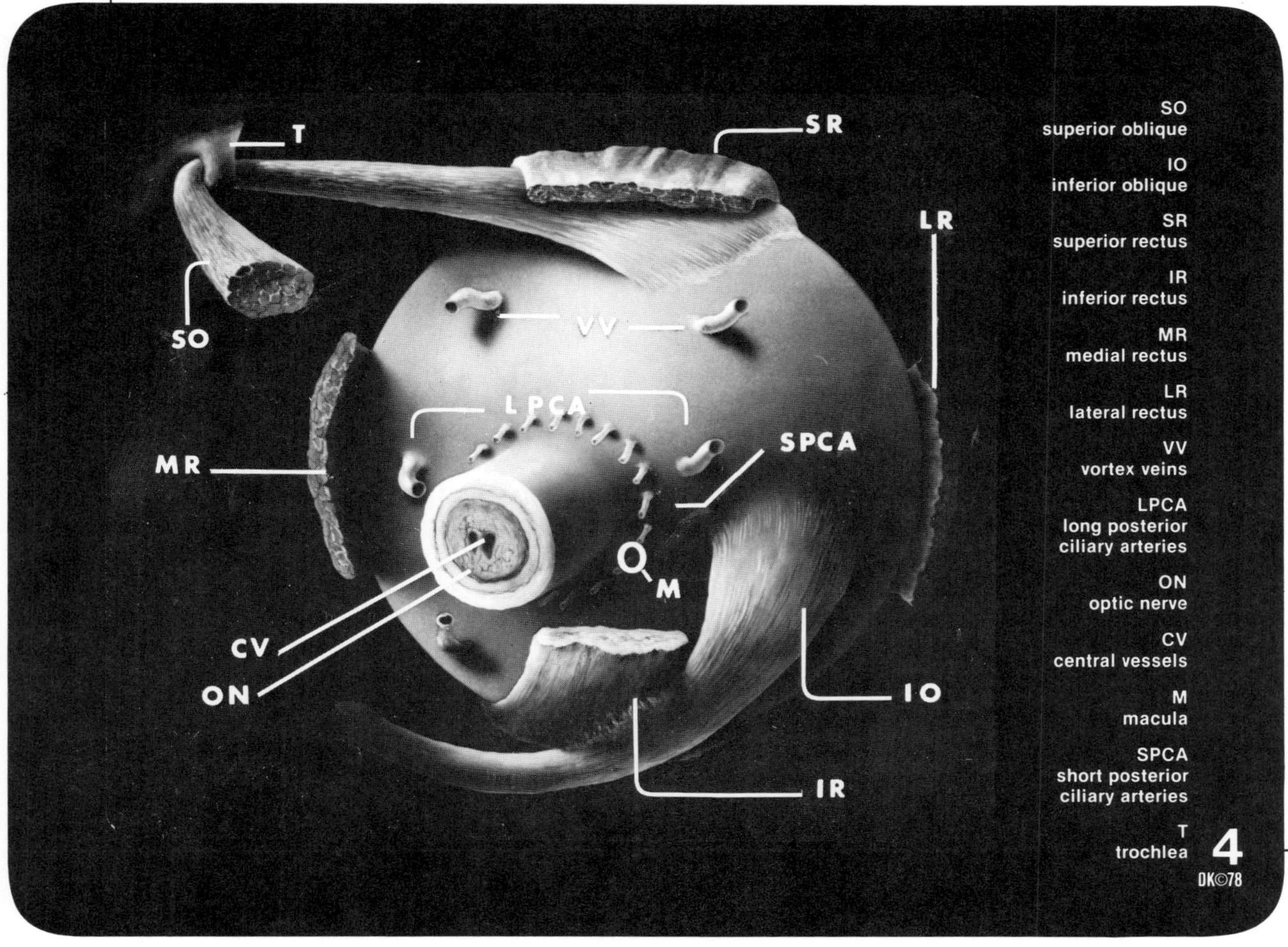

Donald A. Keller

on the sclera. The muscle has the broadest insertion of the four rectus muscles, measuring 10.8 mm wide. The muscle inserts 7.7 mm from the limbus and creates a 23-degree angle with the optic axis. It is innervated by the superior division of the third cranial nerve, which enters the muscle on its undersurface. Primarily, it functions as an elevator when the eye is abducted; secondarily, it provides intortion and adduction.

The inferior rectus muscle, IRM [5] , courses anteriorly and laterally to insert 6.5 mm from the limbus by a tendonous insertion 9.8 mm wide. The muscle creates a 23-degree angle with the optic axis. The inferior division of the third cranial nerve innervates the muscle. The primary action of the inferior rectus muscle is to depress the globe; secondarily, it provides adduction and extortion.

The largest of the extraocular muscles, the medial rectus muscle, MRM [5] , originates medial and inferior to the optic foramen. It extends anteriorly along the medial wall of the orbit to an insertion 10.3 mm in width on the sclera, 5.5 mm from the limbus. Exotropic patients often exhibit a variable insertion which ranges from 3.0 to 5.5 mm from the limbus. This fact must be considered when the surgeon considers muscle recession. A larger recession may be necessary if the insertion is closer to the limbus than 5.5 mm. Like the inferior rectus muscle, the medial rectus muscle is innervated by the inferior division of the third cranial nerve. It functions as a pure adductor.

The origin of the lateral rectus muscle, LRM [5] , bridges the superior orbital fissure, SOF [5] . It passes anteriorly along the lateral wall of the orbit to insert 6.9 mm from the limbus along a tendonous insertion 9.2 mm wide. Unlike the medial rectus muscle, the insertion of the lateral rectus muscle is a fairly consistent distance from the limbus. The lateral rectus muscle receives its blood supply from the lacrimal artery, LA [2] , and it is innervated by the sixth cranial nerve. It serves as a pure abductor.

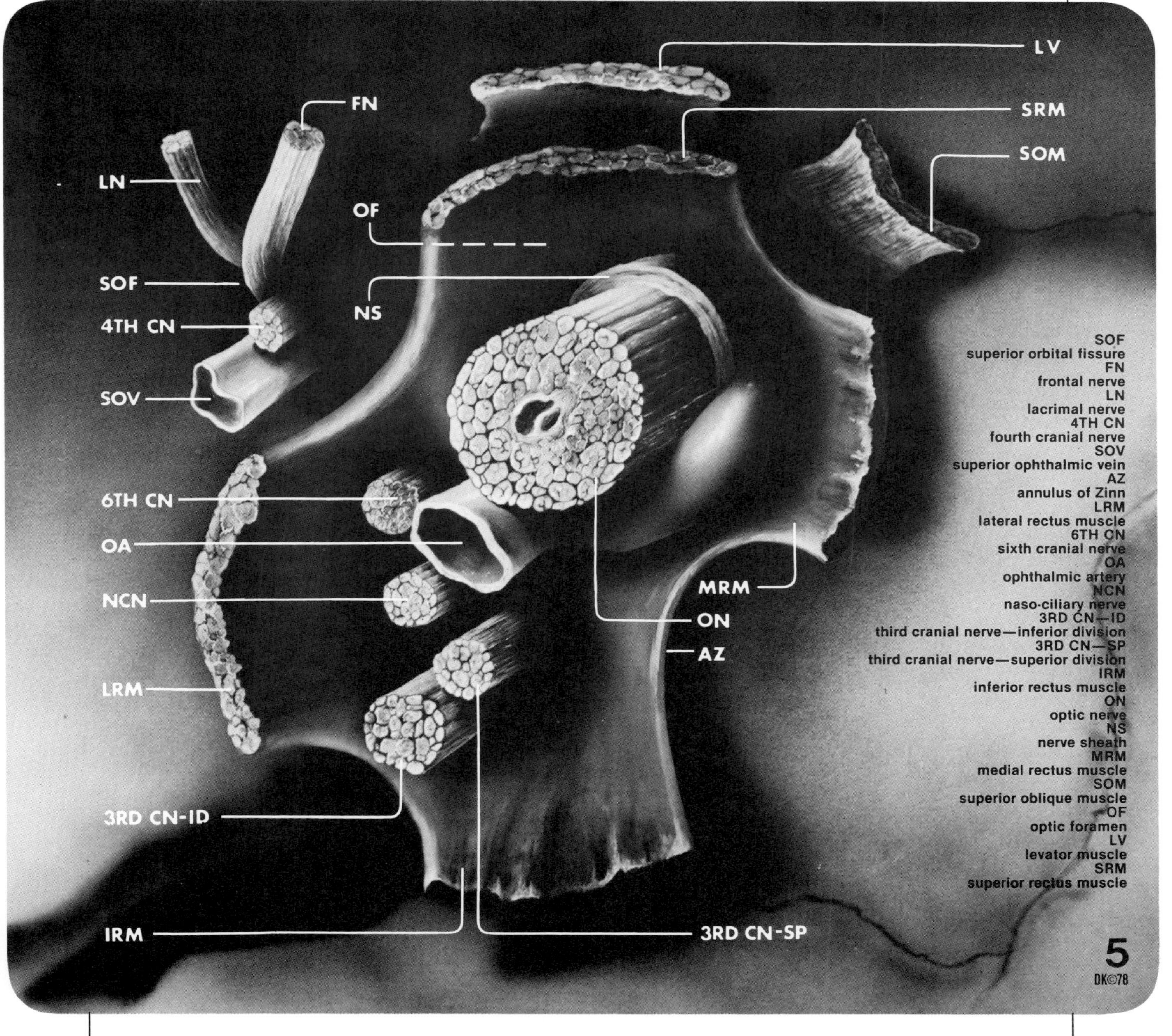

Donald A. Killer

SURGERY OF THE EXTRAOCULAR MUSCLES

The development of binocular vision depends on the fusion of similar optical images into one by the visual cortex. The earlier in life that correct ocular alignment is achieved, the greater is the potential for fusion. The longer a child continues to have an ocular deviation, the greater will be the sensory deprivation. Any child who has a deviation greater than 15 prism diopters that cannot be corrected medically or optically should be considered for surgery.

Children with psychomotor retardation require a more conservative approach. Good cosmetic and occasionally fusional results can be obtained when a consistent angle of strabismus is determined. If ocular measurements show a wide variability, an overcorrection is more likely to occur than in a healthy child.

The goal of surgery is to align the eyes as straight as possible and as soon as possible. Surgery done only for cosmetic purposes should be undertaken by the time the child is of school age. The psychological implications for a child with an ocular deviation must not be overlooked.

No surgery on the extraocular muscles should be started without first performing a forced-duction test on both eyes in all cardinal positions. A positive test is one in which the eye, when rotated with a pair of forceps, shows some limitation or restriction of movement in one or more directions. This usually signals some type of abnormal muscle development (Duane's or Brown's syndrome), scar tissue from previous surgery (adherence syndrome), or other disease process (orbital floor fracture or Graves' disease).

The adequacy of the instruments is far more important than the particular hook or forceps used. A dull pair of scissors, a forceps with bent teeth, or a needle holder that does not release easily are subtle factors that undermine the skill with which the surgeon accomplishes the task in strabismus surgery.

Dexon and Vicryl suture materials are currently popular because of their greater tensile strength, longer absorption times, and less tissue reactivity than catgut, which has been popular for so many years. A spatula needle is usually preferable, since it is specifically designed to produce a lamellar intrascleral suture tract.

With these basic considerations in mind, the common strabismus procedures may now be considered. In the descriptions to follow, rectus and oblique muscle surgery are presented separately. Although the surgery on the rectus muscles concentrates on horizontal deviations, the recession-resection techniques are identical to those recommended for the vertical rectus muscle deviations.

CONJUNCTIVAL INCISIONS

Gary L. Rogers, M.D.
Richard E. Simmons, M.D.

While many techniques exist to make a conjunctival incision, we will describe three of the most commonly used procedures popularized by Swan, von Noorden, and Parks.

In the classic incision described by Swan, the conjunctiva is incised just posterior to the muscle insertion, approximately 10 mm posterior to the limbus. The incision should be approximately 15 mm long and should extend past each border of the muscle. The conjunctiva is elevated with Bishop-Harmon forceps at either the superior or inferior edge of the muscle and is incised with Westcott scissors [1]. The incision is enlarged as the blade of the scissors is passed over the muscle for the desired length [2]. To avoid cutting the muscle, the surgeon elevates the conjunctiva as the scissors is advanced. Tenon's capsule lies exposed in the depths of the incision. It is grasped near the border of the muscle tendon with Bishop-Harmon forceps, lifted, and incised to expose bare sclera [3]. A muscle hook may be introduced beneath the muscle

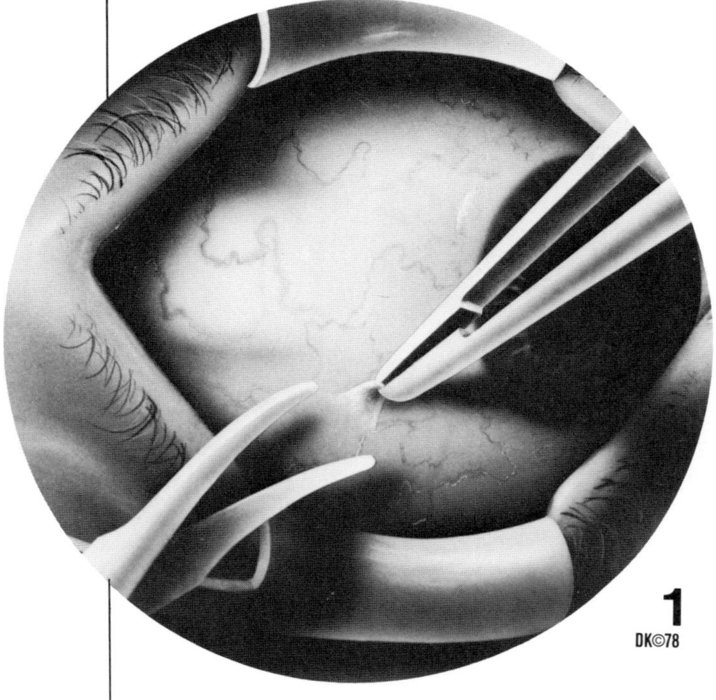

1
DK©78

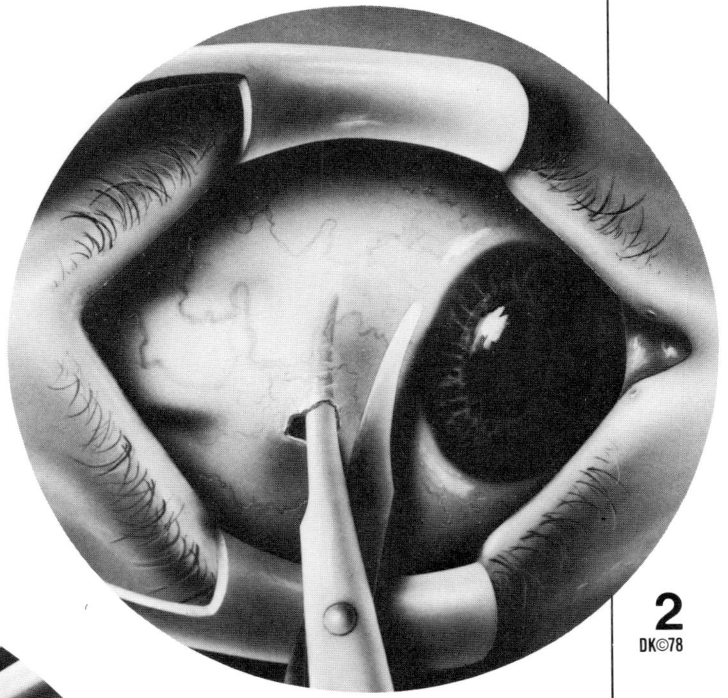

2
DK©78

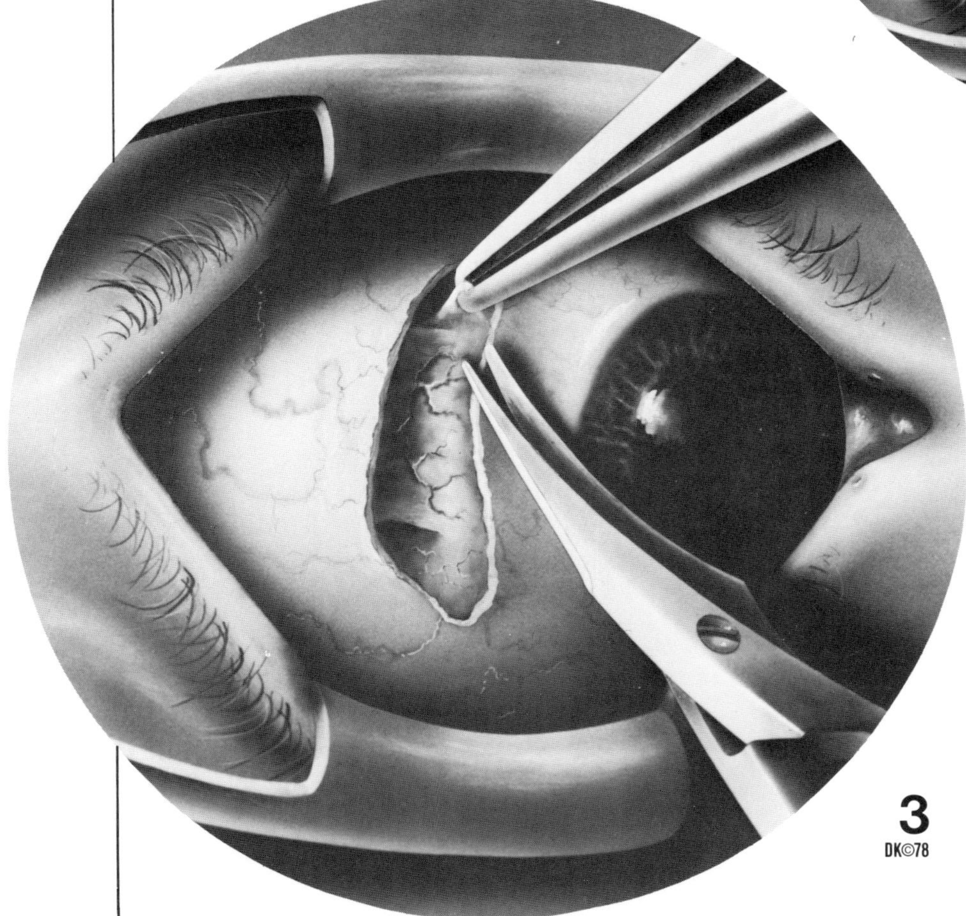

3
DK©78

tendon and advanced until the tip of the hook is visible through Tenon's capsule adjacent to the opposite border of the tendon [4] . A second cut in Tenon's capsule exposes the tip of the hook. Tenon's capsule overlying the muscle may be lifted with forceps and freed of its attachments to the muscle with blunt dissection as the scissors is spread [5] . This completes the exposure. If the muscle is inadvertently cut, considerable bleeding may occur. Postoperatively, usually more tissue reaction occurs because of the sutures required to close the wound [6] .

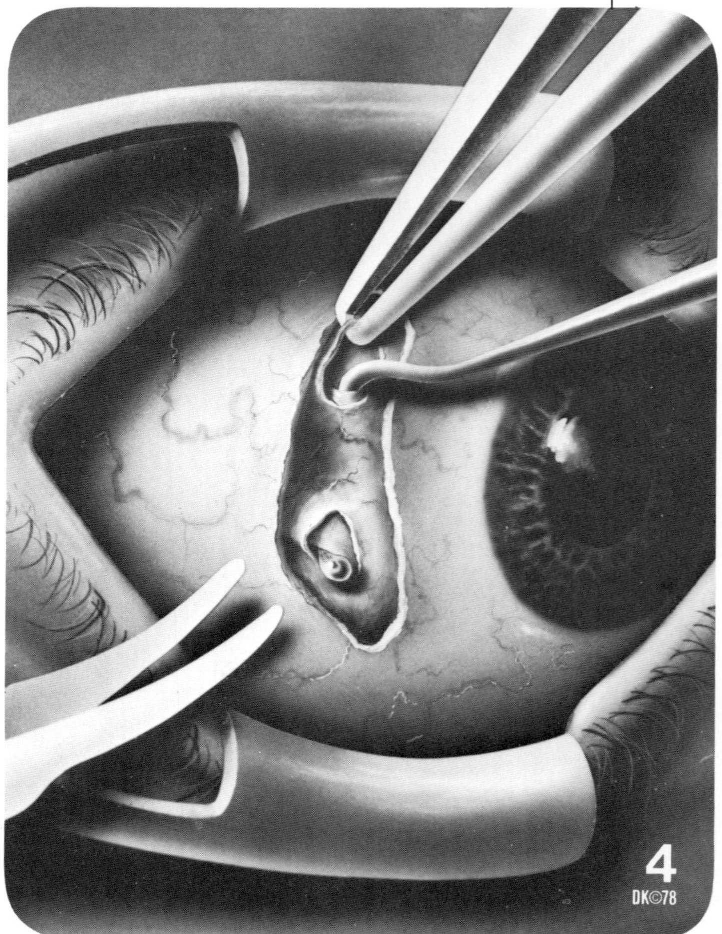

Donald F. Kilar

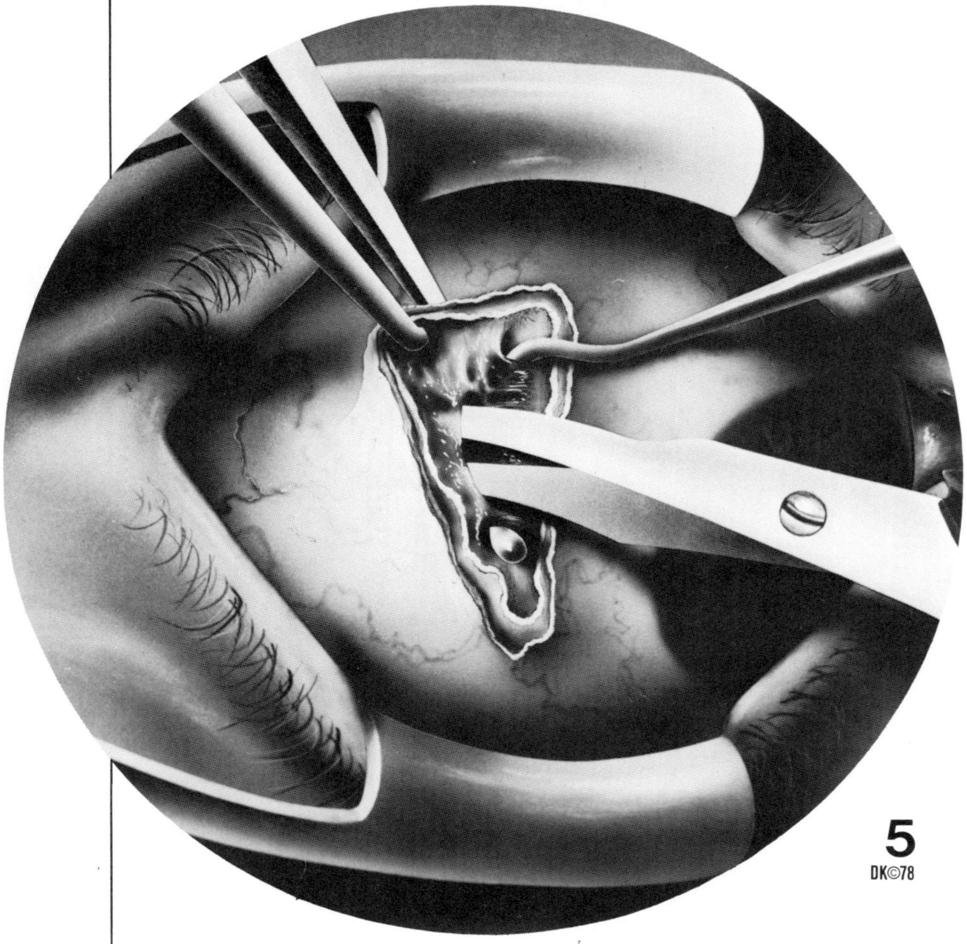

5
DK©78

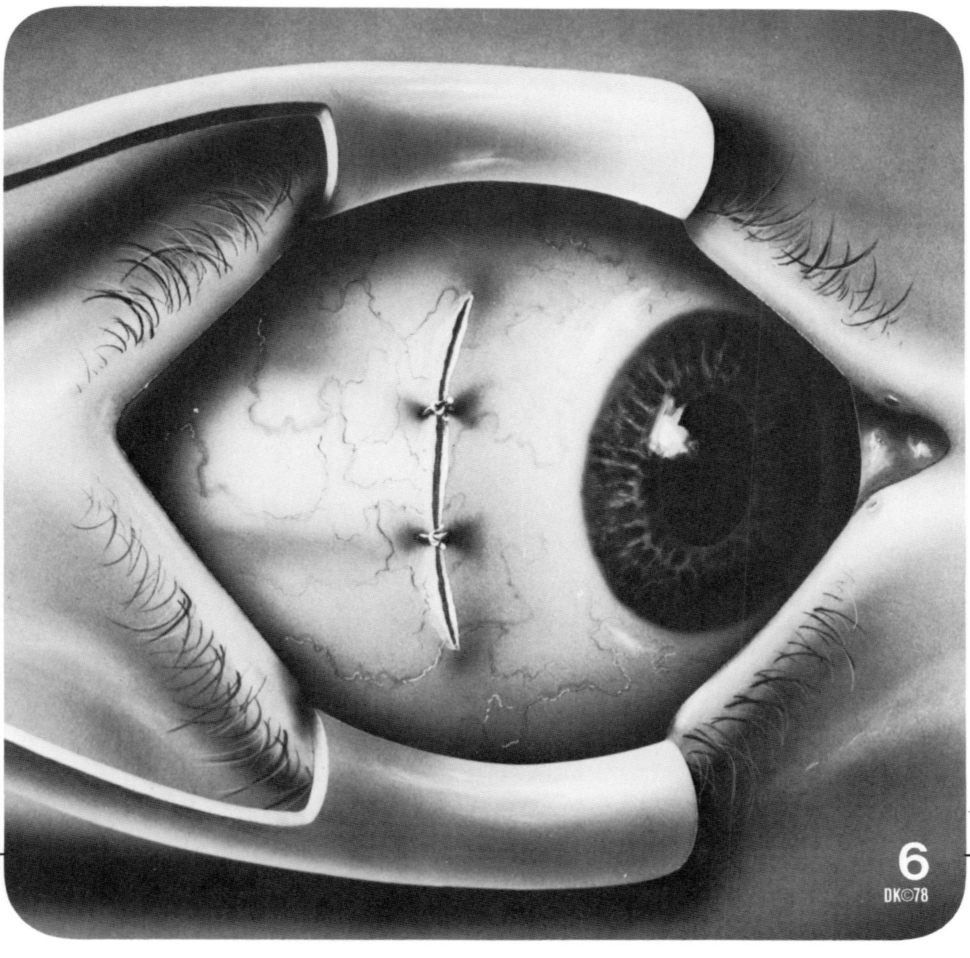

6
DK©78

Donald F. Keller

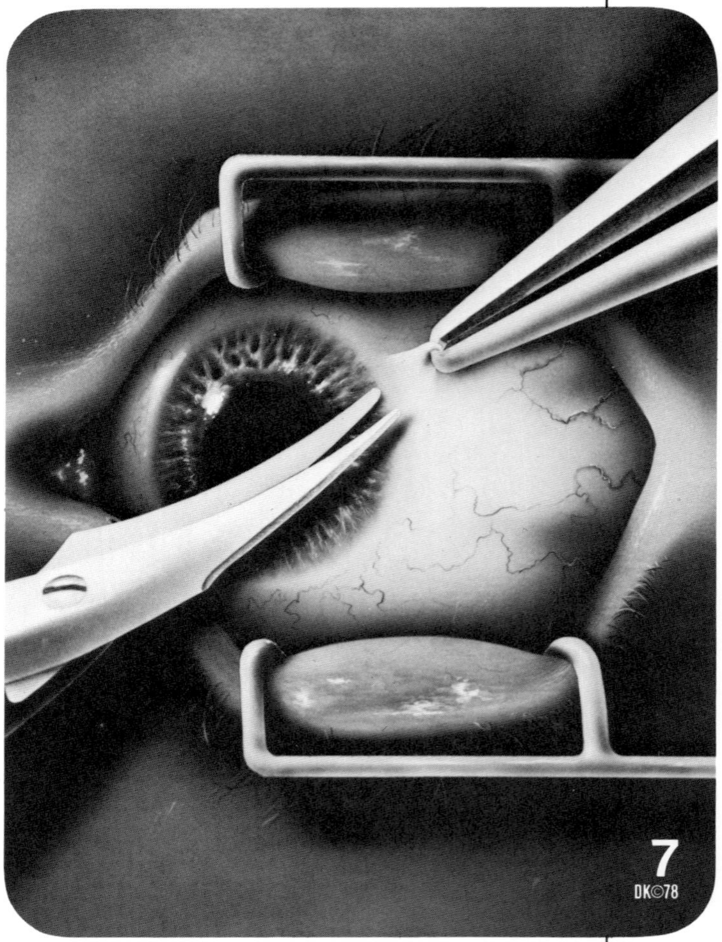

The limbal incision advocated by von Noorden provides maximum exposure since the conjunctiva is removed completely from the muscle insertion. Although the help of an experienced assistant is always desirable, this conjunctival approach may be easier for the surgeon to perform alone in the event that an assistant is not available. A peritomy is performed with Bishop-Harmon forceps and Westcott scissors in the sector of the muscle to be operated [7]. Bare sclera is thus exposed, and the flap is undermined in a manner similar to that used to make a fornix-based flap preceding cataract surgery [8]. Two extensions of the incision on either side of the rectus muscle aid in exposure [9] [10]. The incision is closed with one or two absorbable sutures at the limbus [11]. Occasionally, the patient complains of irritation because of the limbal suture. Should this occur, the suture may be removed safely on the second postoperative day.

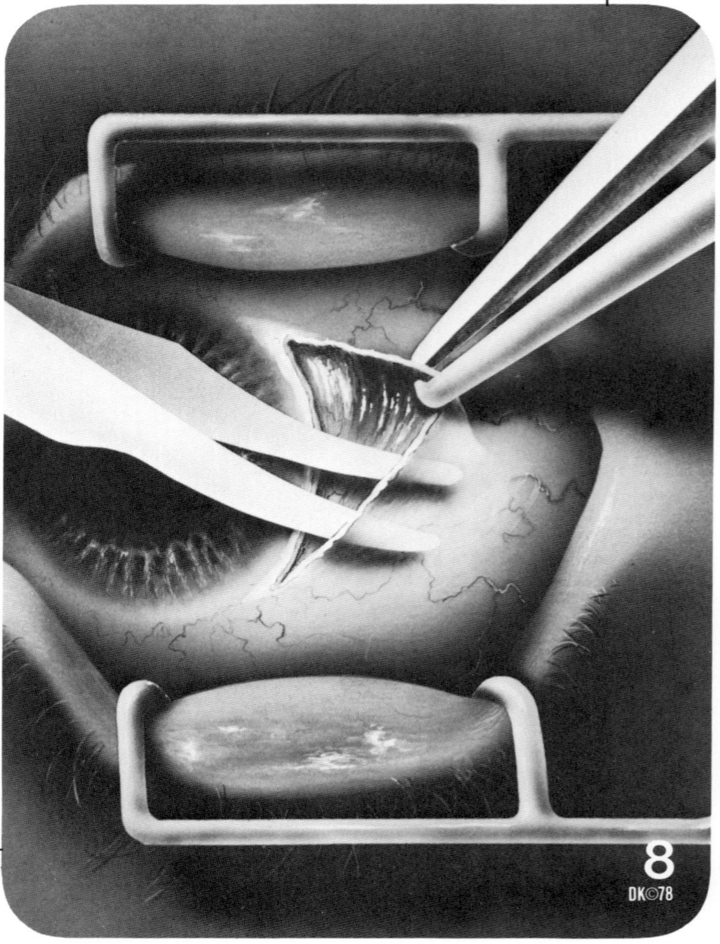

Donald A. Keller

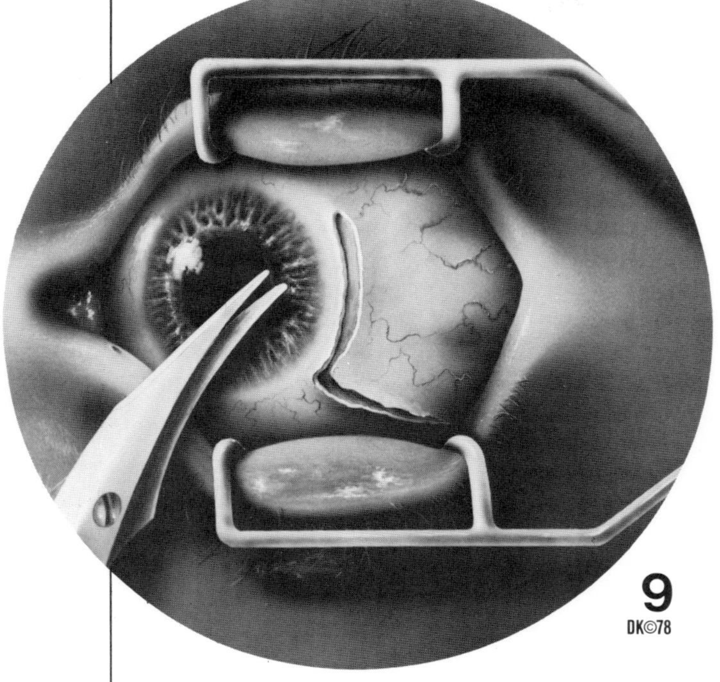

9
DK©78

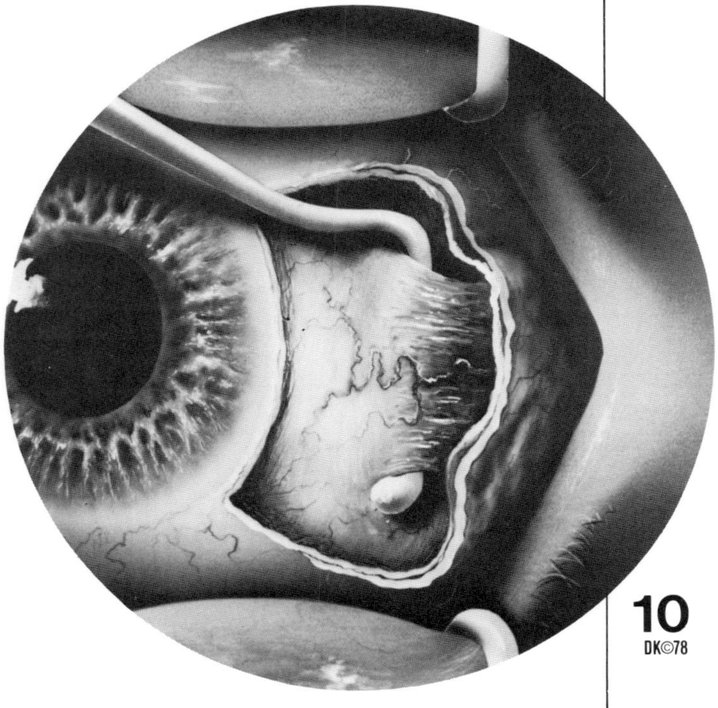

10
DK©78

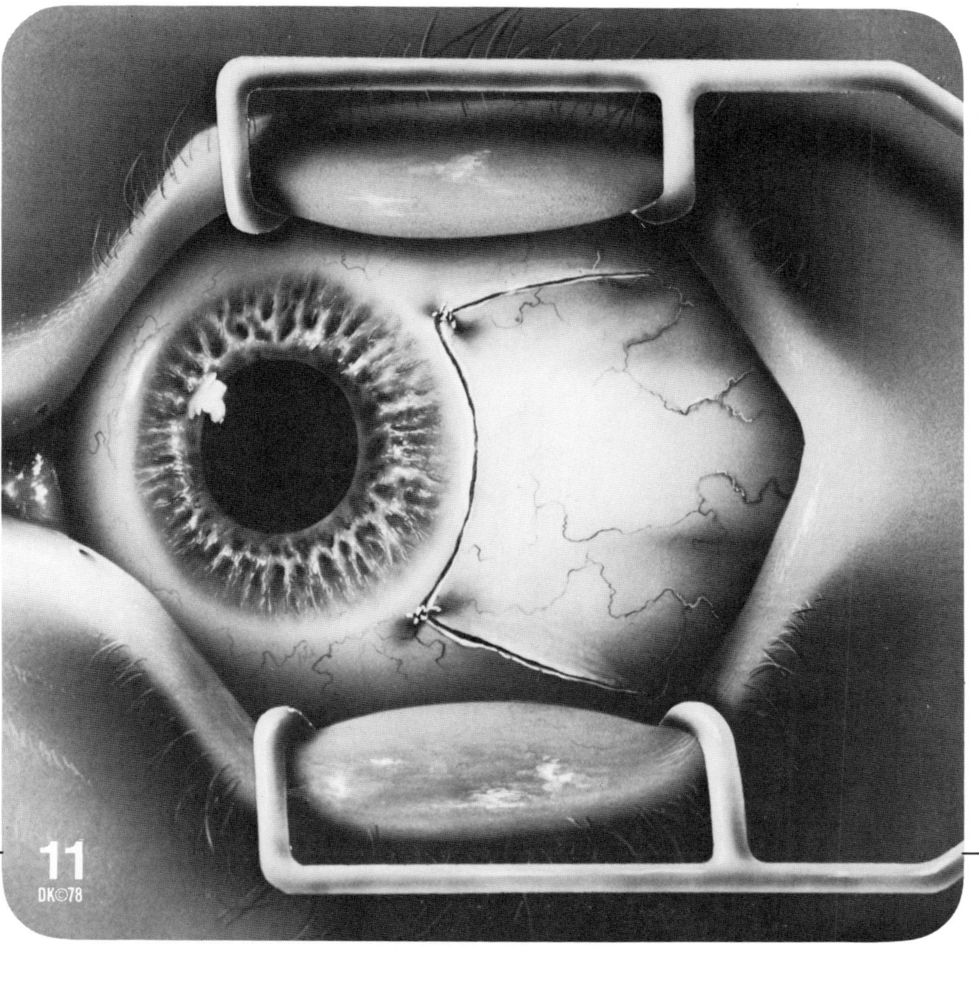

11
DK©78

Donald A. Keller

The self-closing conjunctival incision, as developed by Parks is made near the appropriate cul-de-sac. For example, a procedure on the lateral rectus or inferior oblique muscle would use the inferotemporal quadrant. The inferonasal quadrant would be used for surgery involving the medial rectus muscle. During reoperations, the upper quadrants are frequently used to avoid tough scar tissue. This self-closing incision eliminates the possibility of an allergic suture reaction, since no sutures are used. The help of an assistant is required for this procedure.

The conjunctiva is grasped near the limbus with Bishop-Harmon forceps in the desired quadrant. To expose the incision site, the assistant rotates and immobilizes the eye. Using a second Bishop-Harmon forceps, the surgeon lifts the bulbar conjunctiva and underlying fascia 2 or 3 mm from the cul-de-sac. The incision is made with a Westcott scissors which is directed toward the center of the globe [12]. Since this cut does not usually include all of Tenon's capsule, the remaining layer is grasped, and a second scissors cut is made to produce an opening to the sclera. Spreading the scissors widens the incision. Redundant tissue is then excised.

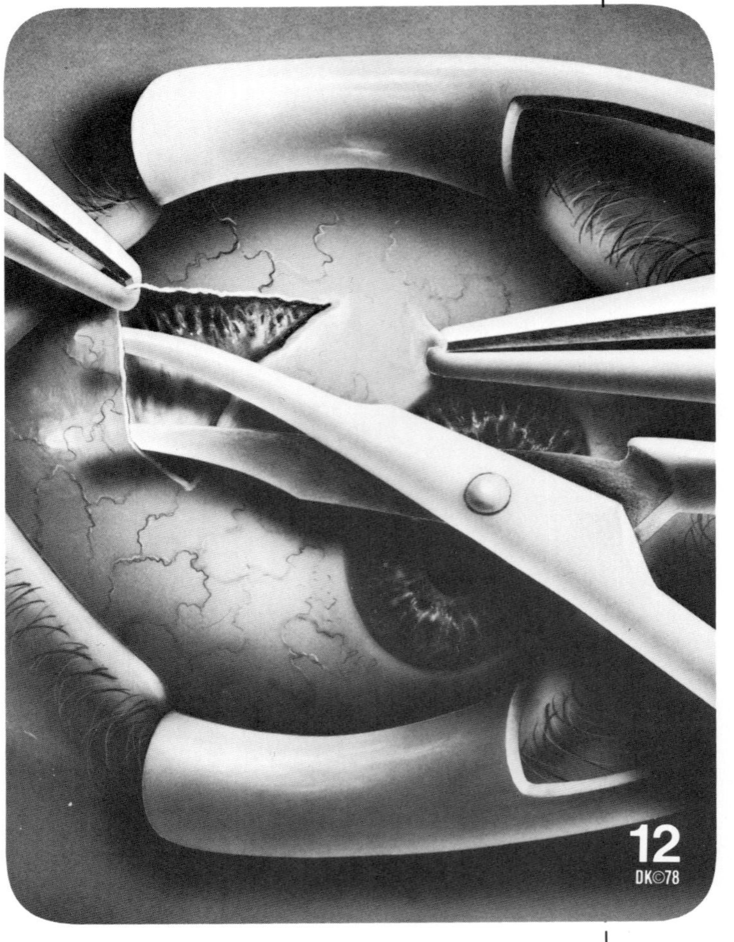

The nasal edge of the incision is elevated with the forceps, and the surgeon passes a small von Graefe hook beneath the inferior belly of the medial rectus [13]. The hook is passed with the tip in contact with the sclera and the heel slightly elevated. This orientation of the muscle hook insures its passage beneath the muscle. A larger Jameson hook is then introduced beneath the muscle to replace the von Graefe hook [14], which is reinserted above the Jameson hook and used to create a plane between Tenon's fascia and the muscle capsule [15]. With a back-and-forth motion of the von Graefe hook, Tenon's capsule and conjunctiva are swept over the top of the larger hook to expose the superior

Donald F. Keller

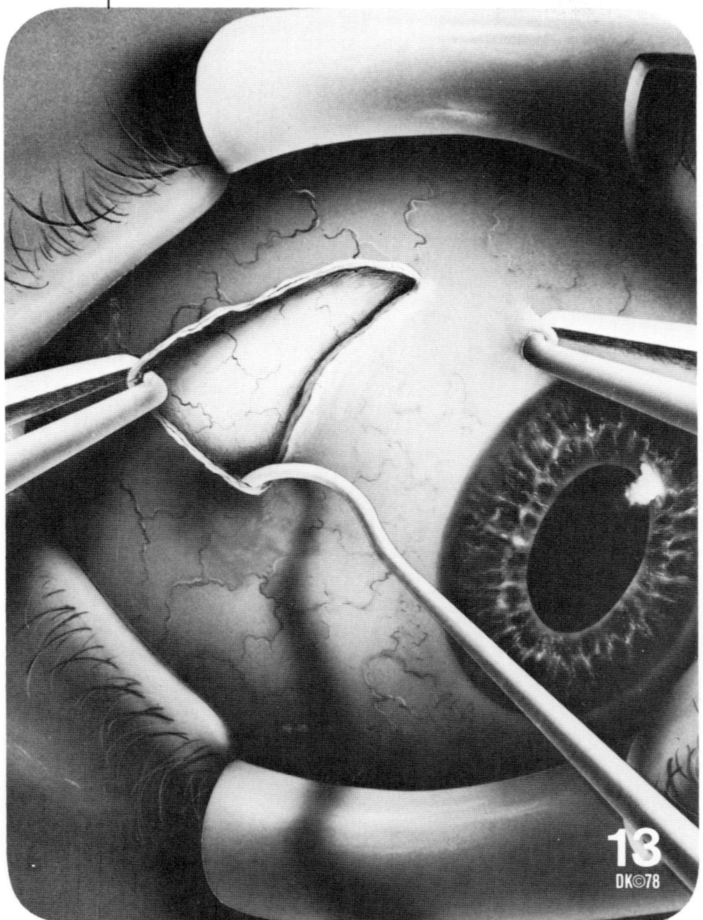

13
DK©78

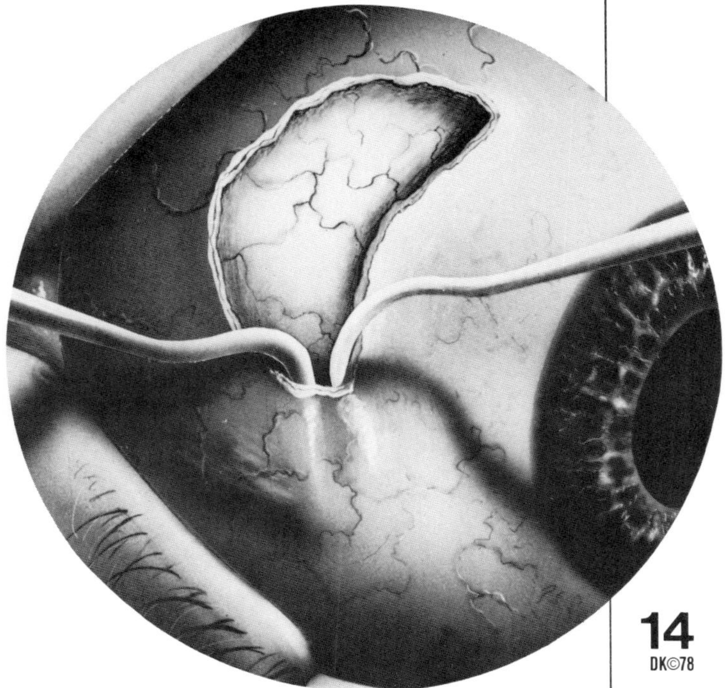

14
DK©78

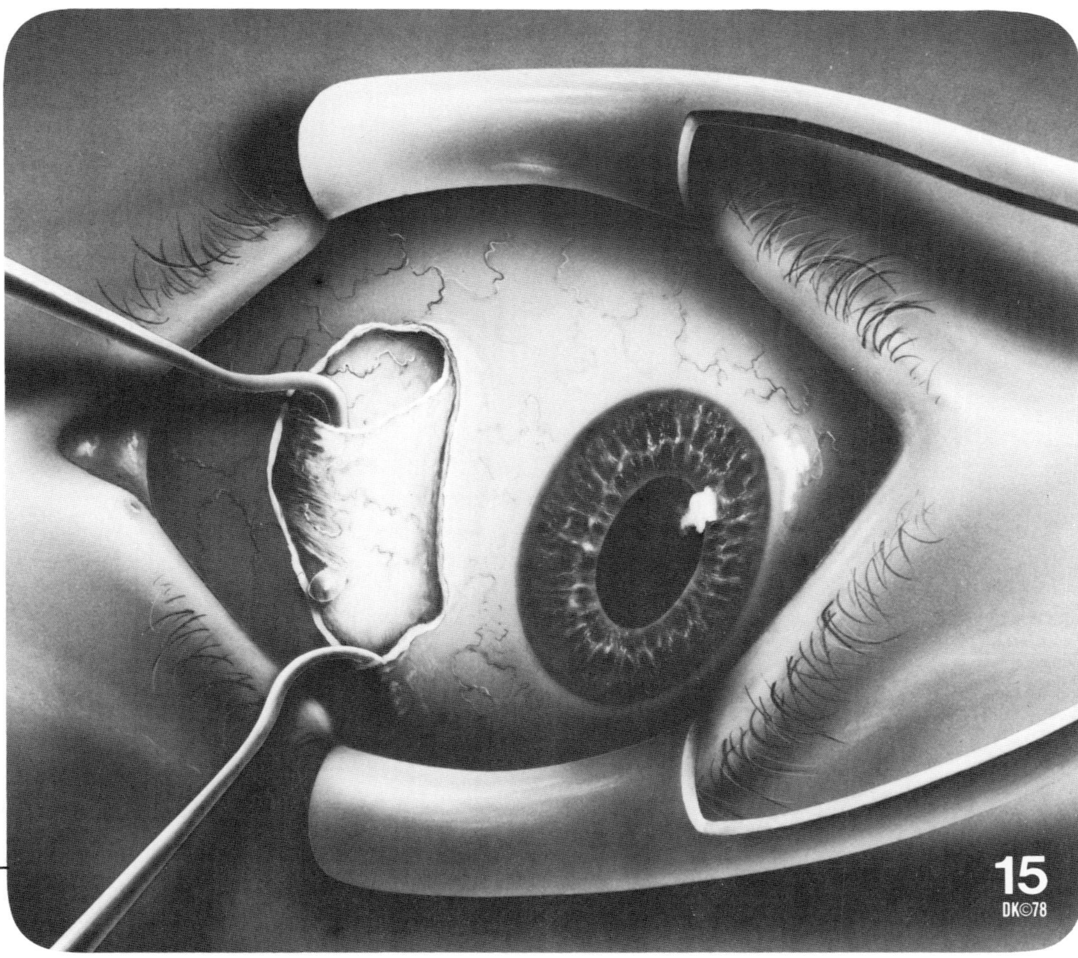

15
DK©78

margin of the muscle. These two muscle hooks are held by the assistant while the surgeon creates a small buttonhole incision through Tenon's fascia that exposes the tip of the Jameson hook [16]. This incision is widened by spreading the scissors until the sclera is visible. The assistant places the tip of the von Graefe hook into the widened incision and retracts it posteriorly and superiorly.

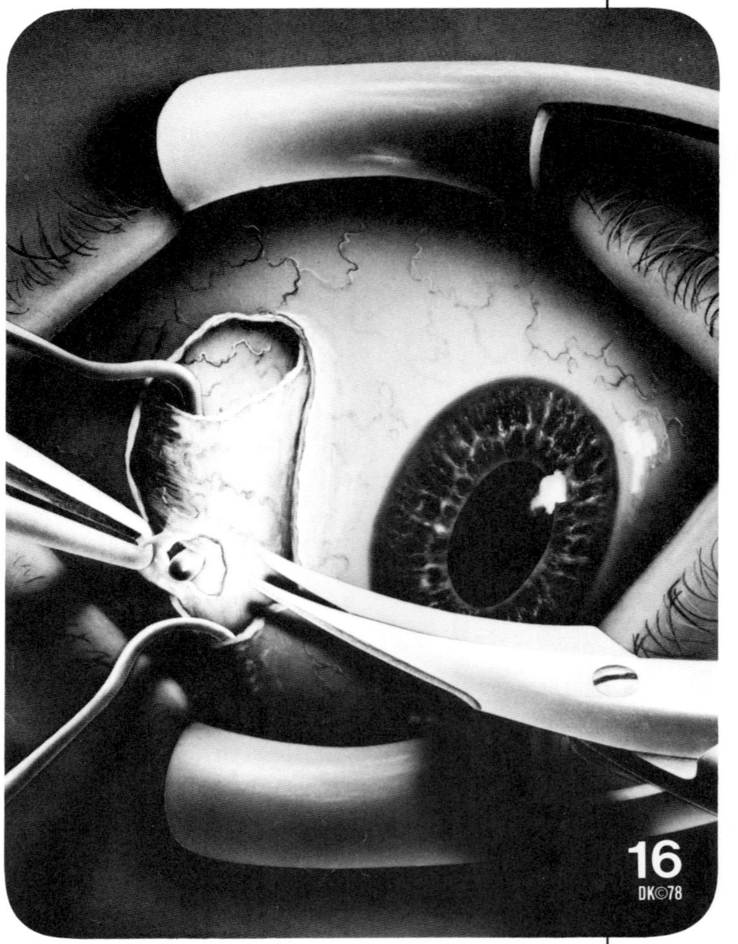

The surgeon introduces a second von Graefe hook into the same incision and sweeps it superiorly around the insertion [17]. If all of the muscle fibers are included on the Jameson hook, this sweep is accomplished without resistance. Tenon's fascia, anterior to the insertion, is retracted with the von Graefe hook and cut with Westcott scissors [18]. This maneuver cleans the distal portion of the muscle in preparation for suturing.

After the muscle has been cleaned anteriorly, the assistant rotates the von Graefe hook, A [19], nasally. A second von Graefe hook, B [19], is inserted in a similar position under the intermuscular septum along the inferior muscle border; it also is retracted nasally. Excision of the exposed fascial tissue completes the muscle exposure.

At the end of the procedure, the conjunctiva is reposited in the cul-de-sac and is self-sealing. This incision provides for minimal postoperative reaction and discomfort. The following procedures use this type of conjunctival incision since it is the one we routinely use.

Donald A. Keller

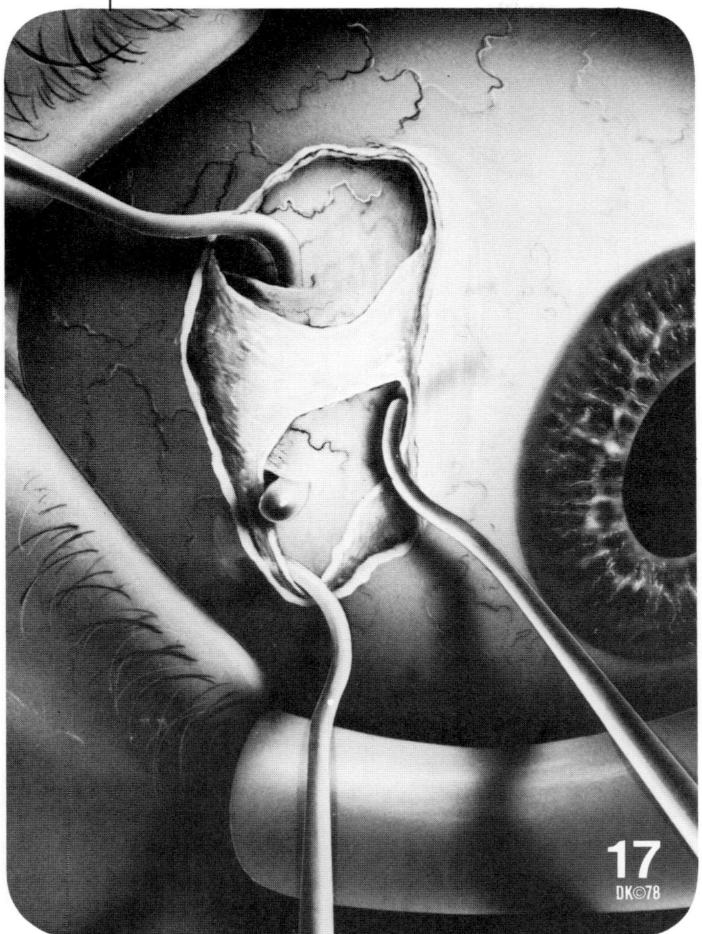

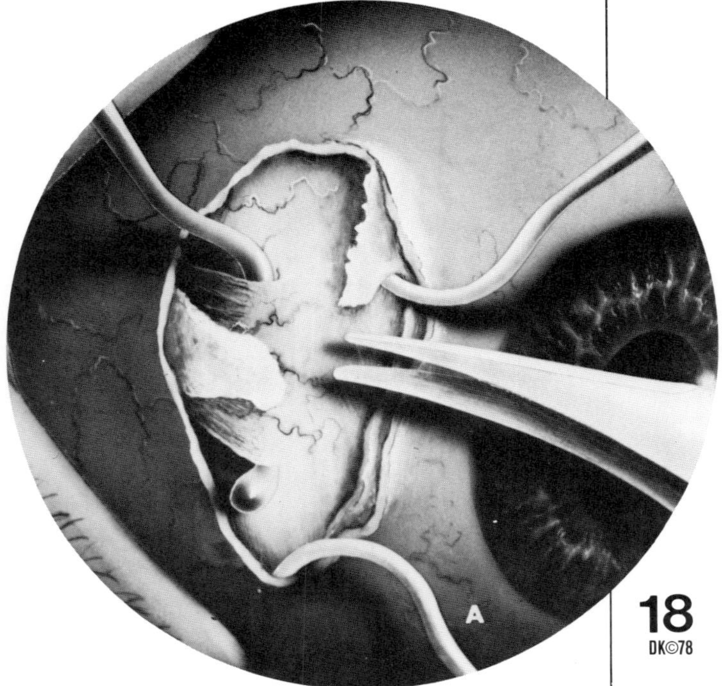

18
DK©78

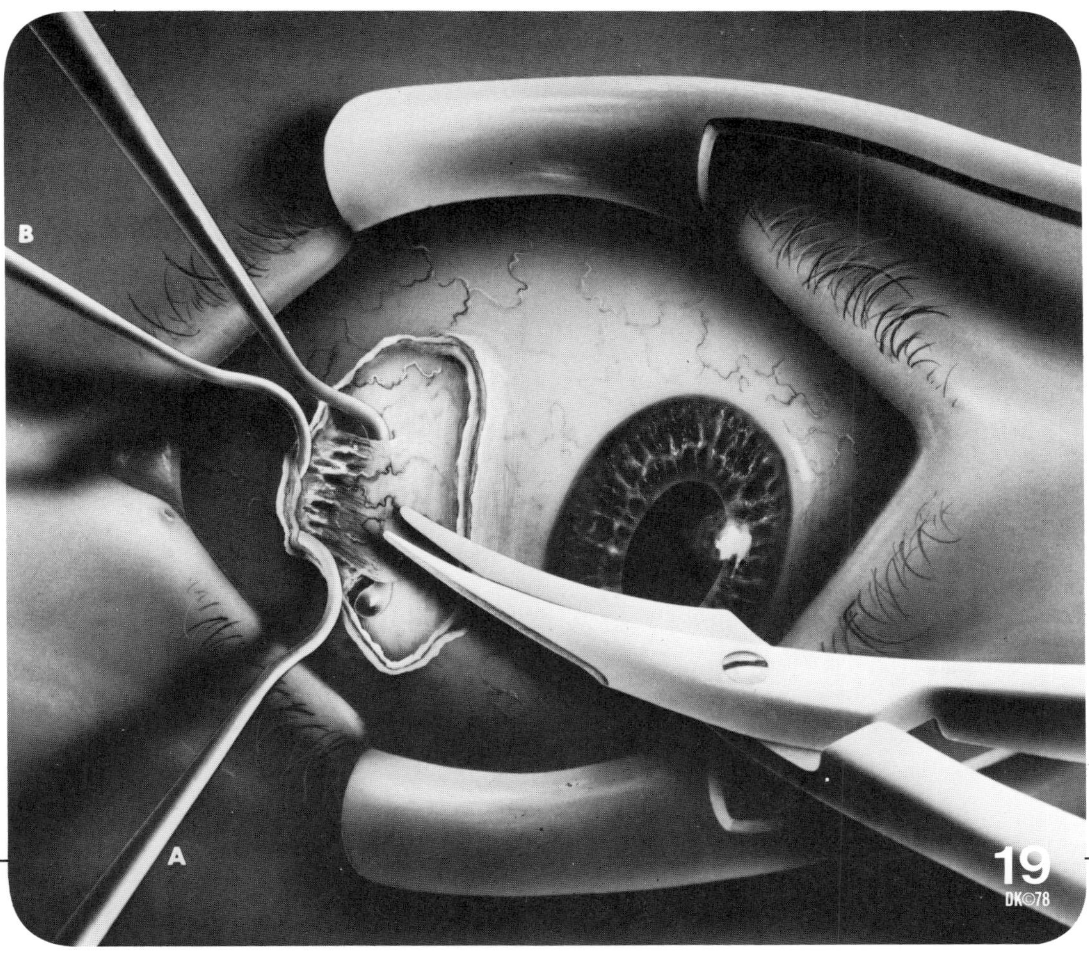

Donald A. Keller

RECESSION OF A RECTUS MUSCLE

Richard E. Simmons, M.D.

The amount and type of surgery recommended for a given deviation vary considerably. We have found the guidelines developed by Parks to be quite useful when planning extraocular muscle surgery. (See table at the bottom of the page.)

Results of the forced-duction test are quite important in the treatment of infants with congenital esotropia. The medial rectus muscles are often tight, and if abduction is restricted somewhat, we recommend increasing the recession. If residual esotropia is present after bilateral medial rectus recession, and the medial rectus muscles are still tight on forced-duction testing, resection of the laterals may not produce the expected correct alignment. Therefore, a further weakening procedure on the medial rectus, such as a marginal myotomy or further recession, may provide a better result.

After exposure of the desired rectus muscle by isolation with muscle hooks and lysis of its fascial attachments, a double-armed 6-0 Vicryl suture is placed through the undersurface of the muscle within 1 mm of its insertion to exit at the superior edge of the muscle [1]. The second arm of the suture is placed in a similar manner. The suture is secured with a lock bite placed at each edge of the muscle.

The tendon is disinserted flush with the sclera by means of short snips with a Westcott scissors [2]. To accomplish this, the surgeon grasps both arms of the suture between the thumb and index finger, and the Jameson hook is grasped between the index and middle fingers of the same hand. The sutures may be tightened so that they will not be cut inadvertently as the muscle is severed from the sclera. During this maneuver, the assistant retracts Tenon's capsule and conjunctiva with a von Graefe hook.

CORRECTION OF ESOTROPIA

Deviation, Prism Diopters	Bilateral Medial Rectus Recession, mm	Bilateral Lateral Rectus Resection, mm	Unilateral Surgery Recession-Resection
15	3.0	4.0	3 + 4
20	3.5	5.0	3.5 + 5
25	4.0	6.0	4 + 6
30	4.5	6.5	4.5 + 6.5
35-40	5.0		5.0 + 7 to 8
45-50	5.5		
55 +	6.0		

CORRECTION OF EXOTROPIA

Deviation, Prism Diopters	Bilateral Lateral Rectus Recession, mm	Bilateral Medial Rectus Resection, mm	Unilateral Surgery Recession-Resection
15	4.0	4.0	4 + 4
20	5.0	4.5	4 + 4.5
25	6.0	5.0	6 + 5
30	7.0	5.5	7 + 5.5
35	7.0	6.0	7 + 6
40 +	8.0		

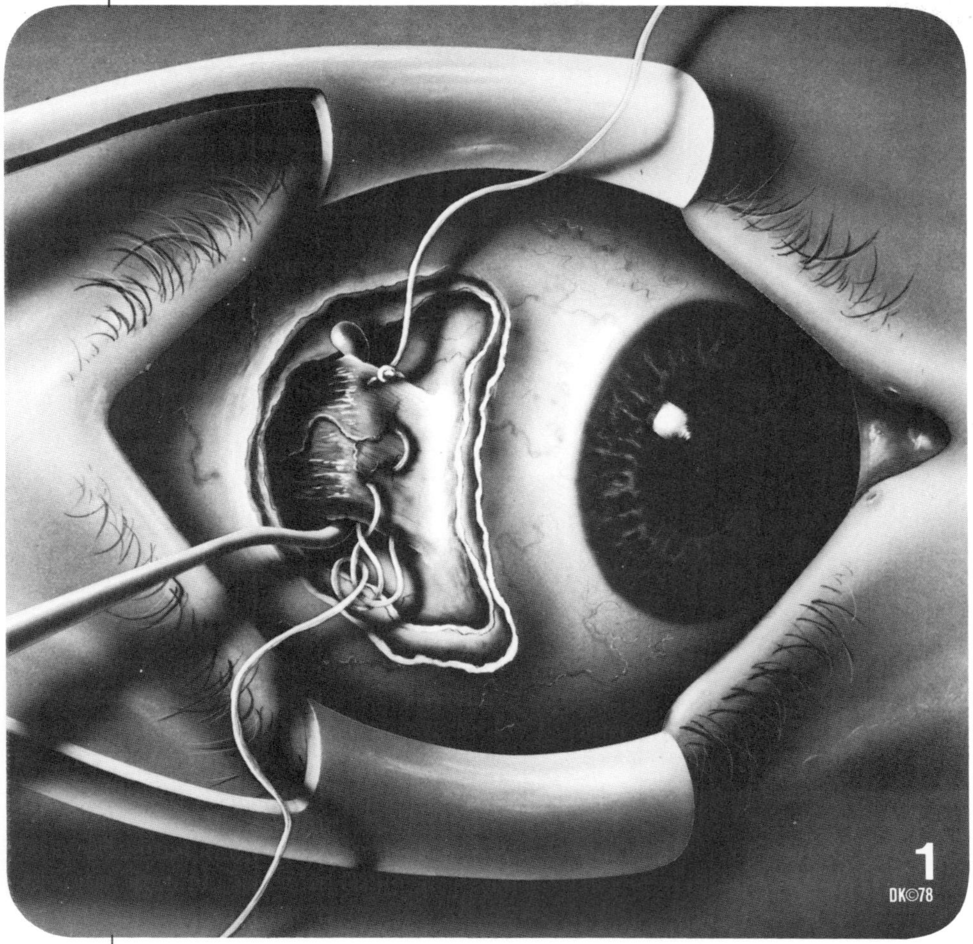

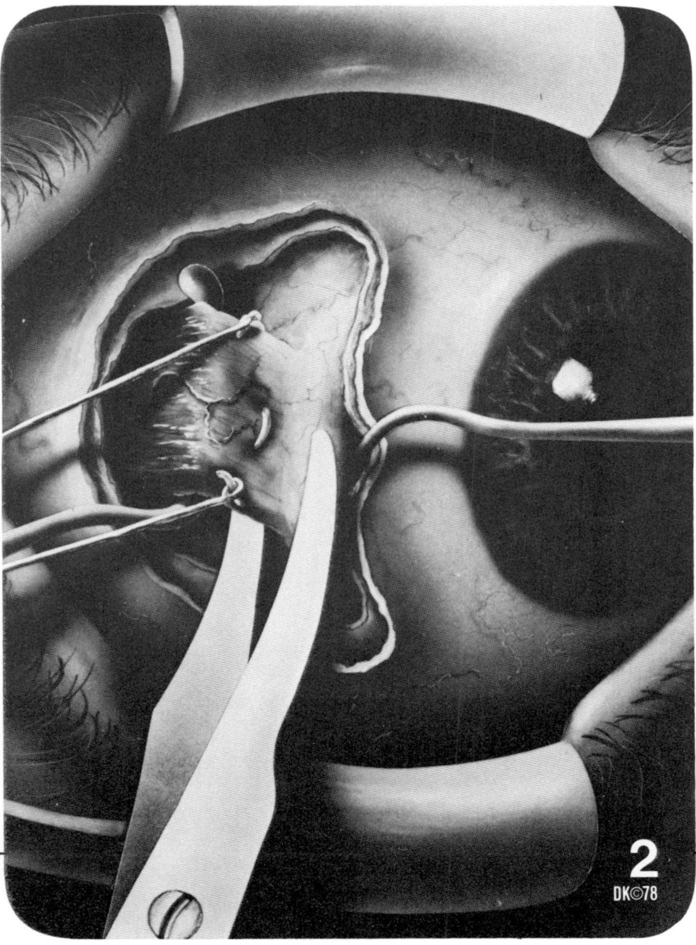

Donald H. Keller

After the muscle has been cut, a caliper marks the desired millimeters of recession on the sclera. Exposure is achieved as the assistant grasps the ends of the stump at the original insertion with two 0.5-mm Castroviejo forceps and rotates the globe. The surgeon holds the measuring calipers in one hand and retracts Tenon's with a von Graefe hook in the free hand [3] .

A superficial intrascleral needle tract is made parallel to the insertion [4] . The initial entrance of the needle should be made with the tip tangential to the globe to avoid accidental perforation. The needles enter the sclera from the opposite ends. Before the suture is reapplied to the sclera, the surgeon should check the severed muscle tendon to be sure that the lock bites have not pulled out. The importance of avoiding crossed sutures cannot be overemphasized; it is better to discover them at this point in the procedure than with a tangled mass of sutures and Tenon's capsule. Similarly, a great deal of frustration will be avoided if care is taken to keep the two arms of suture distinctly separate and not to pass one arm of the suture through a loop in the other arm. The distance between the entry sites should equal the width of the original insertion.

The needles exit from the sclera with a 1- to 2-mm overlap to give a criss-cross appearance to the two opposing intrasclerally placed needles. The sutures are then tied [5] . This "crossed swords" technique creates a new insertion that is parallel to the original one. The conjunctiva is repositioned, and no sutures are necessary.

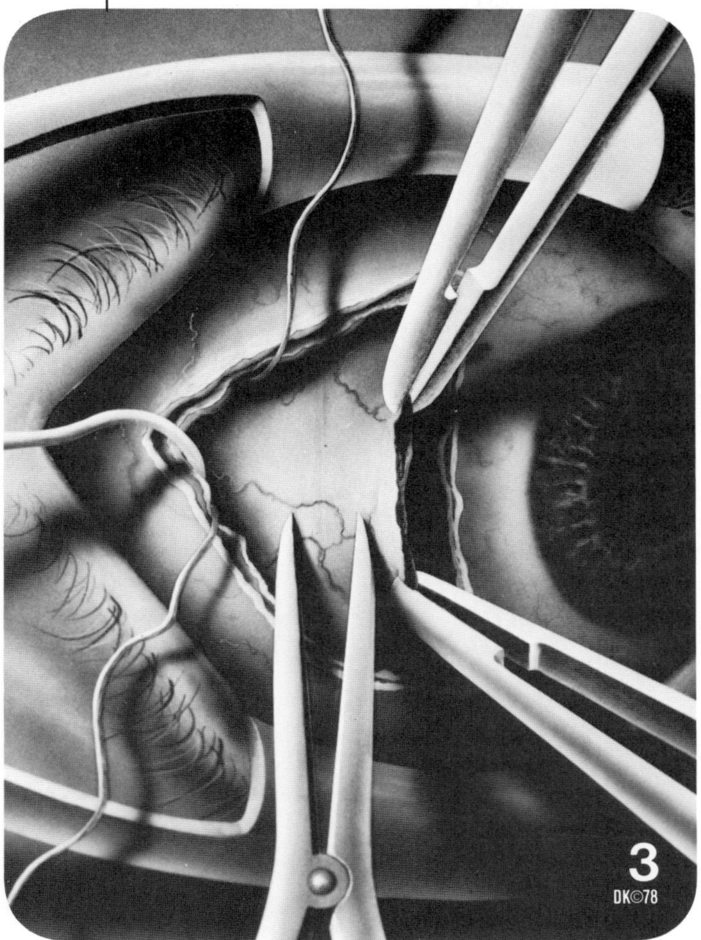

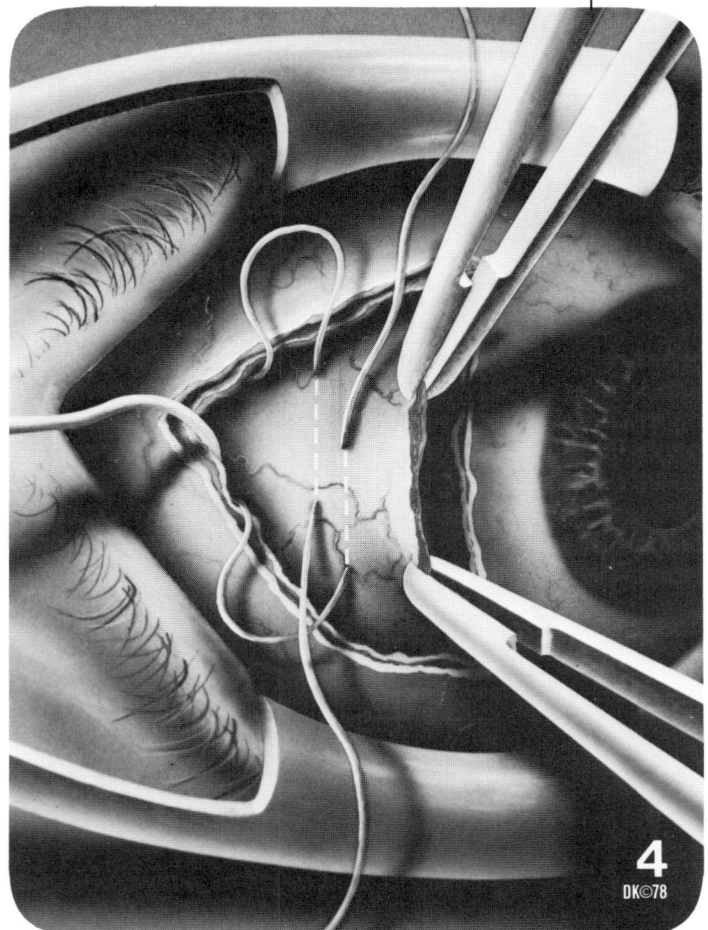

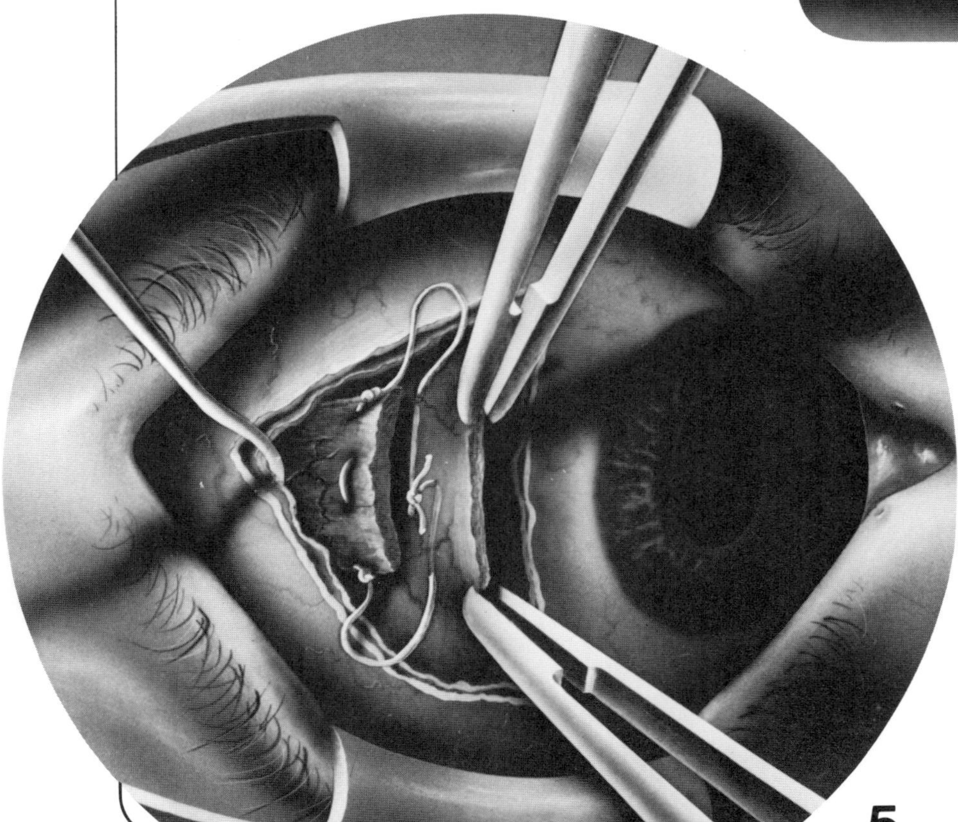

Donald A. Keller

RESECTION OF A RECTUS MUSCLE

Richard E. Simmons, M.D.

After the forced-duction test and conjunctival incision, the muscle is isolated and freed of its fascial attachments in a manner similar to that done in the recession procedure. To provide an adequate surgical field, the assistant introduces a second Jameson hook under the belly of the muscle to stretch it [1]. At the point of the desired resection, a double-armed suture is inserted, and lock bites are placed at each edge of the muscle [2].

To excise the muscle, the surgeon first applies a straight hemostat across the muscle belly, just anterior to the suture [3]. The muscle is disinserted with Westcott scissors, and a small stump is left. Using Bishop-Harmon forceps and a Bard-Parker knife, the surgeon cuts the muscle flush against the hemostat. To bring the muscle forward to the insertion, two intrascleral sutures usually are needed [4]. The assistant grasps each edge of the insertion stump with 0.5-mm Castroviejo forceps to stabilize the globe for suturing. The first needle bite should enter the sclera at the edge of the insertion, traverse the insertion, and exit anteriorly at the mid-point. The surgeon must exercise great care since the sclera is extremely thin in this area.

The hemostat is removed, and to facilitate tying the sutures, the assistant now incorporates the lateral ends of the muscle and insertion with each forceps. This prevents posterior slippage of the muscle as the suture is tied [5]

The basic techniques of horizontal rectus muscle recession and resection, although usually employed in the management of simple esotropia and exotropia, are also useful in the management of several special types of horizontal deviations. Two notable examples are A and V patterns.

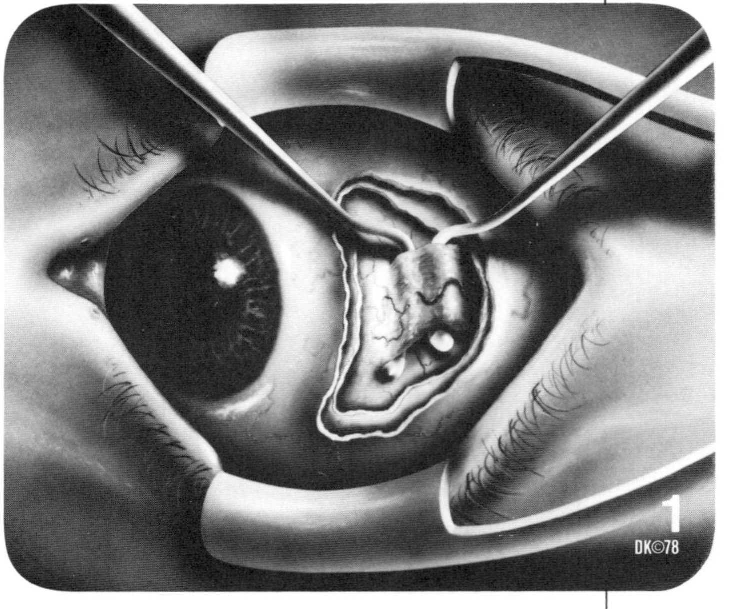

Many patients with a horizontal deviation exhibit a coexisting A and V pattern. This may be secondary to an overaction of one of the oblique muscles. In many cases, however, a significant overaction does not exist. In these patients, we recommend supraplacement or infraplacement of the horizontal muscles according to the following general rule: The degree of movement in horizontal muscles depends on the difference in horizontal deviation between upgaze and downgaze. The examiner should move the insertion 5 mm up or down if the difference is approximately 20 prism diopters. Movement should be as much as 10 mm with larger differences (30 or more prism diopters).

The following table indicates which muscles are infraplaced or supraplaced, depending on the type of deviation that exists.

Disorder	**Correction**
A esotropia	Supraplace medials, infraplace laterals
V esotropia	Infraplace medials, supraplace laterals
A exotropia	Supraplace medials, infraplace laterals
V exotropia	Infraplace medials, supraplace laterals

Donald A. Keller

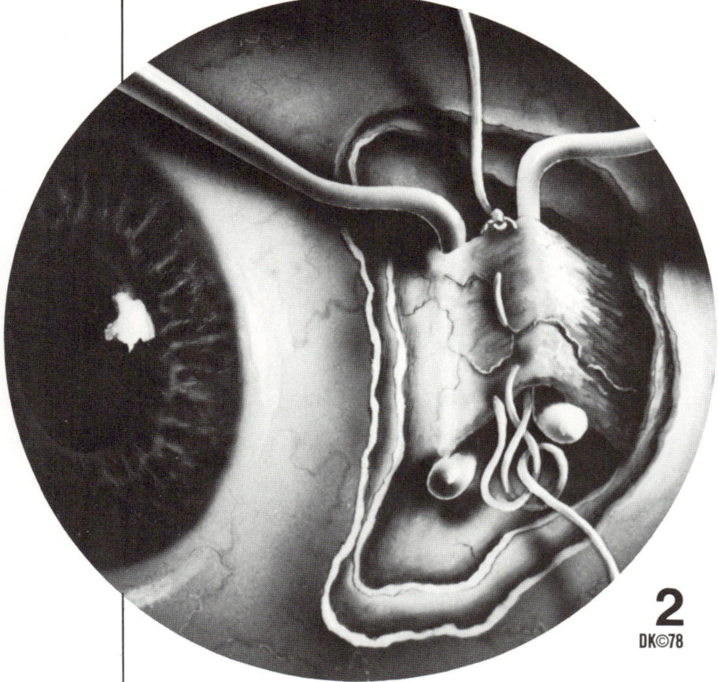

2

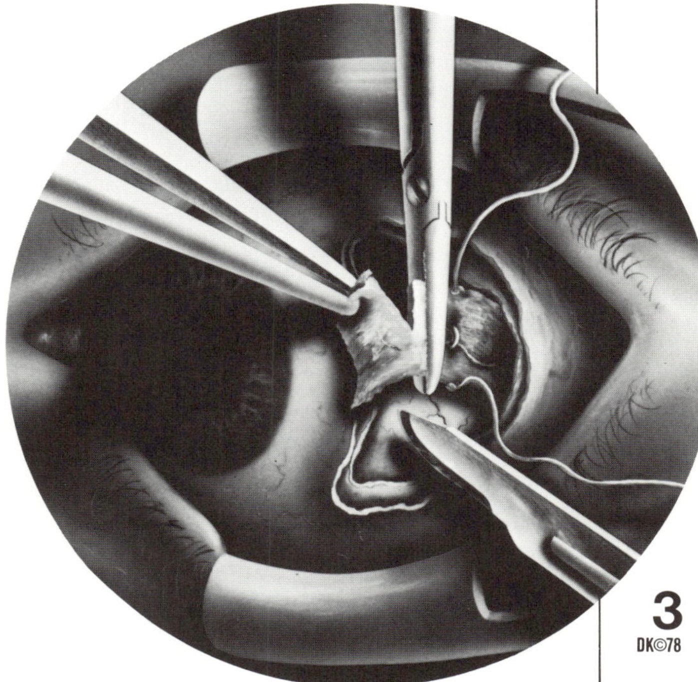

3

DK©78

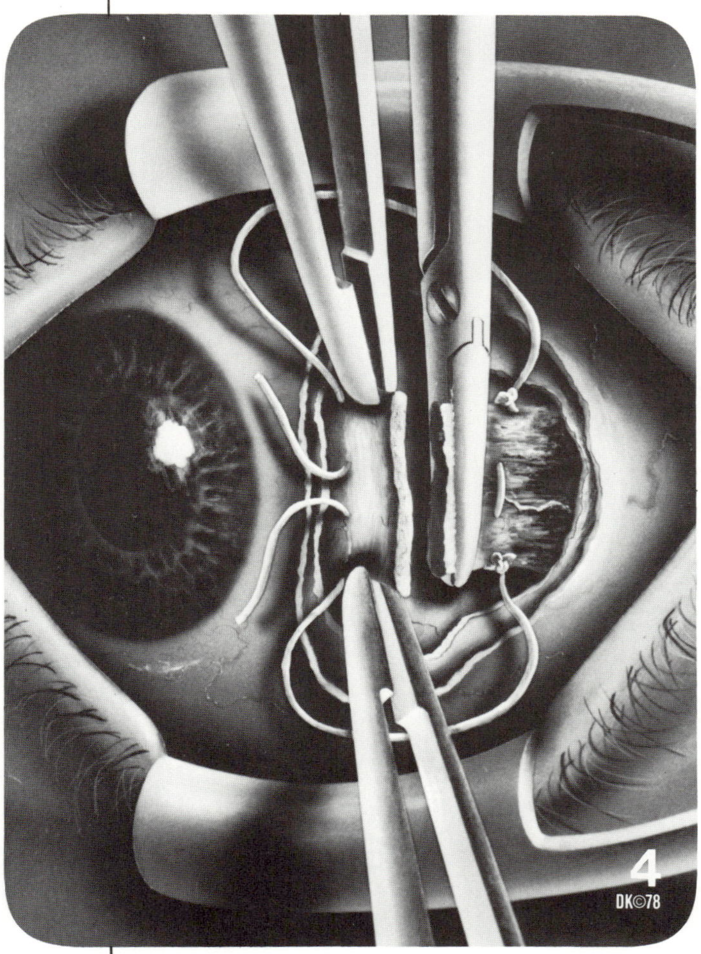

4

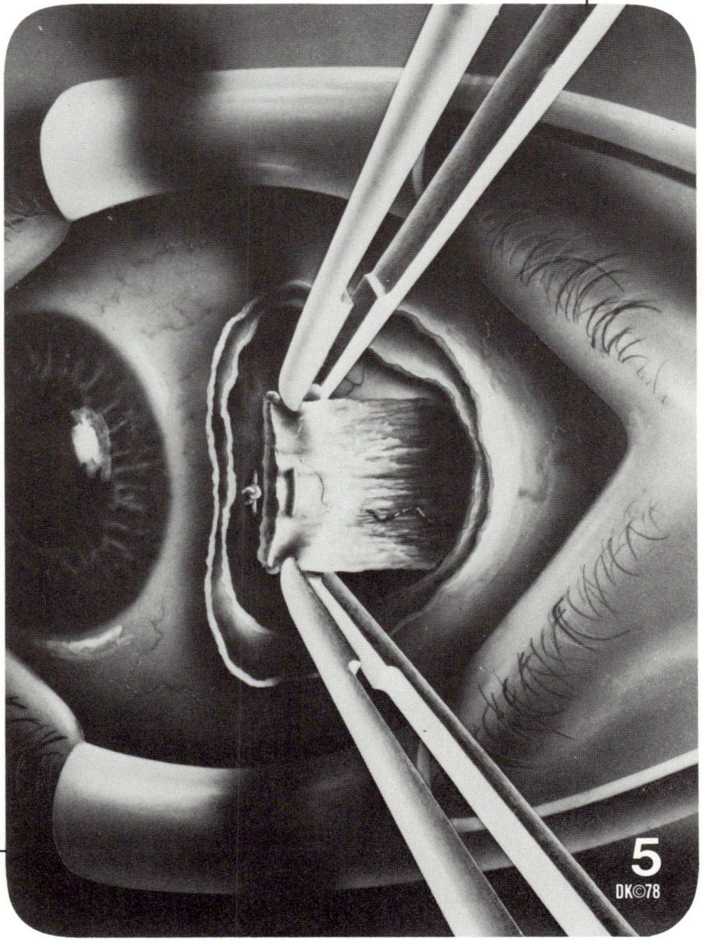

5

Donald A. Keller

MARGINAL MYOTOMY

Richard E. Simmons, M.D.

The final results of marginal myotomy are most unpredictable. It has proved valuable, however, in the following circumstances: congenital esotropia after maximal medial rectus recession where the forced-duction test still shows restriction or tightness of the medial rectus muscles on abduction; exotropic or esotropic deviations with previous large recession and a high AC/A ratio; and in situations where the fissures are too small and the medial rectus muscles are too tight to do a recession procedure.

After the muscle is isolated, a small, curved hemostat is placed on the superior portion of the muscle, 4 mm posterior to the muscle insertion [1]. The amount of muscle included in the bite depends on the amount of deviation present. Another hemostat is placed on the inferior portion on the opposite side of the muscle, 2 mm anterior to the first hemostat [2]. These hemostats crush the tissue and provide hemostasis. When hemostasis is achieved, the hemostats are removed, and the muscle is cut along the line of crushed tissue [3] [4]. It is important to avoid splitting the muscle while isolating it, since this can result in a transection of the muscle when the marginal myotomy is done.

To determine the amount of correction that will be achieved, the following guidelines can be followed. If the hemostats encompass one half of the width of each muscle and the procedure is done bilaterally, 25 prism diopters of correction will be achieved. If the hemostats encompass two thirds of the width of each muscle, 25 to 35 prism diopters of correction will result. If three fourths of the width of each muscle is encompassed, 35 to 40 prism diopters of correction can be expected.

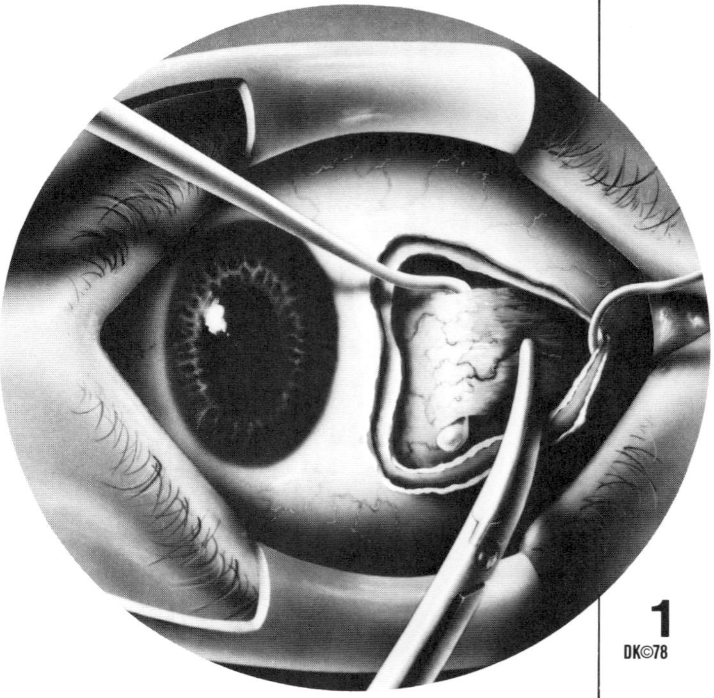

1

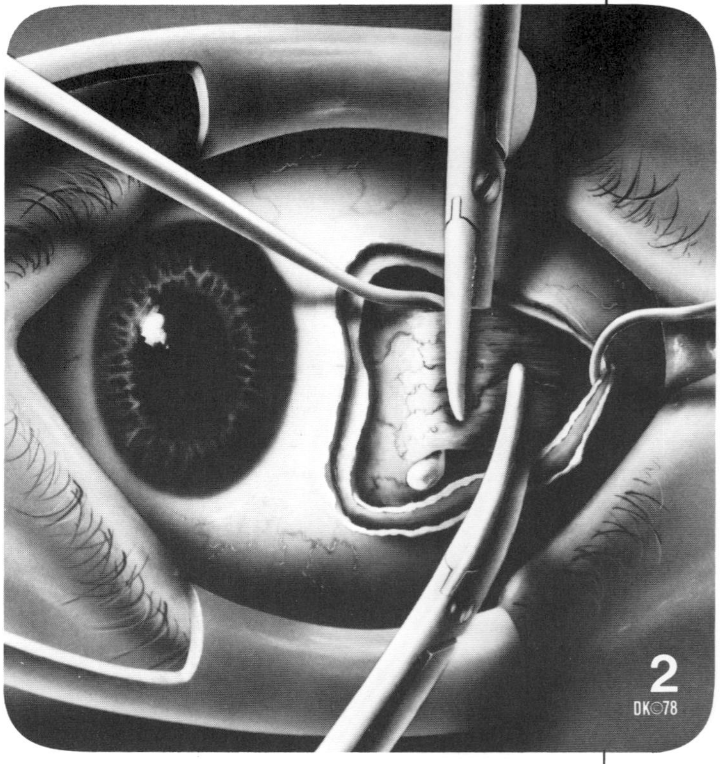

2

Donald A. Keller

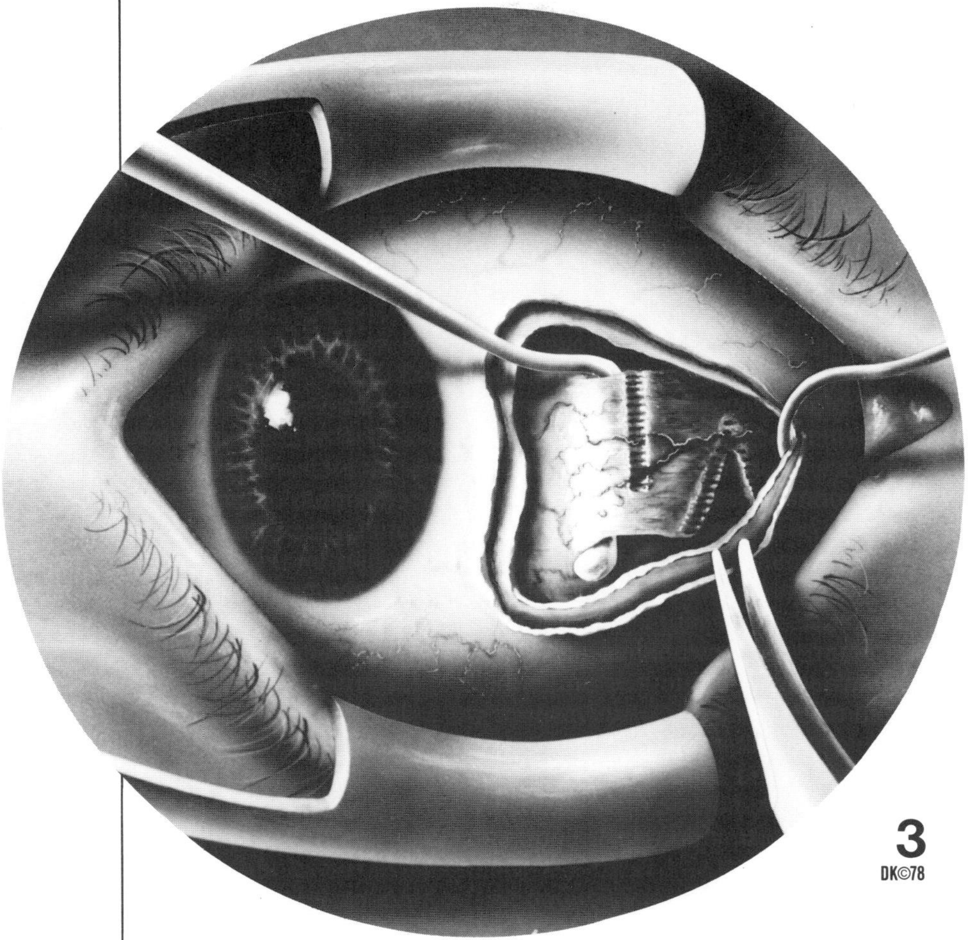

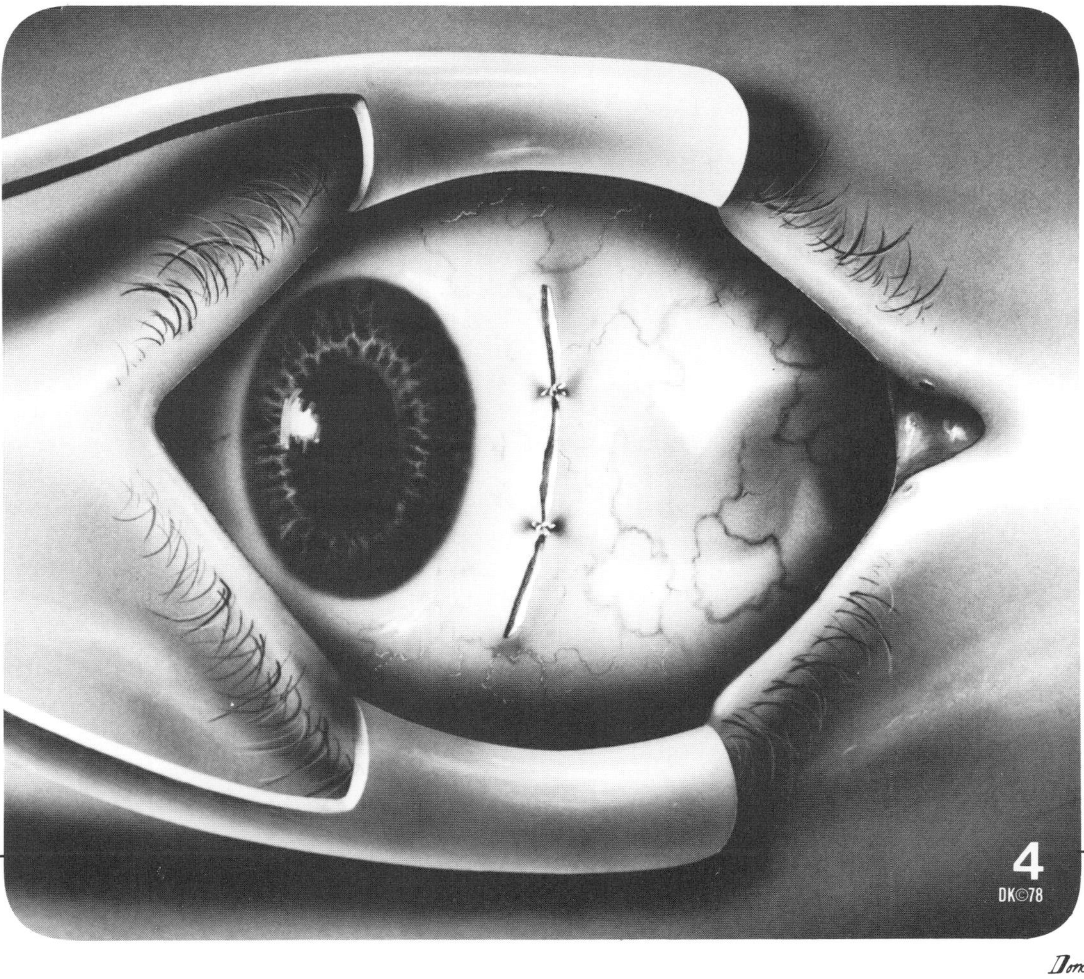

Donald A. Keller

THE BIELSCHOWSKY HEAD-TILT TEST

Gary Rogers, M.D.
James A. Savage, M.D.

The identification of the paretic muscle causing a vertical deviation can be extremely difficult. This problem is compounded since the deviations tend to become more comitant with the passage of time.

The Bielschowsky head-tilt test is a three-step maneuver to identify the paretic muscle when a noncomitant vertical deviation is involved. The first step of the test identifies which four of the eight vertically acting extraocular muscles may be paretic. The second step eliminates two of the four possible muscles. These two remaining muscles are either both superior or inferior and always include both a rectus muscle and an oblique muscle. In the third step, the patient's head is tilted, which finally identifies the paretic muscle.

Initially, the examiner must determine which eye is in hyperdeviation with primary gaze. For example, we will consider a case of right hypertropia [1]. The paretic muscle must be a right depressor (right inferior rectus or right superior oblique) or a left elevator (left superior rectus or left inferior oblique). The patient is instructed to turn his eyes to either side. The examiner observes which gaze demonstrates the greatest hyperdeviation. If, for example, a left gaze increases the right hypertropia [2] [3], the offending muscle must either be the right superior oblique or left superior rectus, since the left gaze puts the eyes in the field of action for these muscles. A right head tilt stimulates intorsion of the right eye (right superior rectus or right superior oblique involvement), and extorsion of the left eye (left inferior oblique or left inferior rectus involvement). These pairs of muscles act synergistically in cycloduction but antagonistically in elevation and depression. In this case the right superior oblique is paretic, and so the vertical deviation is increased with right head tilt [4] [5] due to elevation of the right eye by an unopposed right superior rectus.

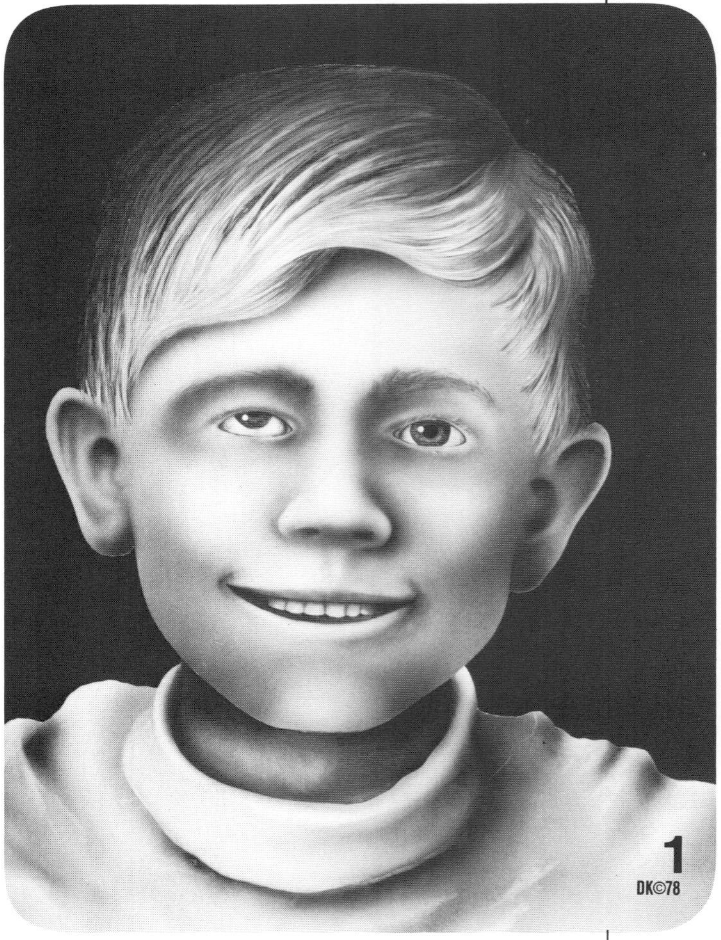

1

In differentiating between the two superior muscles, the hyperdeviation is increased with a head tilt toward the paretic eye. Similarly, when two inferior muscles are involved, hyperdeviation is increased away from the paretic eye.

Donald A. Keller

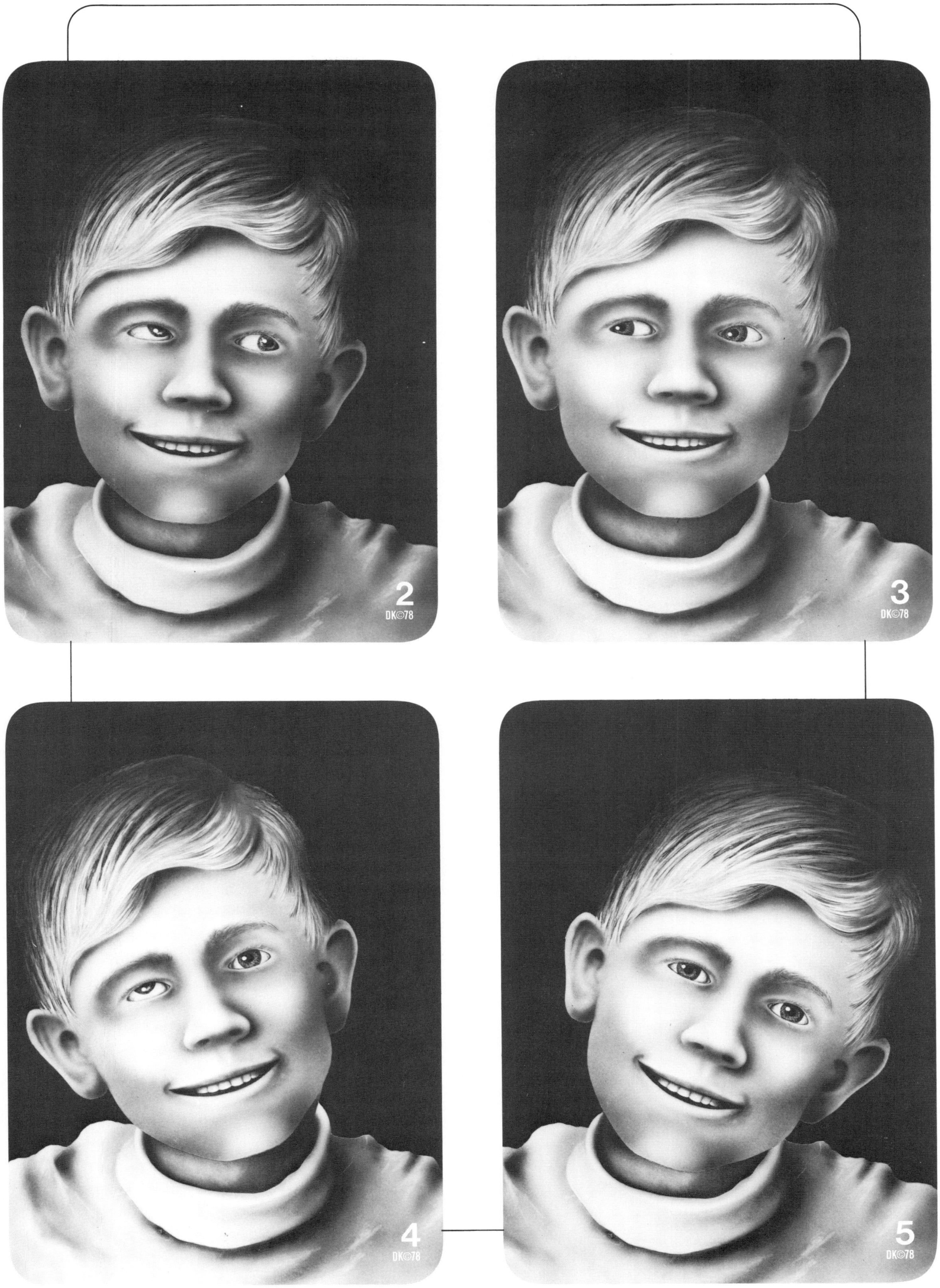

Donald J. Keller

SUPERIOR OBLIQUE TENOTOMY

Gary L. Rogers, M.D.

Malfunctions of the superior oblique muscle often produce cyclovertical symptoms, such as diplopia. In severe cases this may result in abnormal head position.

Brown's syndrome is an inability to elevate the adducted eye past the mid-horizontal plane. It is an excellent example of some of the mysteries surrounding the superior oblique tendon. In spite of a positive forced-duction test, indicating restriction of muscle, no anatomic abnormalities of the sheath, tendon, or muscle have yet been identified. However, in many instances, weakening the tendon does help to relieve the accompanying compensatory head posture. Surgery is indicated when an abnormal head posture is present, either in primary gaze or reading position.

A second indication for weakening of the superior oblique muscle is in A pattern exotropia with accompanying overaction. The procedure should be done only when the following conditions are present: moderate to marked overaction, an A pattern which measures 40 to 50 prism diopters (upgaze versus downgaze), and no overaction of either inferior oblique muscle.

The two most commonly used procedures for weakening the superior oblique muscle are tenectomy and tenotomy. We recommend use of the simpler tenotomy procedure since both yield similar results. Controversy continues over the necessity to expose the tendon in the sheath when a tenotomy is performed. In our experience, the results of weakening the tendon alone or the tendon and sheath together are identical.

Because of the intimate association between the superior oblique tendon, superior rectus muscle, and the levator palpebrae superioris with its fascial attachments, these structures are susceptible to damage when the superior oblique tendon is isolated. We will describe a method that enhances the exposure, thereby minimizing inadvertent damage.

Initially, the surgeon grasps the globe with a Lester forceps at the limbus in the superior nasal quadrant and rotates it inferiorly and temporally. A superior and nasal incision is made in the conjunctiva, approximately 8 mm posterior to the limbus. The incision begins near the nasal border of the superior rectus muscle and is extended for 1½ clock hours nasally [1]. The Tenon's capsule is grasped and incised to expose the underlying sclera. A Stevens tenotomy hook is passed through this opening beneath the superior rectus muscle. A larger Green muscle hook replaces the Stevens hook to provide a more secure hold on the superior rectus tendon. The Tenon's capsule opening is enlarged with the Stevens hook to accommodate the No. 0 Desmarres retractor [2].

The check ligaments are divided between the superior surface of the superior rectus muscle and the Tenon's capsule anteriorly [3]. This exposes the glistening white superior oblique tendon, 2 mm in thickness. The

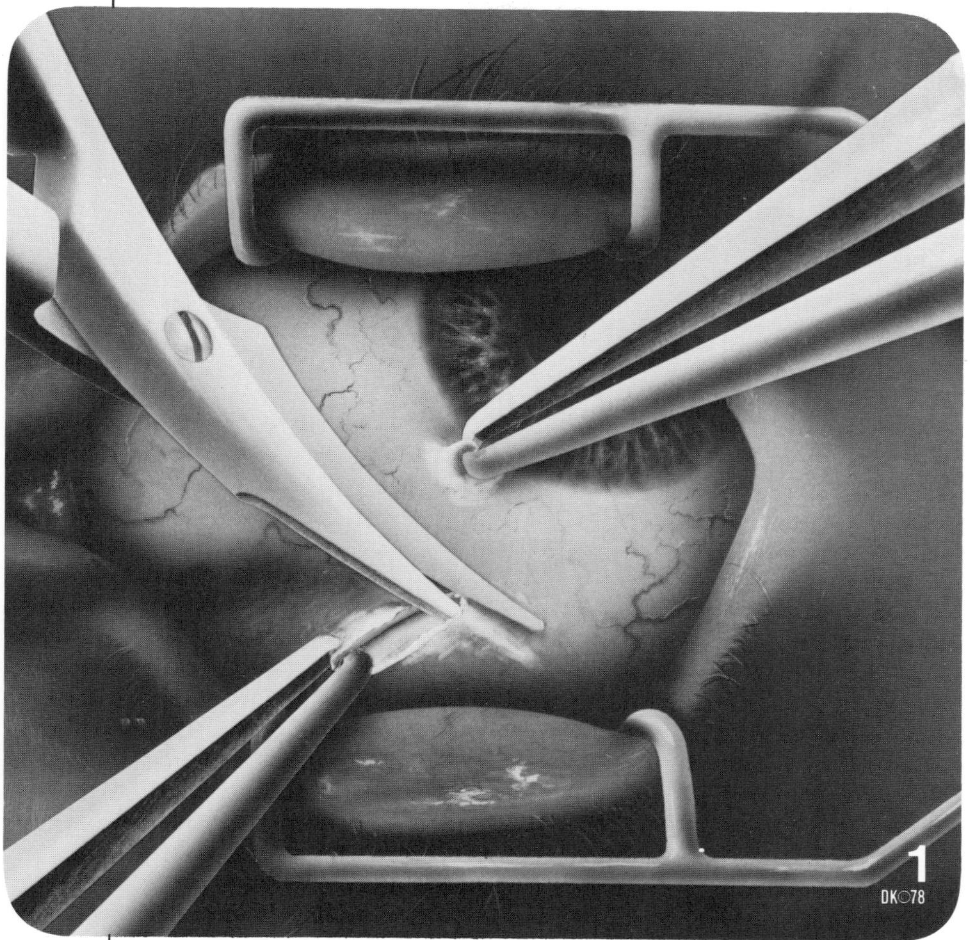

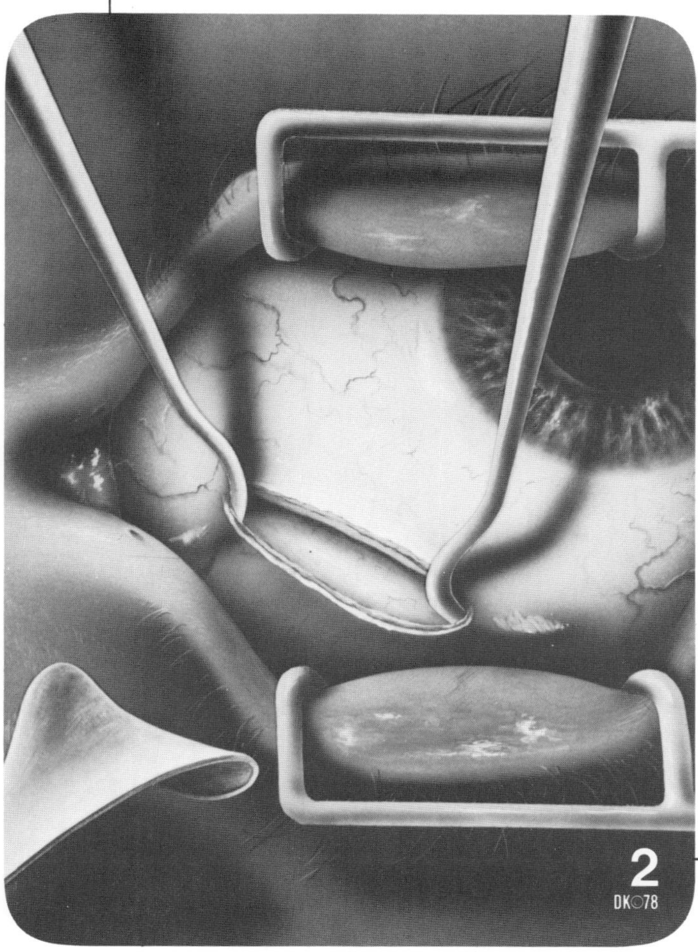

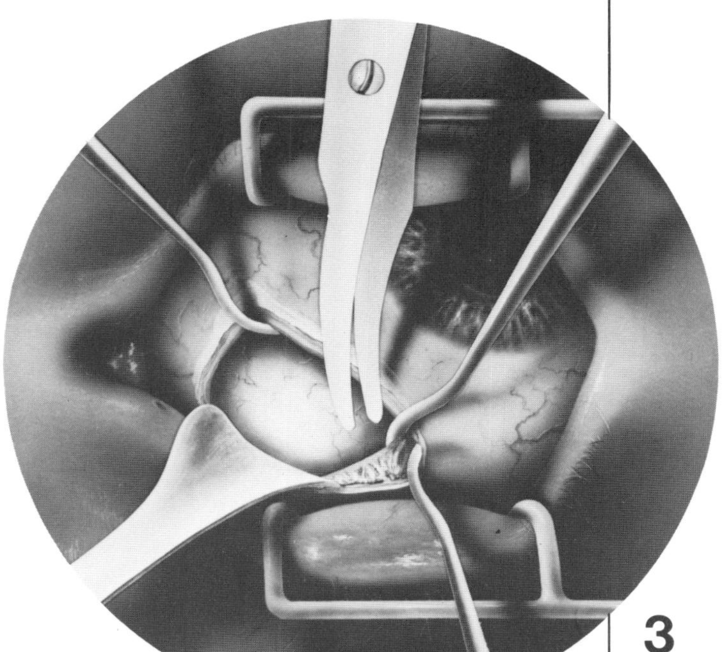

Donald A. Keller

tendon is engaged with a Stevens tenotomy hook and drawn from the incision [4] . A buttonhole is made through Tenon's capsule at the margin of the muscle for passage of the muscle hook [5] . Spreading the tips of the scissors through this opening in the intermuscular septum facilitates the passage of two Green hooks beneath the muscle from

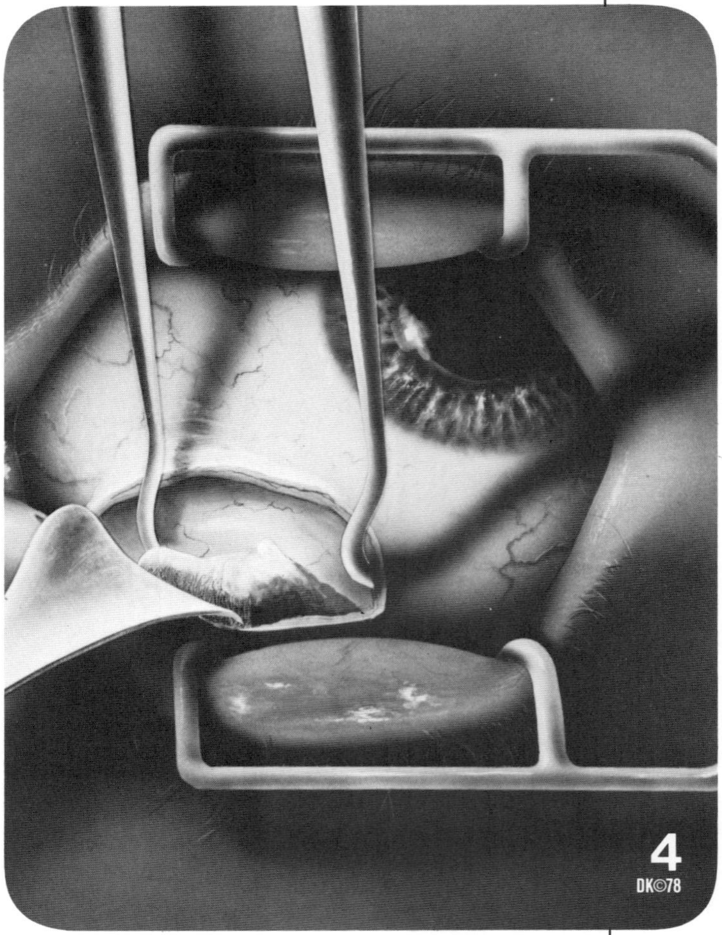

opposite directions [6] . The interface of the orbital septum runs along the course of the superior oblique tendon. If Tenon's capsule is incised in this area, it may result in the protrusion of orbital fat into the operative field. Spreading the hooks gently will expose a length of the superior oblique tendon in its sheath [7] . Once the tendon and sheath are isolated, they are transected [8] .

Donald J. Keller

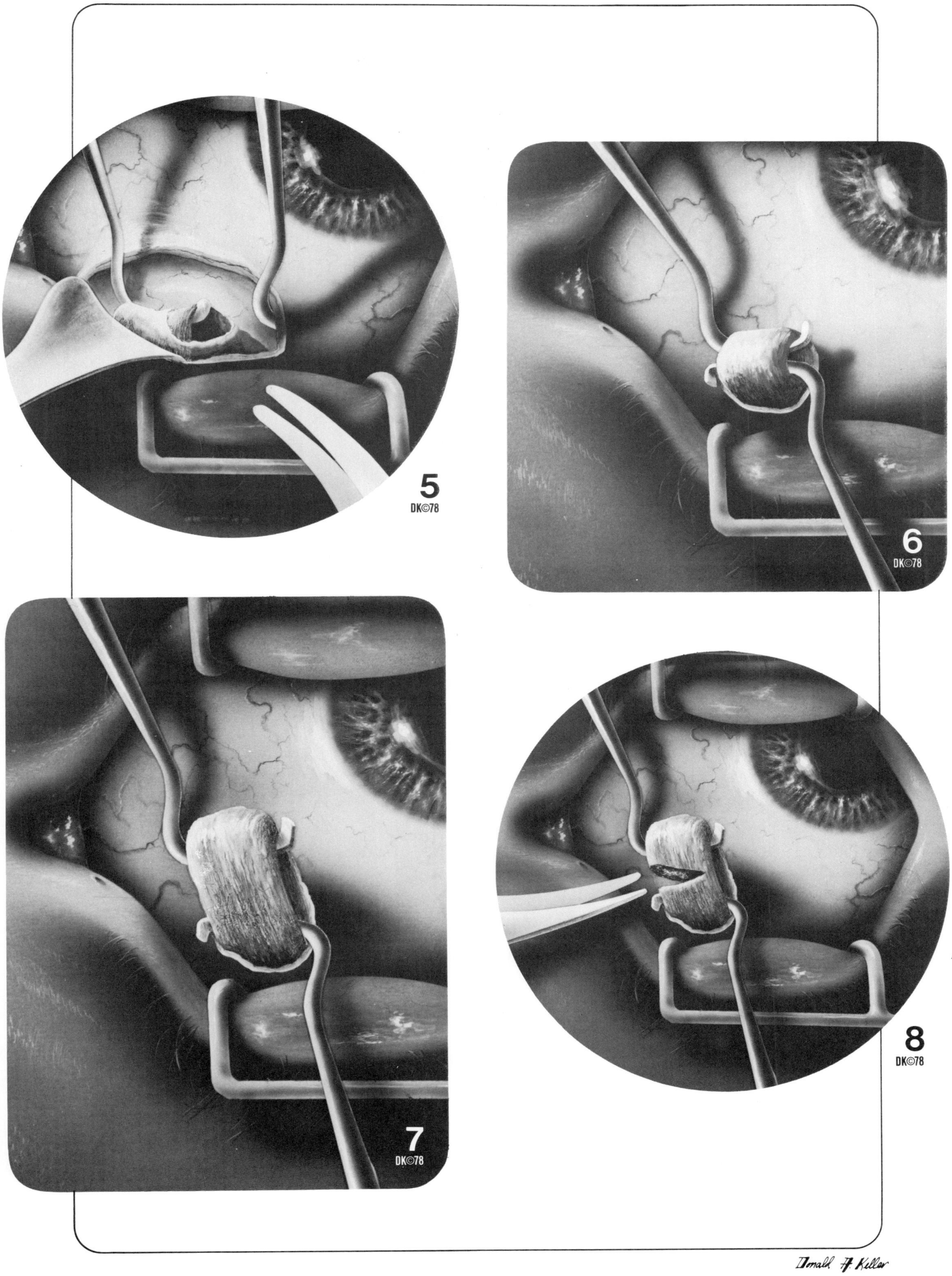

Donald A. Keller

INFERIOR OBLIQUE RECESSION

Gary L. Rogers, M.D.
James A. Savage, M.D.

We believe the surgical procedure that yields the most consistent results when weakening the inferior oblique muscle is the recession. Overactions of the inferior oblique muscle may be divided into primary and secondary types.

In primary overactions, a vertical deviation occurs in adduction but not in primary gaze. It occurs in patients who are orthophoric, esotropic, or exotropic, and most commonly appears in patients between 2 and 4 years of age. It is often associated with a V pattern, and occasionally it is found with bilateral dissociated vertical deviation. Primary overactions may be unilateral or bilateral and exhibit varying degrees of symmetry.

Secondary inferior oblique muscle overaction occurs after ipsilateral superior oblique muscle palsy or contralateral superior rectus muscle palsy. A vertical deviation exists in both adduction and primary position. The patient adopts a head tilt to avoid diplopia, and a positive Bielschowsky test is present. Surgical weakening of the overacting inferior oblique muscle is indicated to improve cosmesis and to eliminate diplopia.

After the forced-duction test, a cul-de-sac incision is made in the inferotemporal quadrant. The surgeon grasps the margin of the incision with Bishop-Harmon forceps, passes a small muscle hook (Stevens or von Graefe) beneath the lateral rectus tendon [1], and replaces this with a larger hook (Green or Jameson). A 4-0 silk suture is passed beneath the lateral rectus tendon [2]; its needle penetrates Tenon's capsule and conjunctiva at the superior border of the muscle. With a hemostat, this "bridle" suture is fastened to the drape over the patient's contralateral brow. This adducts and elevates the globe, exposing the inferotemporal quadrant.

The assistant places a Stevens tenotomy hook in the lateral aspect of the incision beneath the belly of the lateral rectus muscle. A Green hook is inserted inferiorly and retracted [3]. Another Green hook is placed

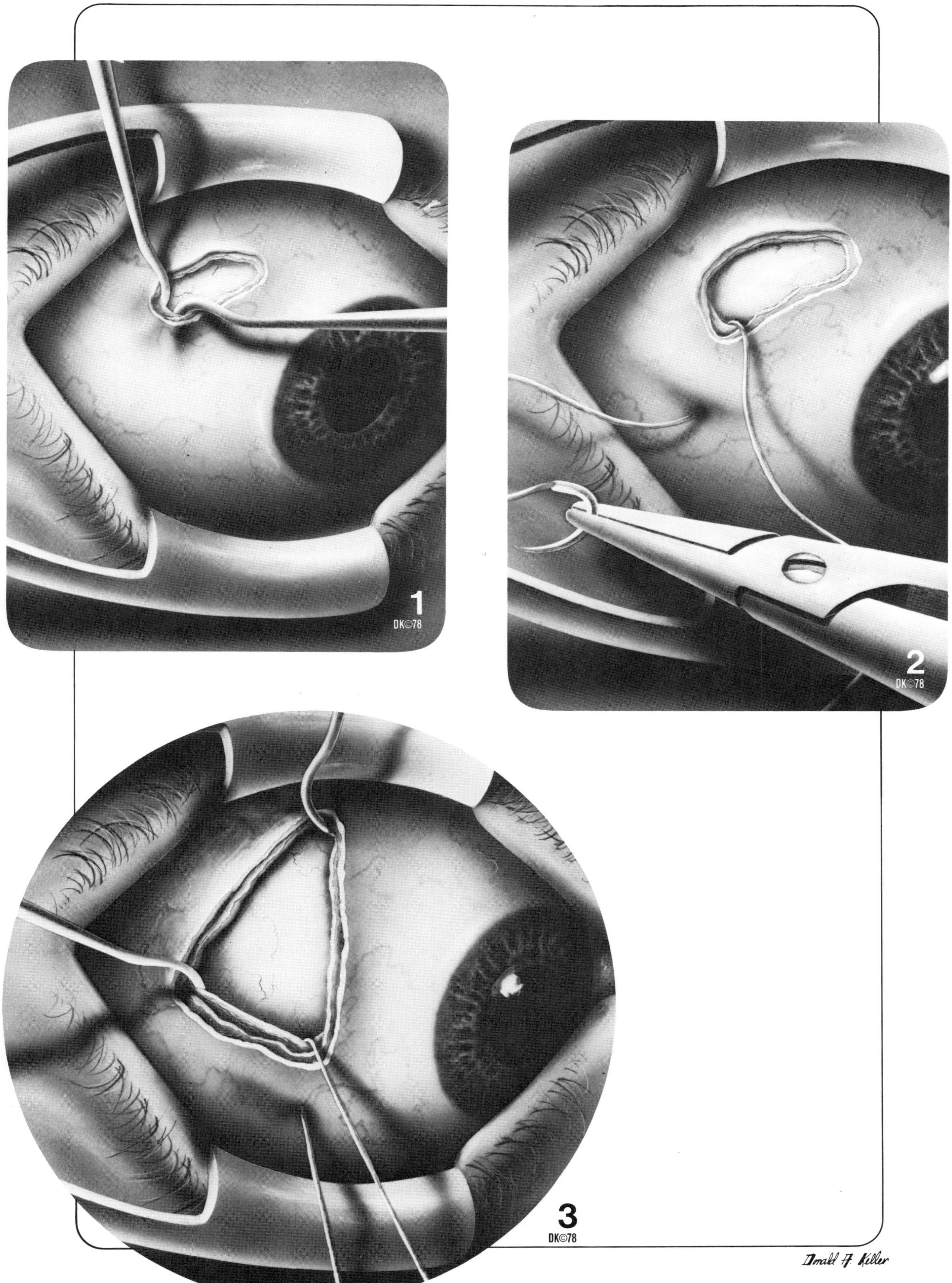
1
DK©78
2
DK©78
3
DK©78

between these two hooks and is retracted inferiorly and laterally [4]. This exposes the inferior oblique muscle in the wall of the surgical wound. Behind the hook held by the surgeon, the muscle will appear as a red band embedded in the white Tenon's capsule. Exposing the muscle in this manner provides direct visualization to avoid damage to surrounding structures such as the inferior and lateral rectus muscles.

A Stevens hook is passed posteriorly and rotated to engage the inferior oblique muscle past its posterior border. It is drawn from the incision [5], and a buttonhole is made in Tenon's capsule with Westcott scissors at the muscle's posterior border [6]. Since the orbital septum is intimately associated with Tenon's capsule in this area, its disruption will cause prolapse of orbital fat into the operative site, which may lead to excessive postoperative scarring. The scissors tips are spread in this incision to expose underlying bare sclera. The scissors beneath the muscle serves as a guide to pass a Green hook from the opposite direction [7]. The Stevens hook is removed. The assistant inserts the inferior retracting hook into this new opening and retracts it laterally while the surgeon retracts the inferior oblique muscle nasally. This maneuver tents the remaining Tenon's capsule, which is cut with Westcott scissors [8]. The inferior oblique insertion is exposed.

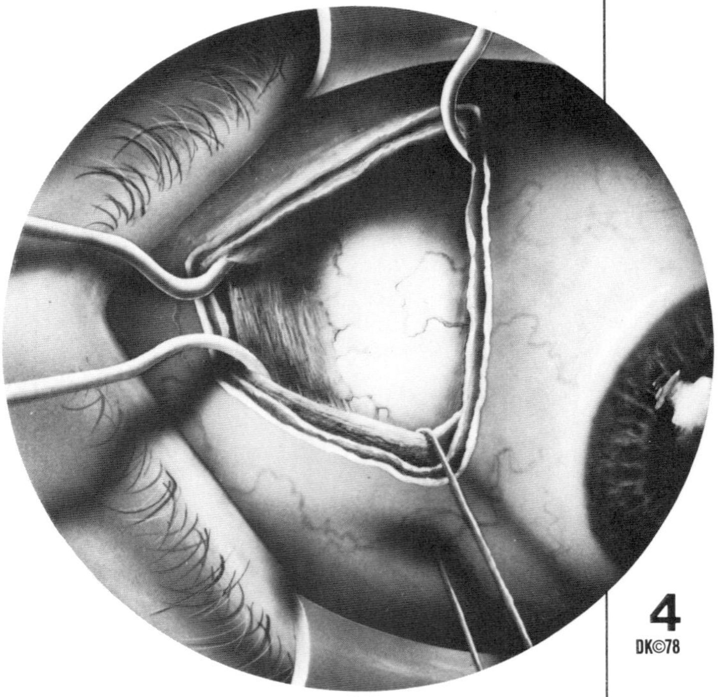

4
DK©78

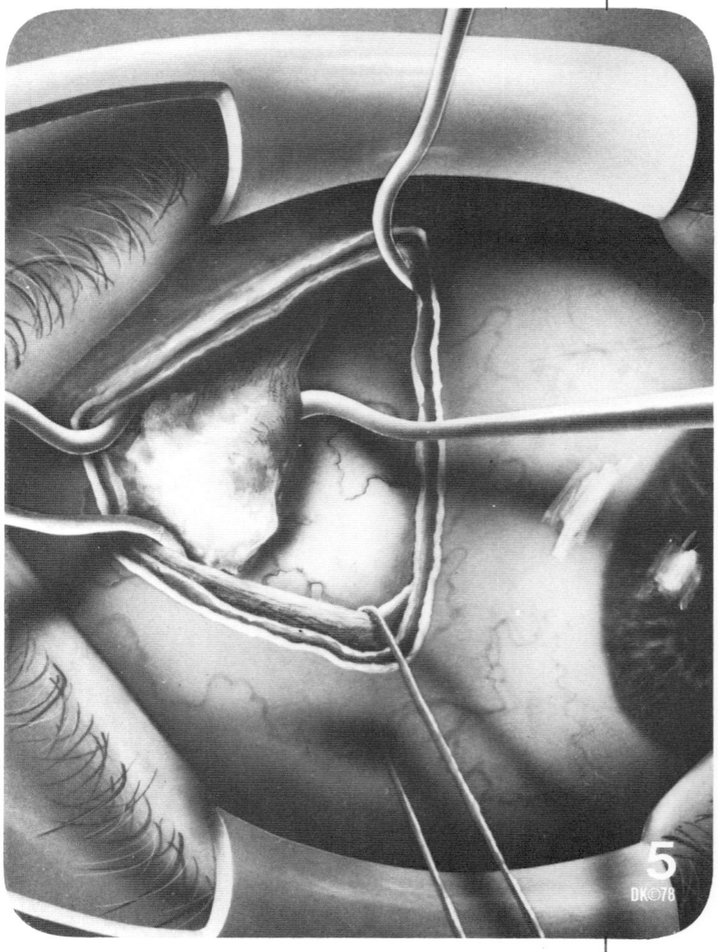

5
DK©78

Donald F. Keller

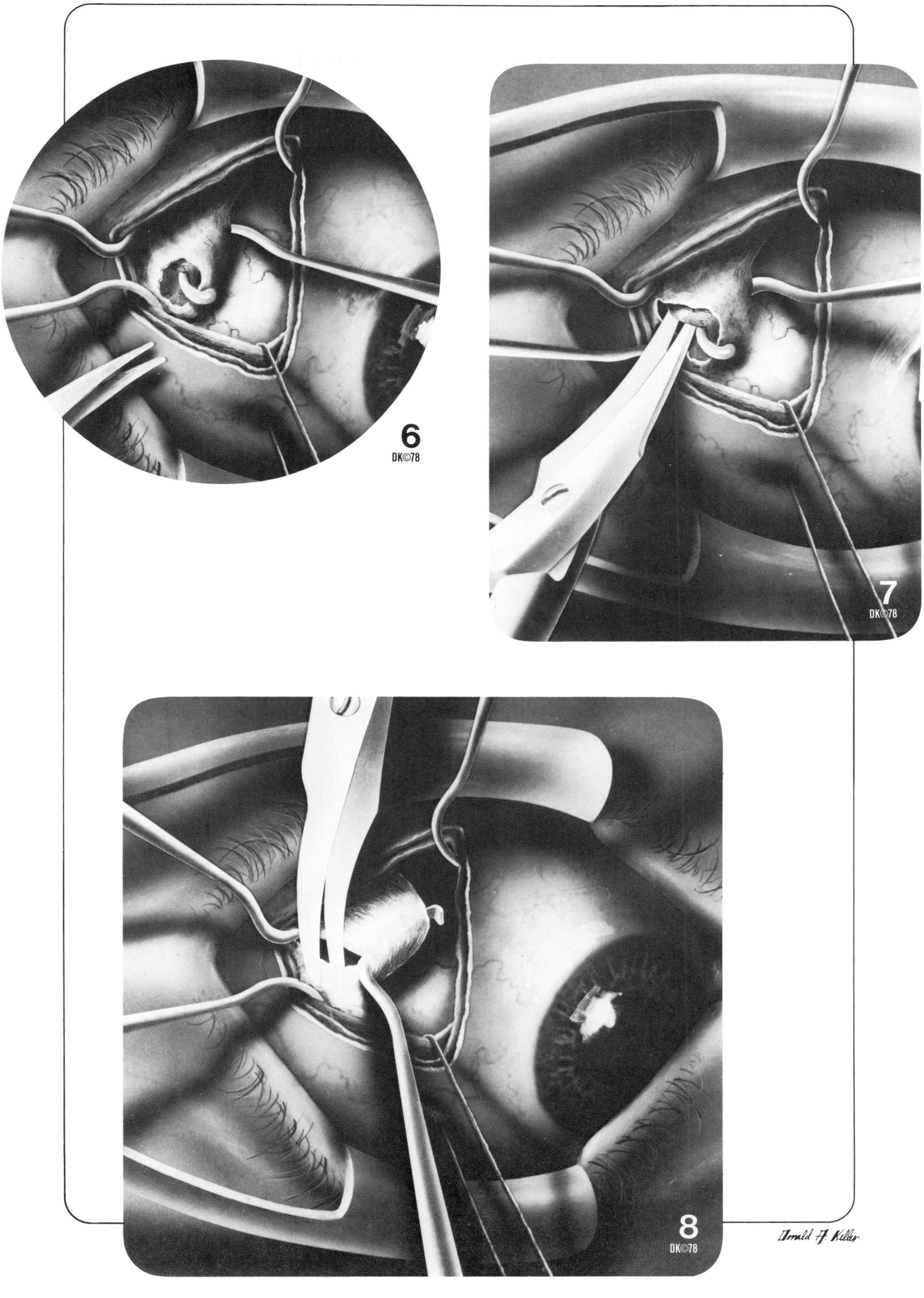
6
DK©78
7
DK©78
8
DK©78

The muscle is disinserted with Westcott scissors [9] , and the bridle suture is removed. While the assistant holds the two ends of the severed tendon with Bishop-Harmon forceps, the surgeon applies a Jameson clamp across the muscle, leaving a small stump for suture placement [10] .

A double-armed 6-0 Dexon suture is applied across the muscle stump, distal to the Jameson clamp, and locked at either end [11] . The clamp is removed. Exposure for application of the sutures is achieved with two large Green muscle hooks. One retracts the inferior rectus muscle superiorly while the other retracts it nasally.

We recommend attaching the anterior margin of the oblique muscle 3 mm posterior and 2 mm lateral to the lateral margin of the inferior rectus insertion (Scheie-Parks point) [12] . This achieves a 10-mm recession. The posterior arm of the suture is placed 5 to 6 mm lateral and 1 mm posterior to this point. Both arms of the suture are pulled and tied to complete the recession.

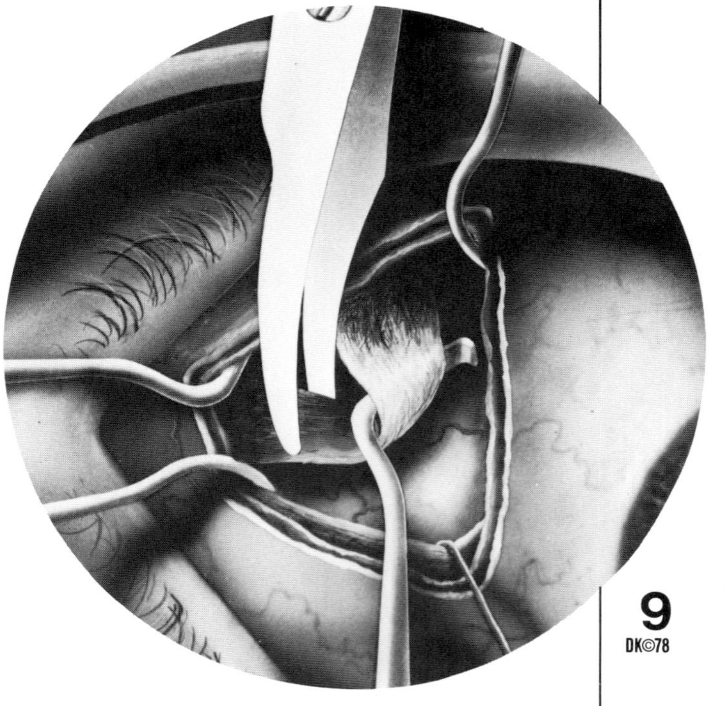

9

DK©78

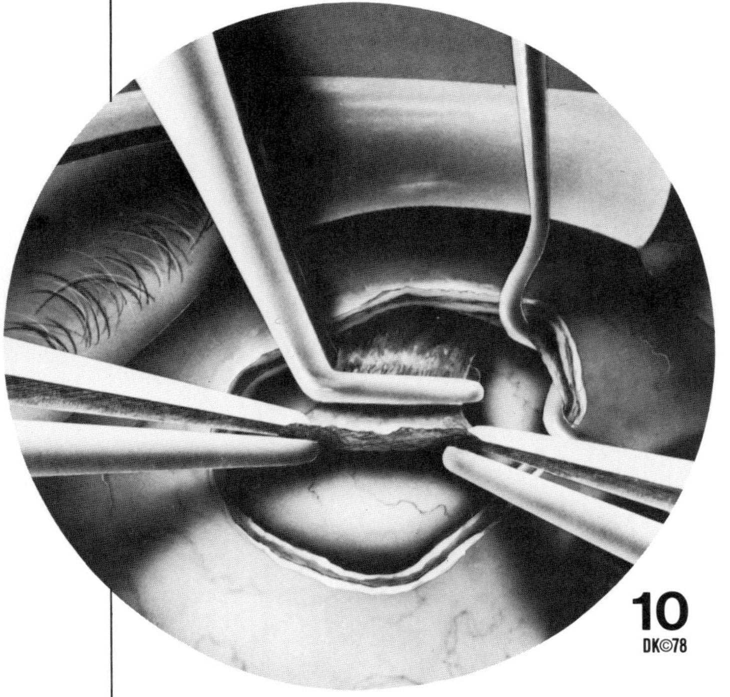

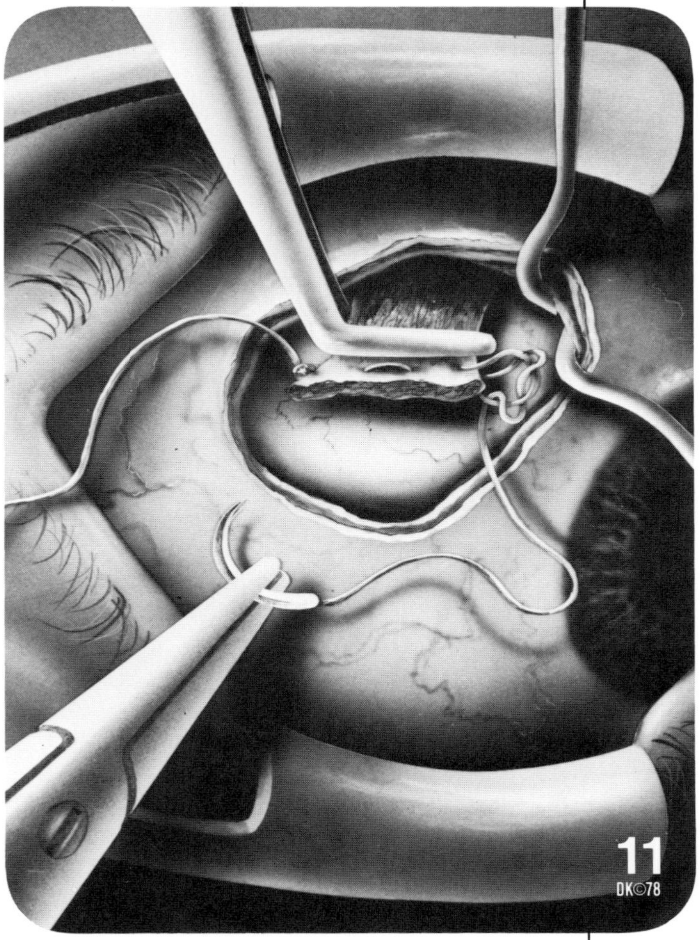

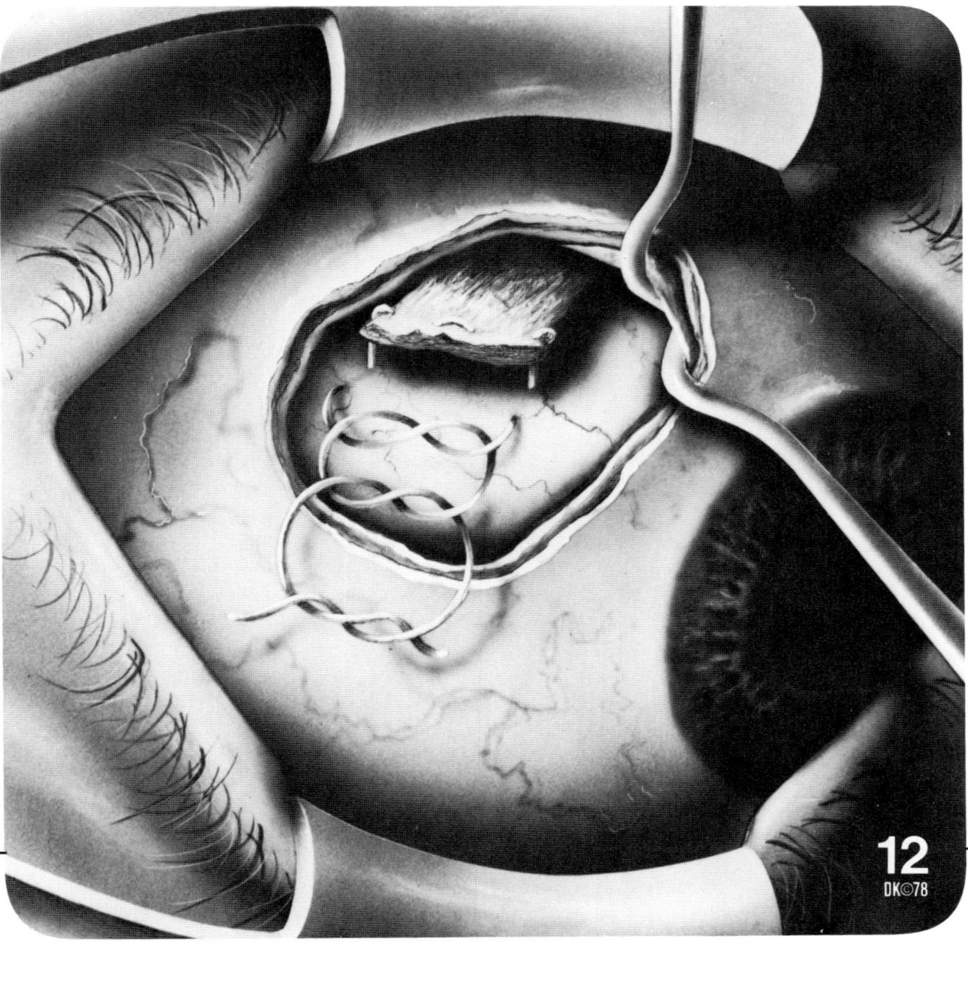

Donald A. Killer

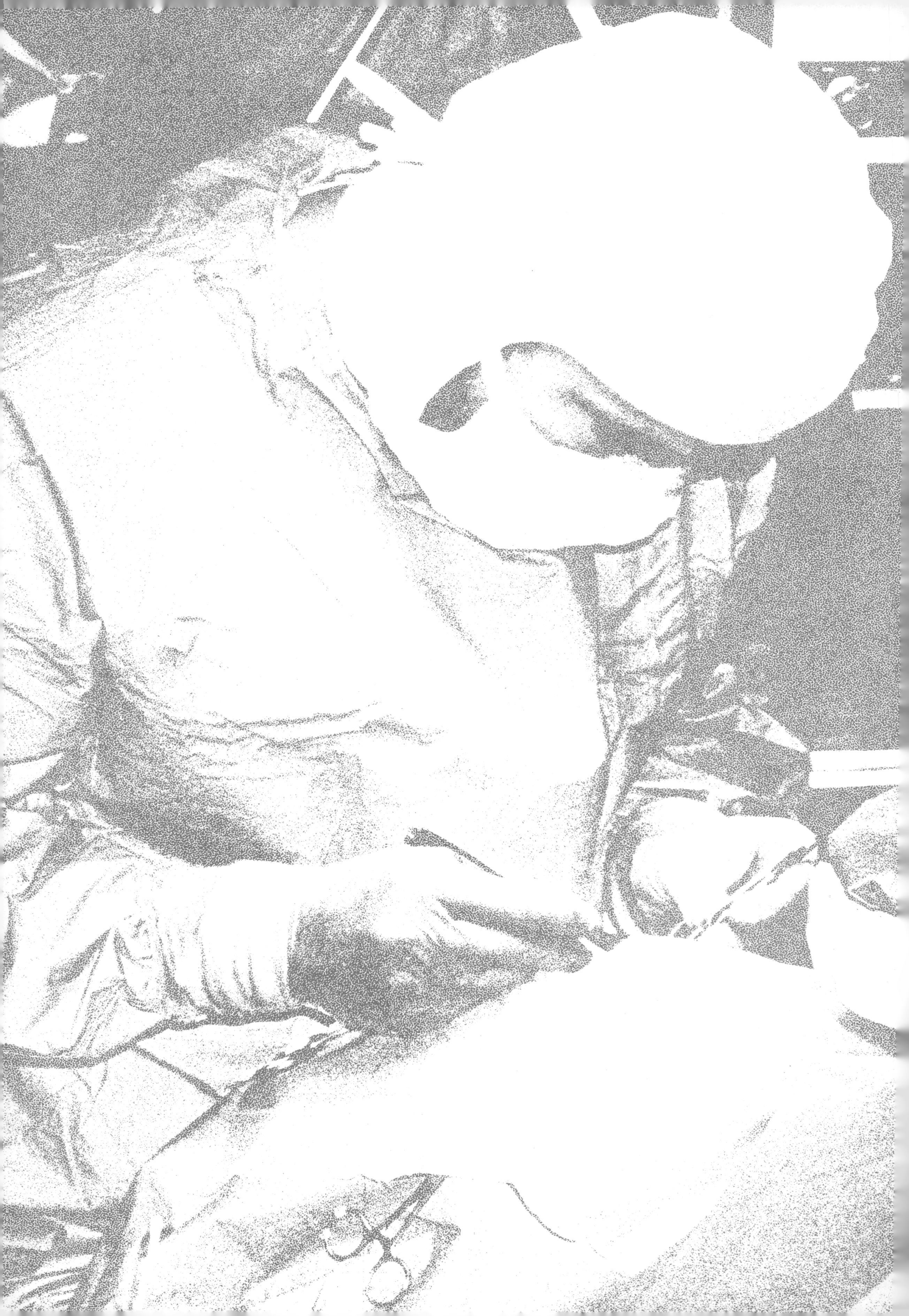

7
EYELID
SURGERY

ANATOMY OF THE EYELIDS

Robert B. O'Dair, M.D.

An understanding of the relationship between structure and function of the eyelids is the starting point in contemplation of repair or reconstruction of an eyelid defect. Any repair must take into account the two basic functions of the lids: proper closure to the eye under all circumstances and proper elevation to permit vision.

To protect the eye, the lids must have reflex closure in the form of the blink and forced closure when dangerous external stimuli demand sustained protection of the eye. The lids also must be capable of the more passive closure in sleep when orbicularis muscle tone exceeds levator muscle tone. The deep surface of the lid must be smooth and moist to protect the delicate cornea.

Adequate elevation of the lid permits vision, of basic concern to the ophthalmologist. In addition, symmetry of the lids is an important consideration.

The discussion of anatomy presented here is necessarily brief. No textbook is a substitute for cadaver dissection under expert supervision.

The eyelids are a unique combination of skin, muscle, hair follicles, fibrous connective tissue, nerves, blood vessels, glandular structures, and mucous membrane surfaces.

The skin [1] within the confines of the orbital rims is very thin and elastic and loosely attached to the underlying orbicularis muscle. The normal redundancy of lid skin increases with age and permits primary closure of fairly large defects. The upper lid is also a plentiful supplier of skin for free grafting, particularly for the opposing upper lid. Since the upper lid skin is thinner than the lower, it does not provide much structural support. Therefore, the thicker retroauricular skin is preferred to repair lower lid defects of larger size. Transverse creases are present in both lids. The most prominent one, usually 4 to 8 mm above the upper lid margin, represents the cutaneous insertion of the levator aponeurosis. Absence of this crease, except in Oriental persons, implies lack of levator function. It is important to note its position in the awake patient, since with the patient under anesthesia, it can be confused with the secondary creases. The site of the upper lid crease in the awake patient becomes the lid fold. Except for the lashes, the lid skin seems hairless, but close inspection reveals many fine hairs. Sebaceous and sweat glands are also present. The lashes arise anterior to the lid margin and project outward from that point. The follicles of the lashes extend backward to the anterior surface of the tarsus.

The circular orbicularis muscle, OM [2], innervated by the seventh cranial nerve, is the sphincter of the eyelids, although it is a skeletal muscle and is under voluntary as well as reflex control. Superiorly, it merges with the frontalis muscle (FM) and inferiorly with the lower facial musculature. Laterally, it is attached to the periosteum of the orbital rim and helps make up the lateral canthal tendon (LCT). Medially, it has attachments to the periosteum of the posterior lacrimal crest, the lacrimal fascia, and the medial canthal tendon (MCT). In incising or repairing a lid, it is helpful to remember the circumferential direction of the fibers, since it is more prudent to divide muscle bundles by spreading, rather than cutting, at right angles to their direction. The orbicularis is usually divided into the orbital portion (OP) and the palpebral portion, PP [2], which is further subdivided into preseptal and pretarsal segments, PS and PT [3]. The preseptal muscles arise from deep heads attached to the posterior lacrimal crest and lacrimal fascia. Their superficial heads are attached to the medial canthal tendon. Laterally, the preseptal muscles fuse at the palpebral raphe. The pretarsal muscles also arise from deep and superficial heads medially. The deep heads are attached to the periosteum of the posterior lacrimal crest, Horner's muscle (HM) or tensor tarsi, and the lacrimal fascia. The superficial heads arise from the medial canthal tendon (MCT). Laterally, the pretarsal orbicularis fibers unite to form the lateral canthal tendon (LCT). Riolan's muscle is a part of the orbicularis located at the lid margin.

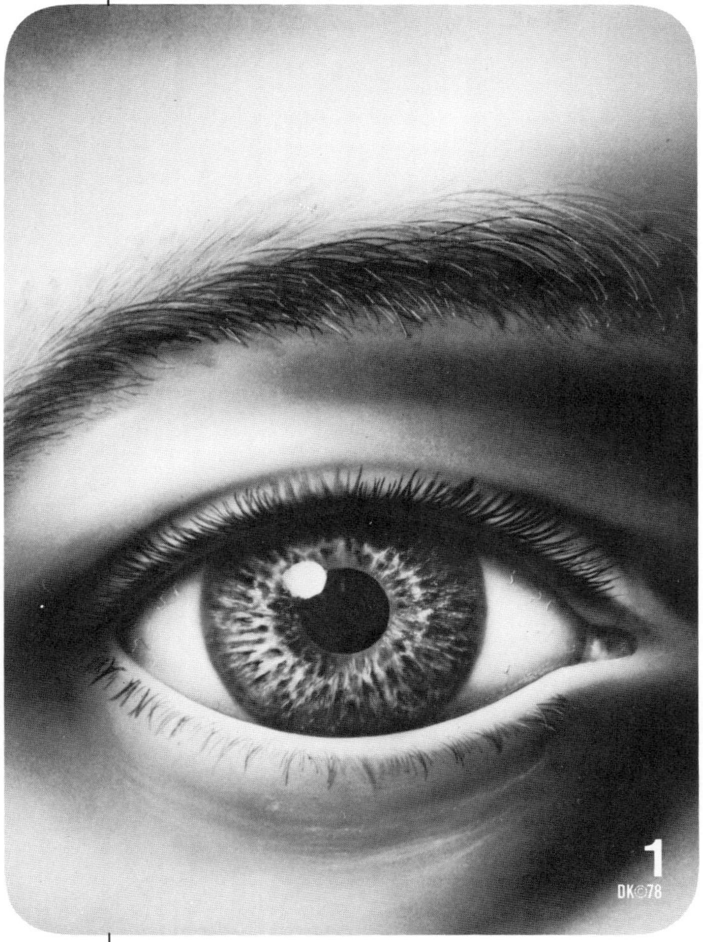

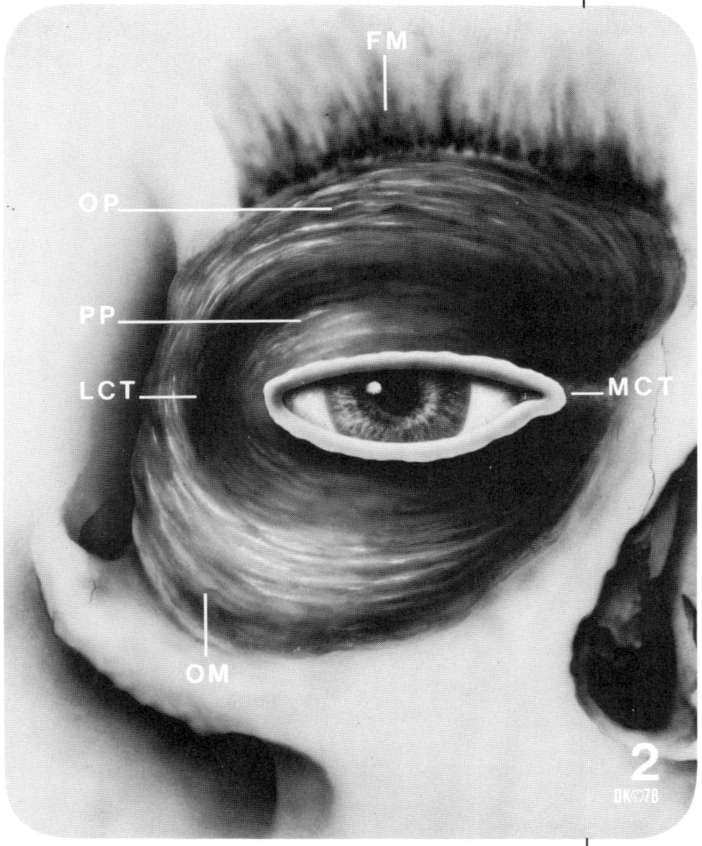

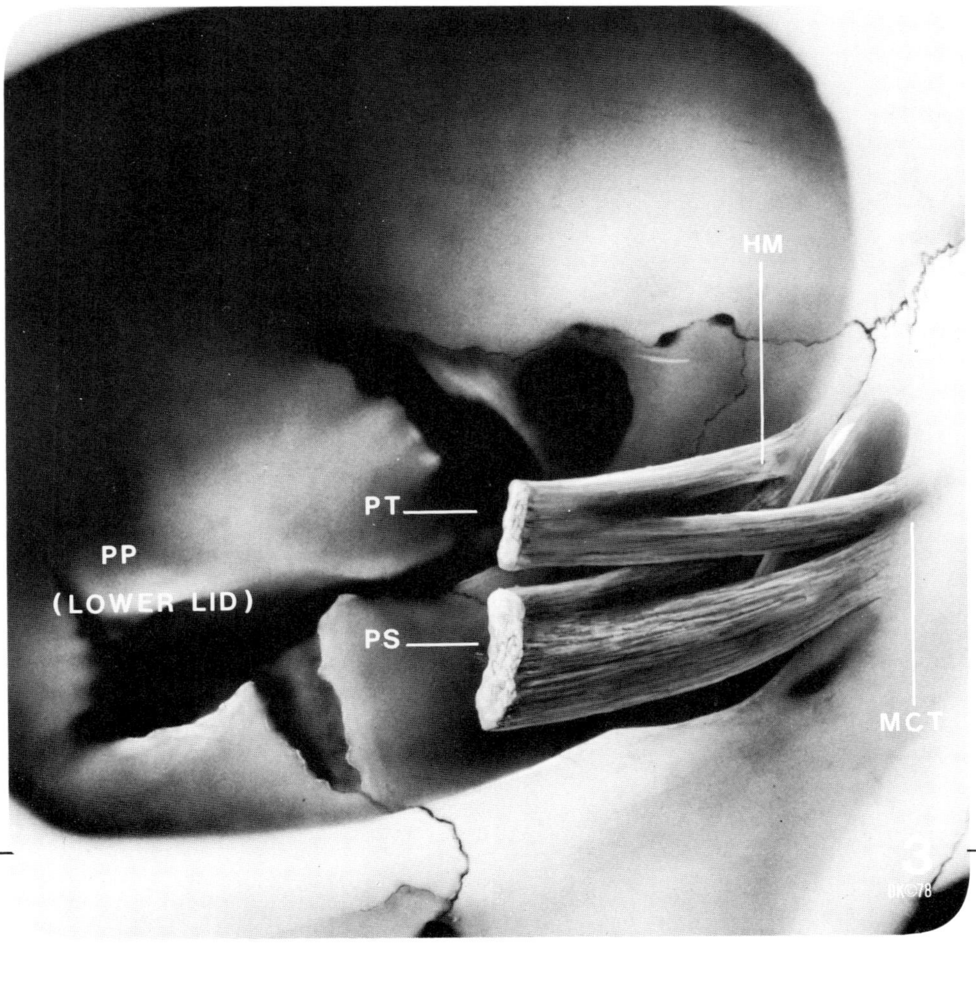

Donald F. Keller

The orbital septum, OS [4], separates the lids from the posterior orbit and tends to limit the spread of hemorrhage and infection. The orbital septum arises from the periosteum of the orbital rim and attaches to the levator aponeurosis. It is rather strong in the upper lid and may appear to be in several layers during dissection. Once the orbital fat is visible, the surgeon may be sure that the septum has been properly divided. In the lower lid, the orbital septum arises from the inferior orbital rim and attaches to the lower tarsal border. It is weaker, particularly nasally, than the upper orbital septum.

The tarsal plates are firm, fibrous structures that provide the framework of the lids. The upper tarsal plate, TP [5], is larger than the lower tarsal plate, TP [6] and, at its greatest convexity, has a vertical dimension of about 10 mm. The lower plate measures about 5 mm vertically. Horizontally, both are 25 to 30 mm long. The Meibomian glands, MG [5] [6], numbering 25 to 30 in the upper lid and 20 to 25 in the lower lid, are contained within the tarsal plate and span the entire vertical length of the plate. Their orifices are visible just in front of the posterior margin of the lid. Laterally and medially, the tarsal plates fuse with the orbicularis muscle to make up the canthal tendons. In the upper lid, the terminal fibers, TF [5], of the levator aponeurosis, LA [5], attach to the upper 4 mm of the anterior surface of the tarsus. The pretarsal space (PTS), between upper tarsus and levator aponeurosis, is a useful surgical landmark. The conjunctiva on the deep tarsal surface is closely adherent to them. In the lower lid, the orbital septum, OS [6], is attached to the inferior tarsal border. In addition, fibrous extensions from the inferior rectus muscle (IRM) and inferior oblique muscle (IOM), comprise the inferior aponeurosis and attach to the lower border of the tarsus. Deep to the inferior aponeurosis is the inferior tarsal muscle (ITM) which also attaches to the lower tarsal border.

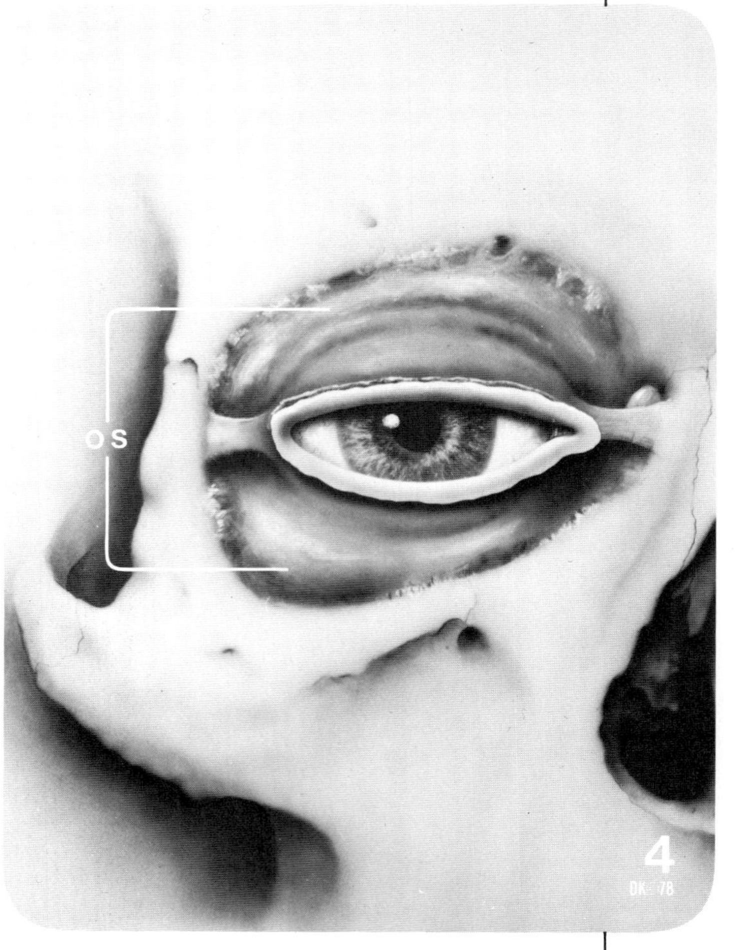

The relationship of the levator palpebrae superioris muscle and its tendon, the aponeurosis, is of vital importance in the surgical treatment of ptosis. The muscle arises posteriorly from the periorbita above the annulus of Zinn. It comes forward in the superior orbit, separated from the periosteum of the roof by orbital fat. Below it and connected to it by fibrous bands lies the superior rectus muscle. The skeletal portion, about 40 mm long, widens as it comes anteriorly and fans out as it becomes the fibrous aponeurosis. The fibrous portion has two terminal insertions, a thinner one anteriorly, which interdigitates with the orbicularis muscle, OM [5], and attaches to the skin, creating the lid fold,

Donald A. Keller

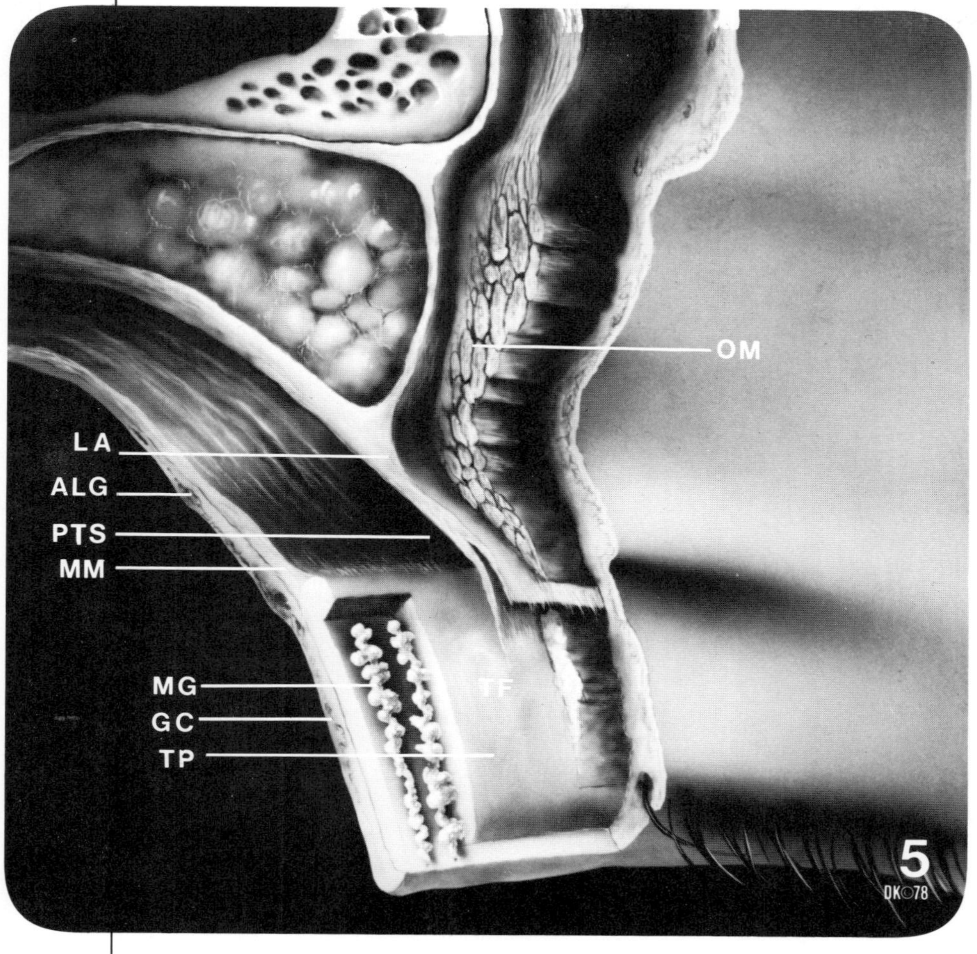

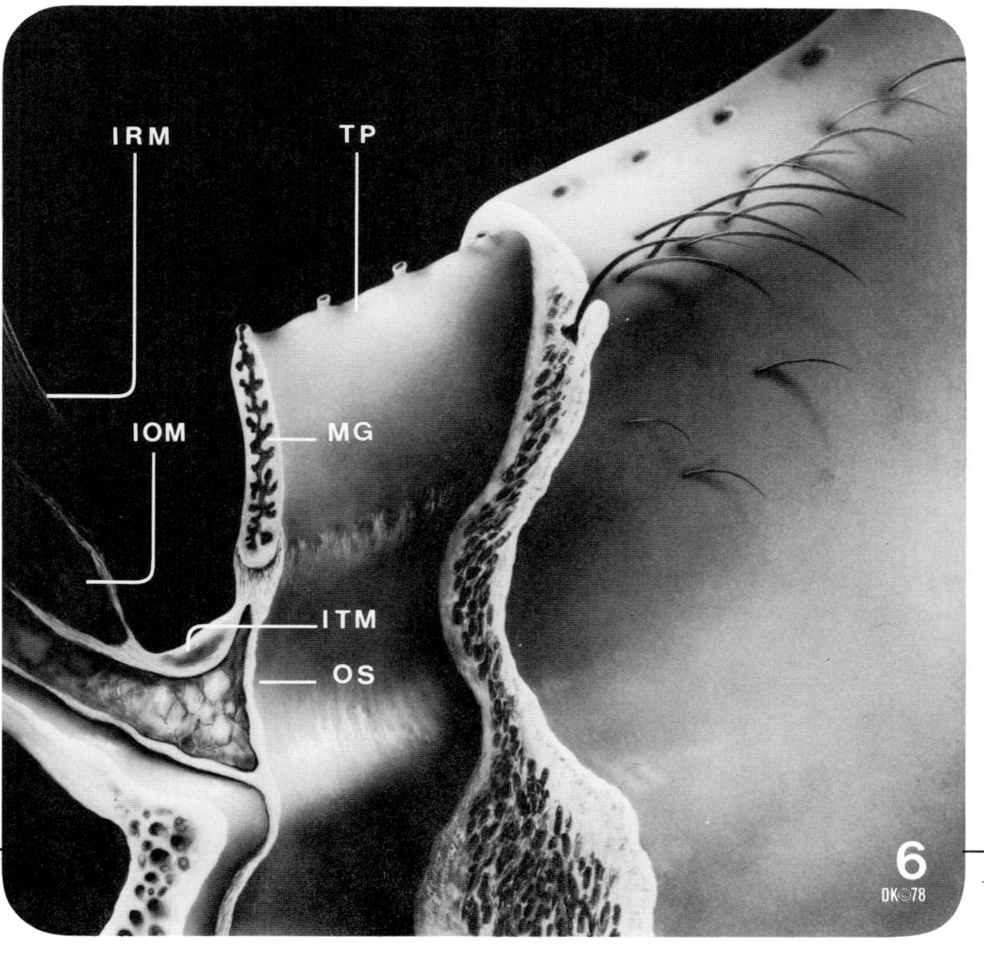

Donald A. Keller

and the thicker posterior attachment, which inserts on the anterior border of the tarsus, about 3 to 4 mm from its upper border. The medial horn passes over and is attached to the superior oblique tendon, SOT [8], which should be considered carefully in division of the tendon during ptosis surgery. The medial horn then attaches to the posterior limb of the medial canthal tendon. The lateral horn divides the lacrimal gland, LG [7], into its orbital and palpebral lobes, and the ducts of the orbital portion pass around the lateral horn as they enter the palpebral portion. The horn continues to attach laterally to the lateral canthal tendon. The orbital septum fuses to the anterior part of the levator aponeurosis, usually 3 to 4 mm above the upper tarsal border. This important landmark is identified by the orbital fat that lies behind the septum and anterior to the aponeurosis. This insertion can be quite variable, as can other aspects of levator anatomy. The superior check ligament of the levator muscle consists of a condensation of fibrous tissue on the superior sheath of the levator muscle at the level of the equator of the globe. It attaches medially to the fascia over the trochlea, T [8], and laterally to the capsule of the lacrimal gland. Superiorly, it inserts on the periosteum of the rim behind the attachment of the orbital septum. The nerve to the levator muscle, which also supplies the superior rectus, is a branch of the superior ramus of the third cranial nerve and enters from below, at the junction of the middle and posterior thirds.

Müller's muscle, MM [5], a nonstriated muscle, is innervated by the sympathetic nervous system and is important in the diagnosis and treatment of ptosis. It arises from the posterior aspect of the levator muscle, descends behind the aponeurosis, and inserts on the upper tarsal border. It is about 12 mm long and 0.5 mm thick. Posteriorly, it is firmly adherent to the conjunctiva. In the lower lid, the inferior tarsal muscle, ITM [6], is less prominent. It arises from the inferior aponeurosis and attaches to the lower tarsal border.

The conjunctiva is the deepest layer of the lids and contains mucin-secreting goblet

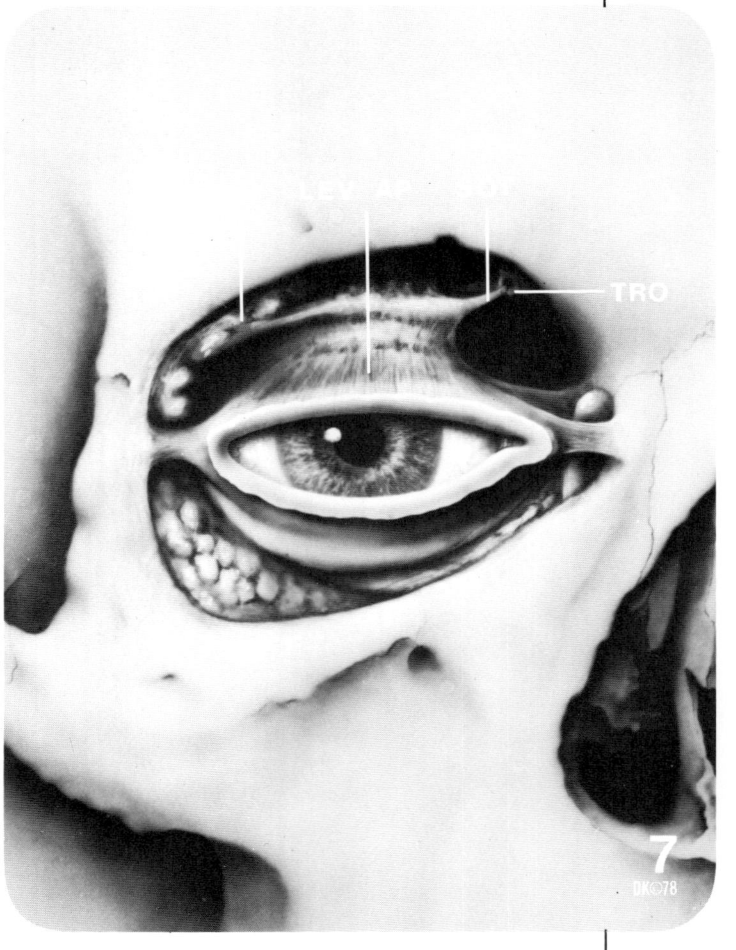

cells, GC [5], and the accessory lacrimal glands, ALG [6], of Krause and Wolfring. Its preservation, when possible, may prevent the unfortunate complication of dry eye. It is closely adherent to the tarsus and loosely attached as it lines the lids and merges in the fornices with the bulbar conjunctiva.

Arterial supply to the lids comes chiefly from the ophthalmic branch of the internal carotid artery, as well as collateral circulation from branches of the external carotid. As these vessels approach the lids, they divide into marginal and peripheral arcades, MA and PA [9]. The peripheral arcade occurs anterior to the tarsus near its upper border, while the marginal arcade is found 1 mm from the lid margin on the anterior surface of the tarsus. The rich blood supply is of great help in promoting healing and resisting infection. The venous drainage of the lids is through tributaries of the ophthalmic vein and superficially through the angular and superficial temporal veins.

Donald A. Keller

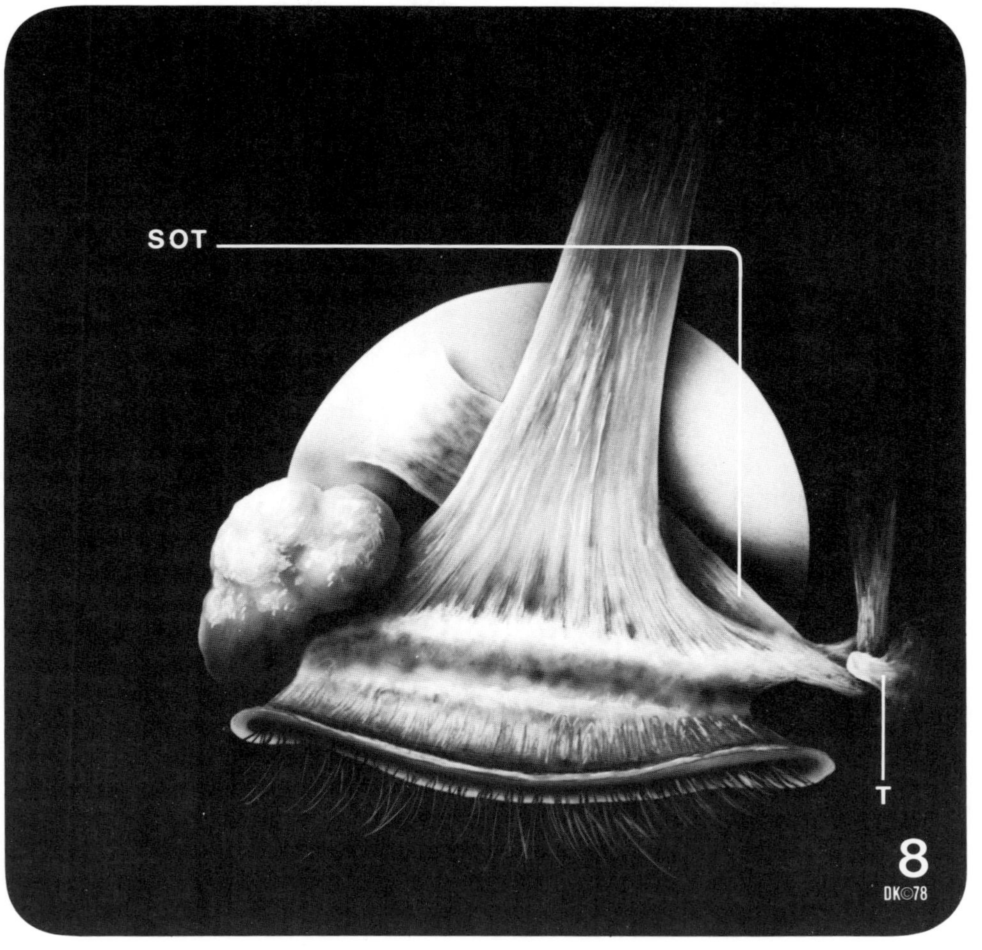

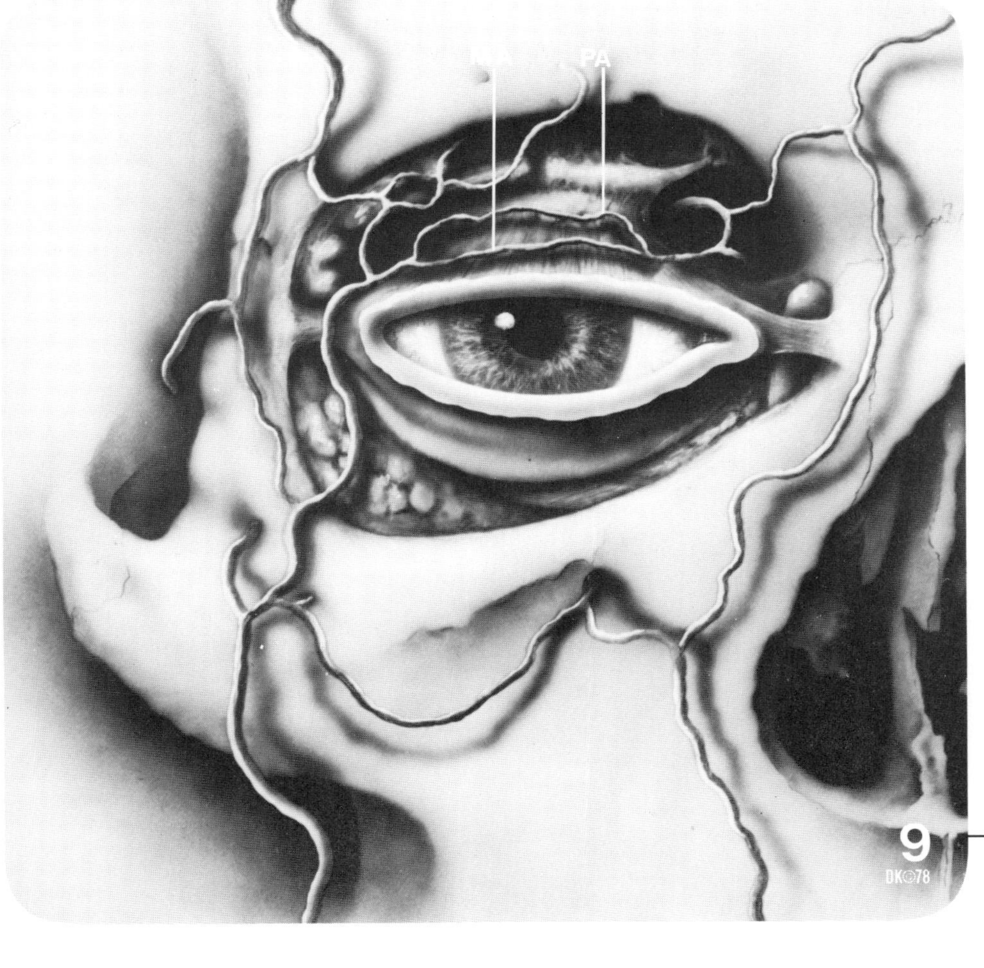

Donald F. Keller

BLEPHAROPTOSIS

John A. Burns, M.D.

When planning ptosis surgery, the three most important factors that the surgeon must consider are the etiology, amount of levator function, and amount of ptosis.

It is important to determine whether the ptosis is congenital or acquired and if the amount of ptosis is stable or intermittent and progressive. Few patients with intermittent or progressive ptosis are surgical candidates. Patients with congenital ptosis have a decreased density of striated muscle fibers in the levator muscle. As the amount of striated muscle decreases, levator function decreases, and the amount of ptosis increases. In congenital ptosis, an associated weakness of the superior rectus muscles may also be present and must be considered in the preoperative evaluation.

Acquired ptosis may be divided into four categories: 1) myogenic, including senile ptosis, chronic progressive external ophthalmoplegia, and myasthenia gravis; 2) neurogenic, including supranuclear ophthalmoplegia, peripheral lesions involving the third nerve, and Horner's syndrome; 3) traumatic, including eyelid lacerations, orbital trauma, foreign bodies, and postsurgical; and 4) mechanical, including neurofibromatosis, hemangioma, and blepharochalasis.

After the etiology has been established, the amount of levator function must be determined. Levator function is the amount of lid excursion from maximum downgaze to maximum upgaze produced by the elevators of the lid without use of the frontalis muscle. Normal levator function is approximately 15 mm. Abnormal function is rated as good (8 mm or more), fair (5 to 7 mm), or poor (4 mm or less).

To evaluate the degree of levator function, the patient looks down as far as possible while the examiner holds a millimeter ruler against the brow across the lid margin [1]. The examiner's thumb must be held firmly against the patient's brow to prevent use of the frontalis muscle. The level of the lid margin is noted. The patient then looks up [2]; the distance the lid moves up the ruler indicates the amount of levator function.

The amount of ptosis must also be measured. To determine the amount of unilateral ptosis, the examiner measures the vertical fissure on the normal side and compares it with the opposite side [3] [4]. The difference between the measurements is the amount of ptosis. About 25 percent of the time, congenital ptosis is bilateral, and the amount of ptosis is measured against an arbitrary determination of normal. In primary gaze, the upper lid normally covers the upper 2.0 mm of cornea. The degree of ptosis can be found if the amount of cornea covered by the upper lid is measured in primary gaze, and 2 mm are subtracted [5] [6]. The amount of ptosis is classified and defined as mild (2 mm or less), moderate (3 mm), or severe (4 mm or more).

Additional criteria must be evaluated before surgery is considered. In patients with unilateral ptosis, the location and configuration of the lid fold in the fellow eye must be measured carefully to insure that the lids will match postoperatively. If a redundancy of upper lid skin is anticipated, a therapeutic blepharoplasty may be done at the same time as the ptosis surgery.

Visual acuity, fusion, and extraocular muscle function must be evaluated because they are frequently abnormal in the ptosis patient.

The presence or absence of a Bell's phenomenon should be noted. Its absence indicates that, postoperatively, the patient will be more susceptible to corneal exposure.

In elderly patients, the Schirmer test and evaluation of the fluorescein-stained tear film are recommended. Because of the increased corneal exposure after ptosis surgery, if either test indicates the existence or possibility of keratitis sicca, surgery is probably contraindicated.

The preoperative examination must include photographs for operative planning and medicolegal reasons. They should be taken with the patient looking in primary gaze and in maximum up- and downgazes.

The Tensilon test (edrophonium chloride) is done if myasthenia gravis is suspected. The Neo-Synephrine test (phenylephrine hydrochloride) can be administered to determine the functional level of Müller's muscle.

After all necessary evaluations have been made, the surgeon is prepared to select the appropriate procedure.

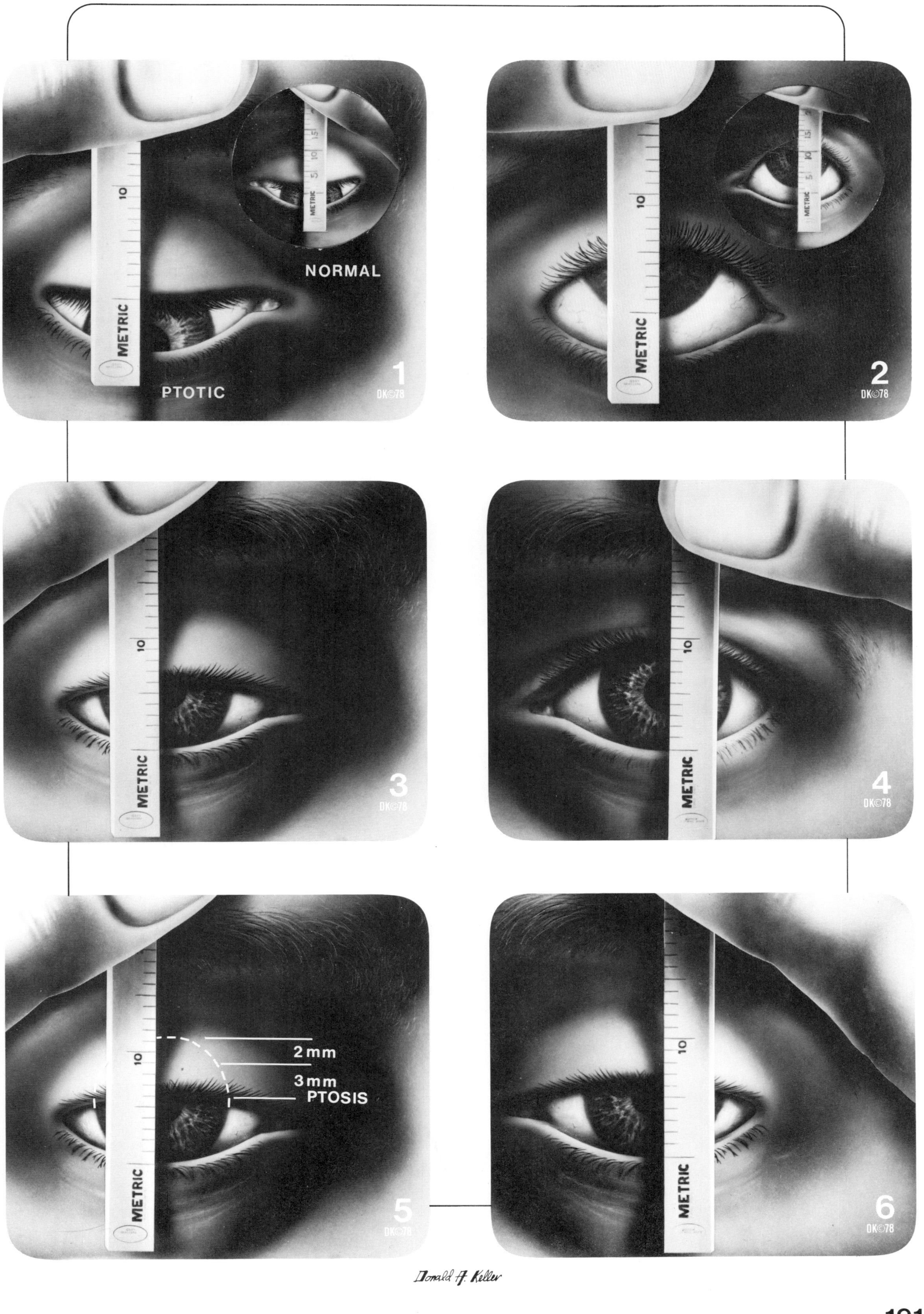

Donald A. Keller

FASANELLA-SERVAT TRANSCONJUNCTIVAL TARSAL RESECTION

John A. Burns, M.D.

The Fasanella-Servat tarsal resection is technically the simplest ptosis procedure and is indicated to correct mild degrees (1.5 mm or less) of both congenital and acquired ptosis with good levator function. The lid lift is achieved by resecting the tarsal plate and Müller's muscle. Before this procedure is chosen, a Neo-Synephrine test should be done to help the surgeon decide whether this procedure is appropriate. Two drops of 10 percent Neo-Synephrine are placed in the affected eye. Within two to five minutes, the abnormal lid should elevate to approximate the height of the normal lid. If this does not happen, the procedure will probably result in undercorrection.

In the adult patient, the operation may be performed under local anesthesia, by infiltration of the upper lid, or regional block of the superior orbital nerve.

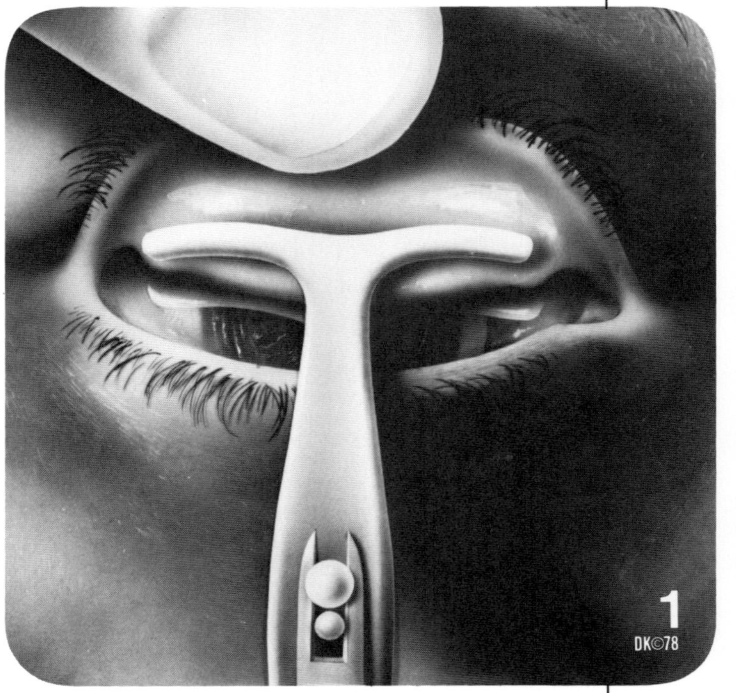

1

Initially, a corneal protector is positioned in this and all other ptosis procedures. The lid is everted to expose the patient's tarsal plate [1]. We recommend the use of a Putterman ptosis clamp which is centered on the tarsal plate 4 mm above the lid margin. Included in the clamp are the upper two thirds of the tarsal plate, the lower part of Müller's muscle, and both conjunctival surfaces [2]. Alternatively, two curved hemostats may be used to clamp the lids. If they are placed too centrally, however, a cosmetically unacceptable dome-shaped defect in the lid arch may occur. Because of its design, the Putterman ptosis clamp obviates this problem.

After the clamp is positioned, a 6-0 plain catgut suture is passed through the skin surface in the lid fold on the temporal side of the lid and exits 1 mm superior to the lateral edge of the clamp on the tarsoconjunctival surface [3]. The suture will hold the lid together when the tarsus, conjunctiva, and Müller's muscle have been excised; therefore, it must

Donald F. Keller

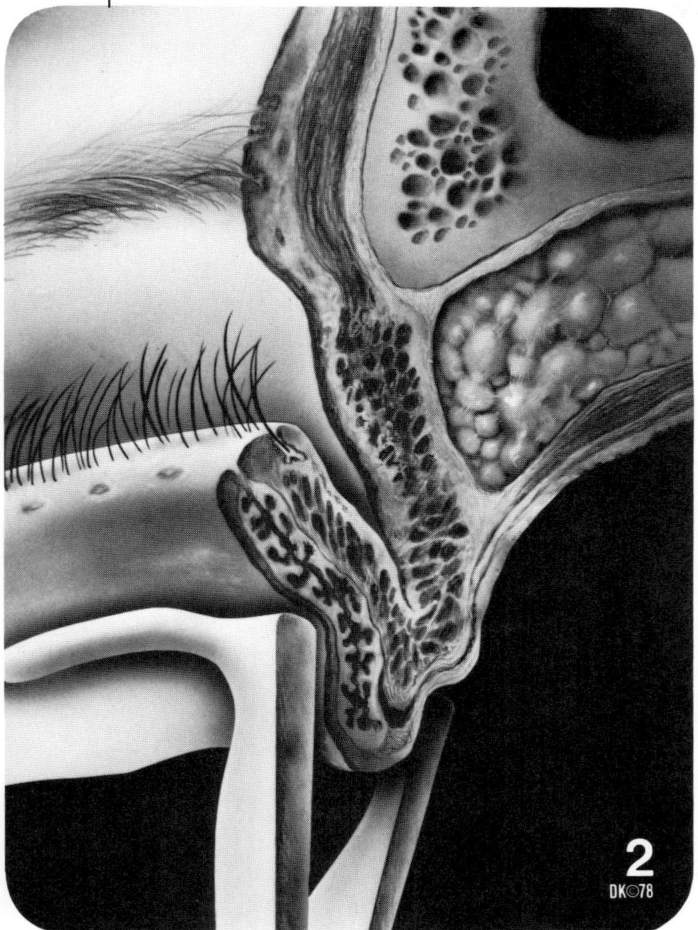

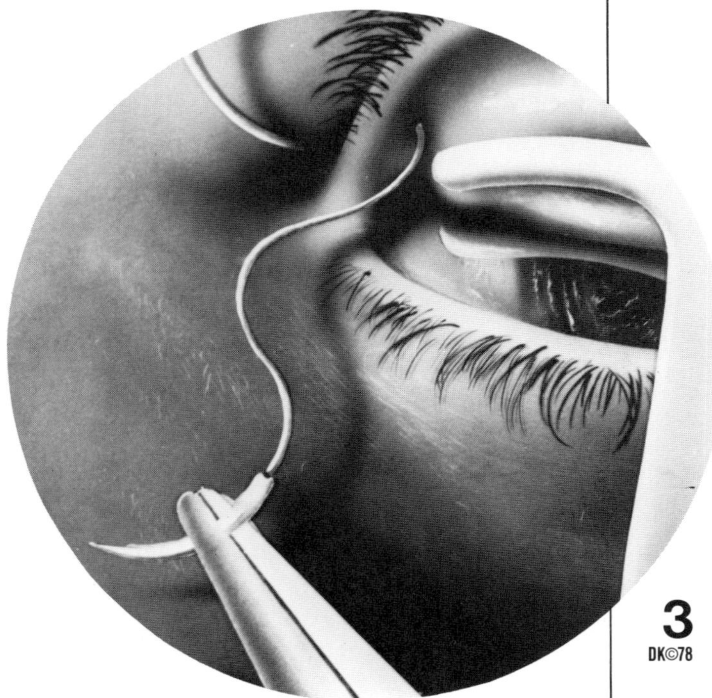

3
DK©78

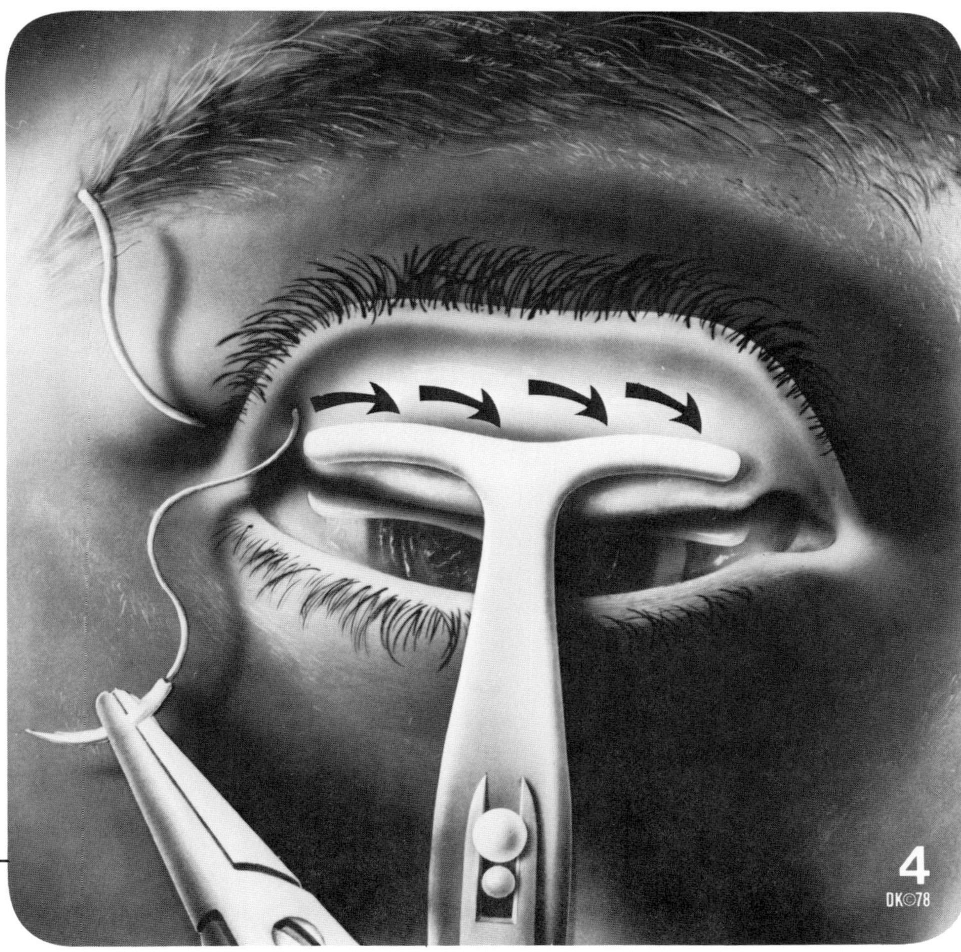

Donald A. Keller

traverse the entire width of the lid in the area resected [4].

The second bite [5] enters 5 mm nasal to the exit site, just above the edge of the clamp. The needle passes through the full thickness of tissue held in the clamp, which includes the tarsal conjunctiva, tarsal plate, and Müller's muscle, and exits on the palpebral conjunctival surface. The third bite [6] begins 5 mm nasal to the previous exit site and is brought back through the same layers to exit through the tarsoconjunctival surface. This process is repeated along the entire width of the clamp, which usually requires five bites (25 mm). The final bite exits 1 mm superior to the nasal edge of the clamp on the tarsoconjunctival surface and is left uncut [7].

The tissue held in the Putterman clamp is excised with a small scalpel [8], and the clamp is removed. The previously placed suture now holds the two sides of the lid together, and the conjunctival surface of the wound is closed with the nasal portion of the same 6-0 catgut suture [9]. The conjunctival bites also are made with a running stitch placed 5 mm apart to reduce corneal irritation [10]. After the conjunctiva is closed, the suture is brought to the skin surface, as close to the original entry site as possible, where it is tied and cut.

Should corneal irritation develop, we recommend the use of a soft contact lens for five days to protect the cornea. If the irritation continues after this time, sufficient healing has occurred, and the suture may be removed. As the lid heals, another 1 mm of correction occurs in addition to that seen in the immediate postoperative period. The maximum effect of the procedure is apparent after 30 days.

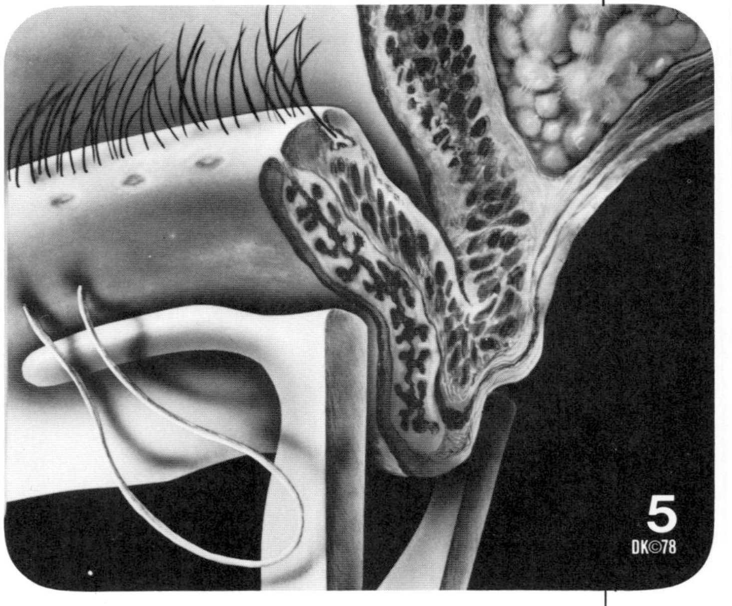

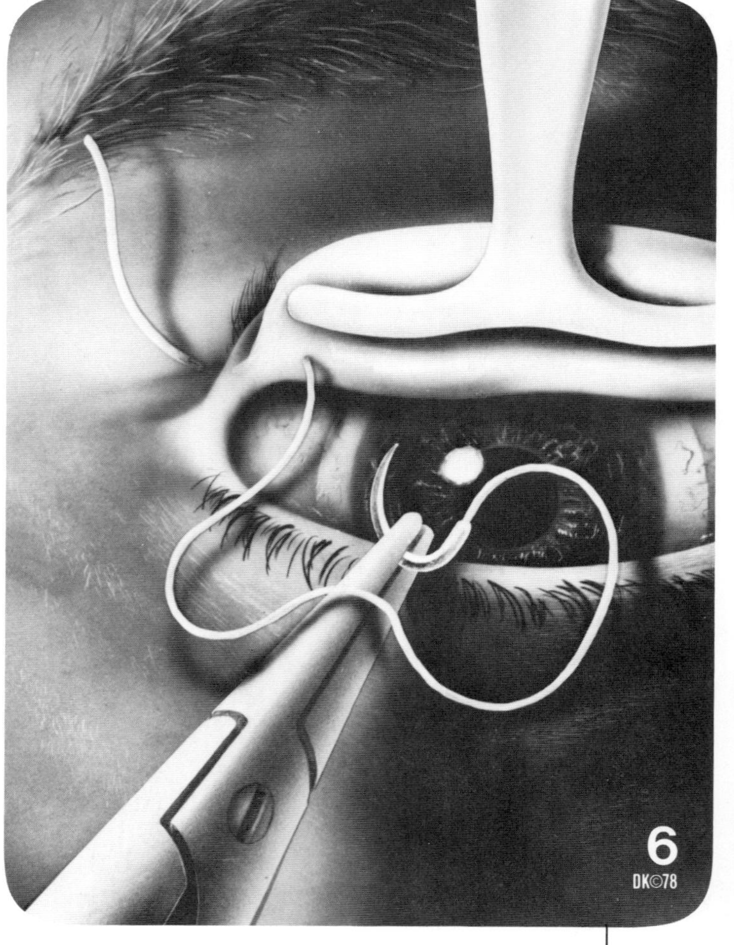

Donald F. Keller

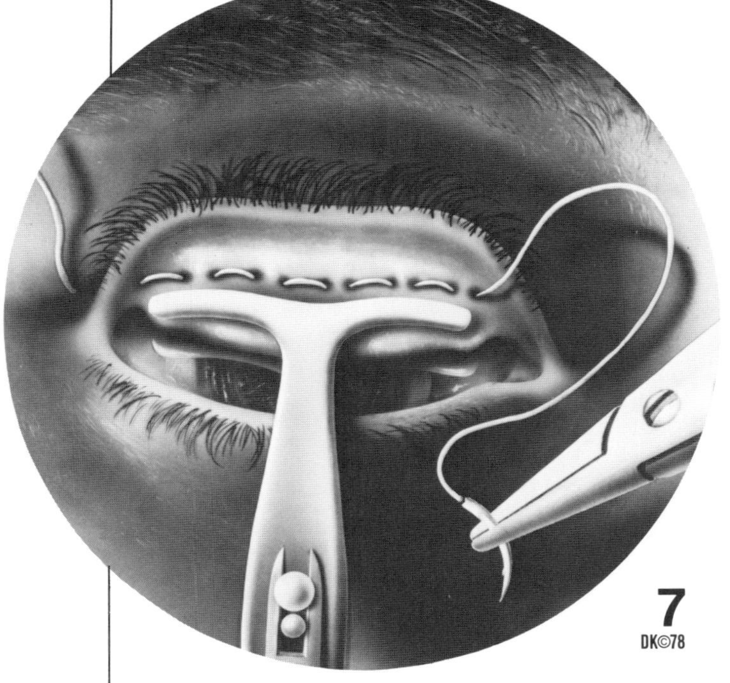

7
DK©78

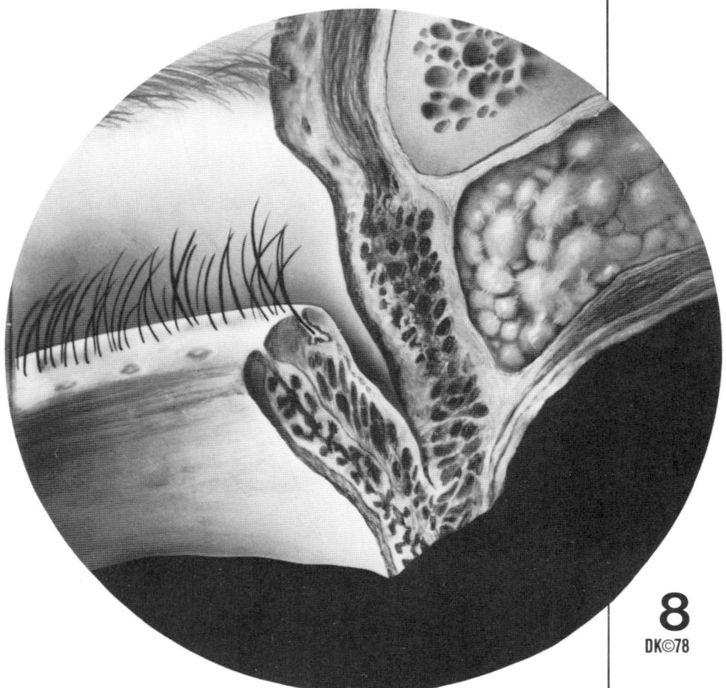

8
DK©78

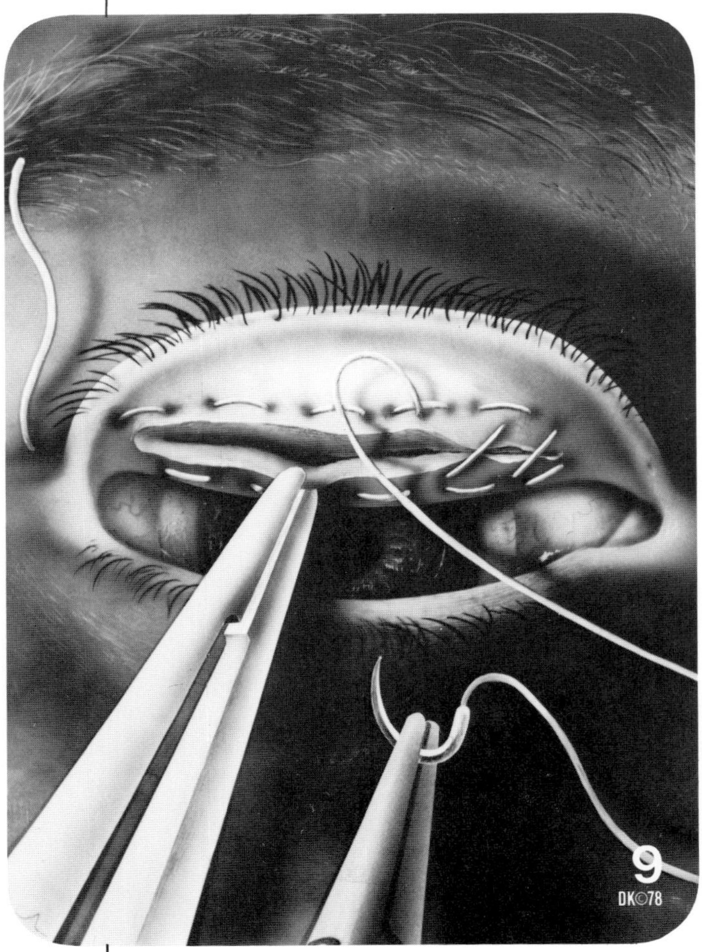

9
DK©78

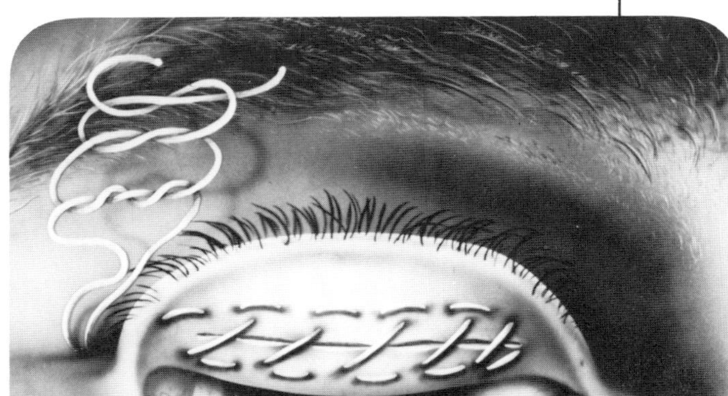

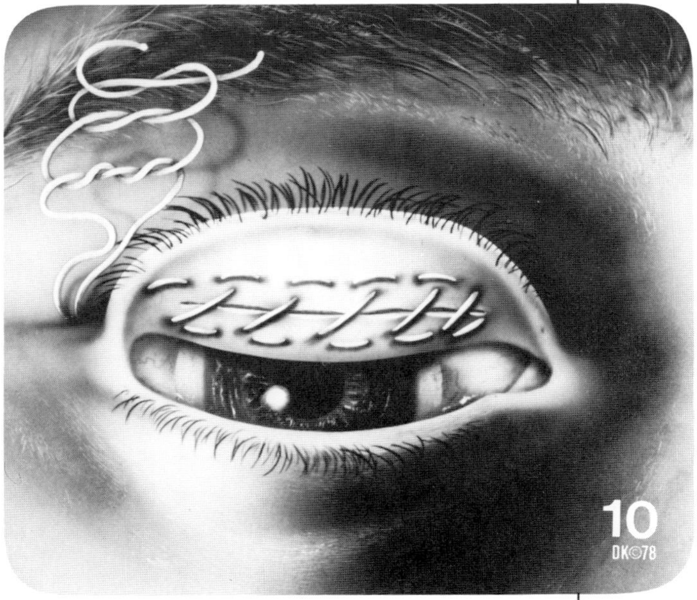

10
DK©78

TRANSCUTANEOUS LEVATOR RESECTION

John A. Burns, M.D.

Transcutaneous levator muscle resection is the most versatile of the ptosis procedures. It can be used with both congenital and acquired ptosis, and satisfactory results can be obtained when the levator function is good, fair, and in some cases, poor.

The skin approach to levator resection offers several advantages. Better exposure permits easy identification of the anatomic landmarks and more accurate resection. In addition, the surgeon may create a new, specifically located lid fold. A longer length of levator muscle can be exposed; therefore, more severe cases of ptosis can be corrected. Finally, the surgeon may excise excess skin above or below the incision to correct either dermochalasis or lash ptosis.

The surgeon first determines the amount of levator muscle to be resected. Ancillary procedures, such as resection of skin, are considered at the same time. Mild congenital ptosis with good levator function can be corrected with a small levator resection, usually 10 to 13 mm. A moderate amount of congenital ptosis with fair levator function may require a larger resection, 18 to 22 mm. Severe ptosis with poor function can sometimes be corrected with maximum resection of 23 mm or more of muscle. The maximum possible resection is approximately 28 mm.

These amounts of resection are for congenital ptosis only. If a levator resection operation is to be carried out on an acquired ptosis, the amount of resection must be reduced to avoid overcorrection. It is rarely necessary to perform more than 12 to 14 mm of resection on an acquired ptosis.

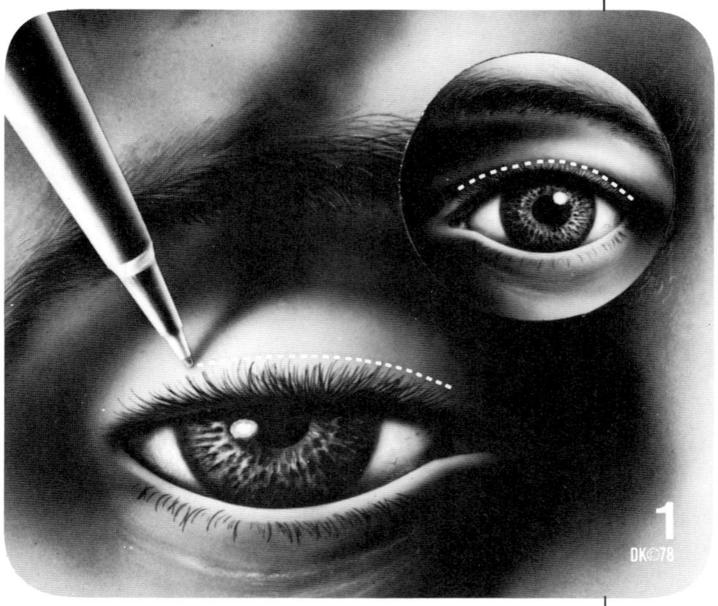

The location of the incision and the placement of the lid fold greatly affect the ultimate results. In patients with unilateral ptosis, it is critical to match the normal eye. Before anesthesia is administered, the surgeon marks the planned lid fold site on the lid with a marking pencil while the patient is in a sitting position [1]. To insure symmetry, the site of the normal lid fold is marked as well since it is impossible to locate it accurately with the patient in the supine position. Children require general anesthesia; a local anesthetic is adequate for adults.

The skin incision is made with a small scalpel through skin only along the previously marked lid fold site [2]. The incision extends from the medial canthal region to just medial to the lateral canthus. The skin is separated inferiorly from the pretarsal orbicularis, POR [3], with Westcott scissors to just above the lash line [3]. Only 2 to 3 mm of skin undermining is necessary superiorly. A vertical scratch incision is made through the pretarsal orbicularis down to tarsus, T [4], at the center of the lid from the lash follicles to the top of the tarsal plate.

The divided muscle is undermined from the surface of the tarsal plate and excised [5].

Donald A. Keller

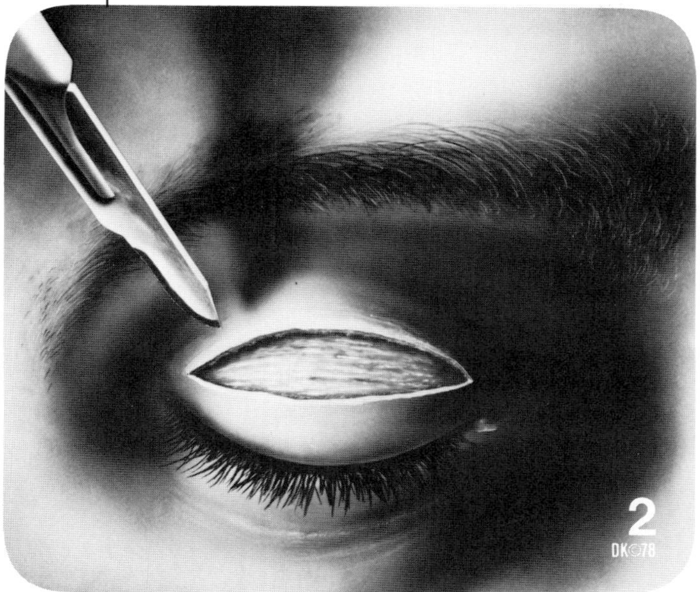

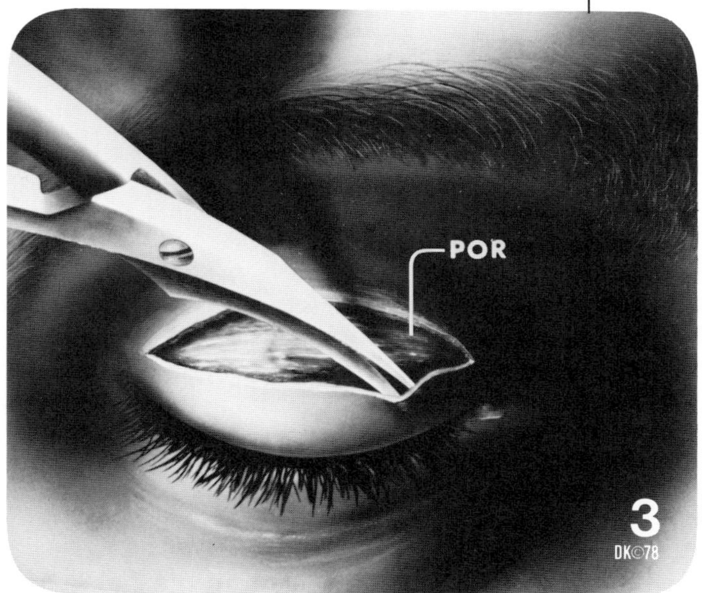

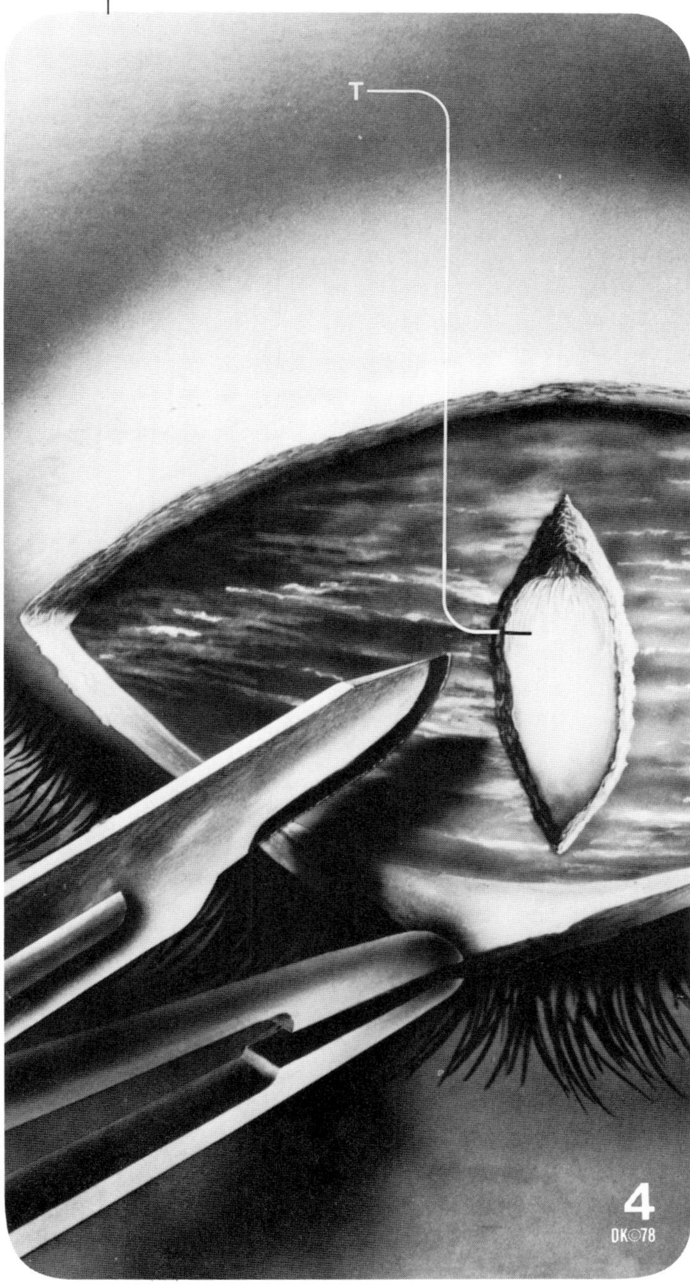

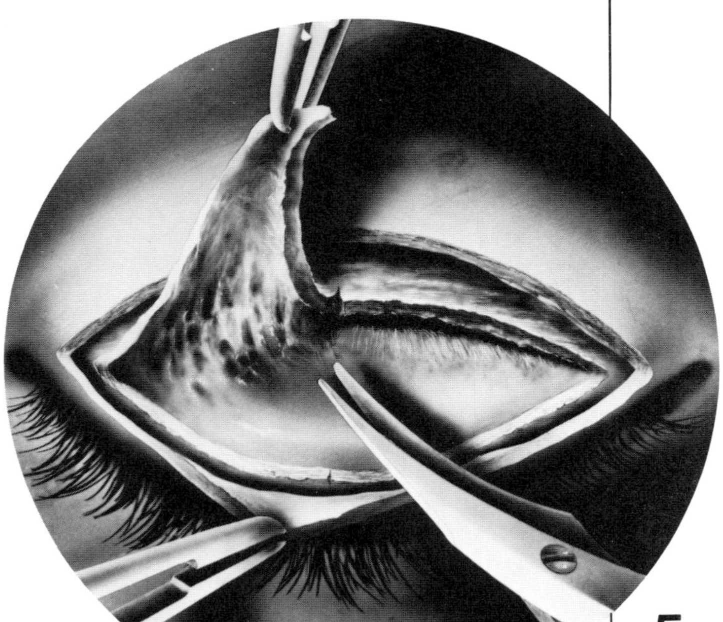

5
DK©78

Donald A. Keller

With Westcott scissors, medial and lateral vertical incisions 25 mm apart are made at the upper edge of the tarsal plate. These incisions extend through the full orbicularis OM , levator aponeurosis (LA), Müller's muscle (M), and conjunctiva, C [6] . One blade of the ptosis clamp is passed through the incisions, and the clamp is locked. With a scalpel, the surgeon cuts the tissue held in the clamp from the upper edge of the tarsal plate [7] .

The sandwich of tissue in the clamp is everted to expose the palpebral conjunctival surface, which must be dissected from Müller's muscle [8] . A 37-mm, 25-gauge needle on a 2.5-ml syringe filled with saline is passed from the lateral edge just below the clamp between conjunctiva and Müller's muscle [9] . If the needle is not faintly visible through the conjunctiva, it has been placed too deeply. The subconjunctival injection of saline balloons the conjunctiva, which facilitates subsequent dissection. A Westcott scissors undermines the conjunctiva to separate it from Müller's muscle [10] . The conjunctiva is then severed at the upper edge of the ptosis clamp. The cut margin is resutured to its ori-

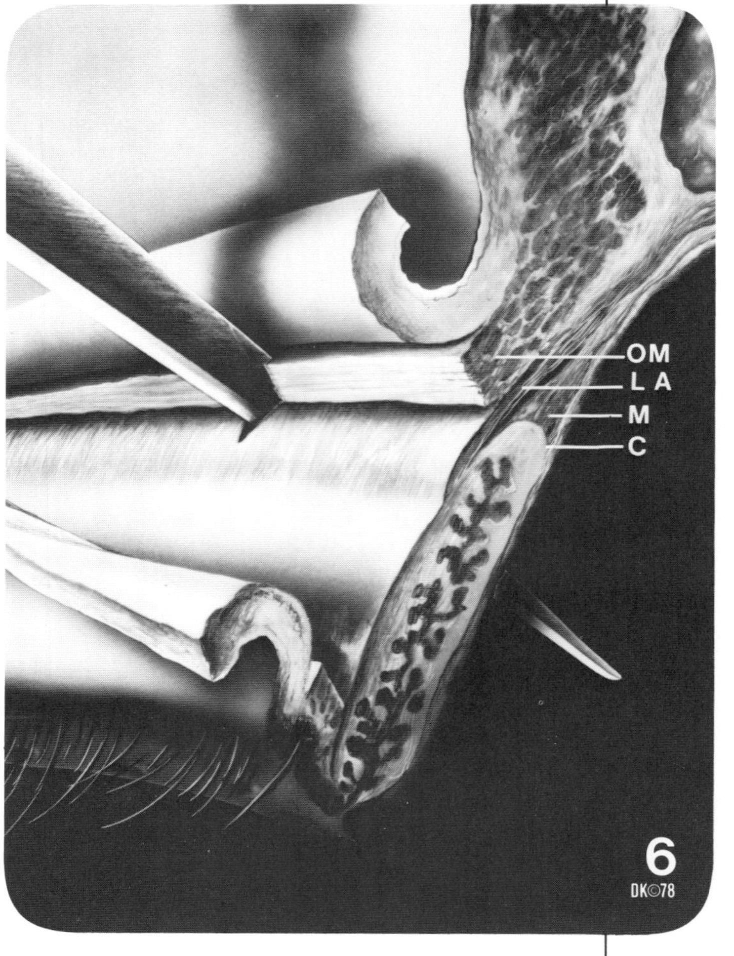

6

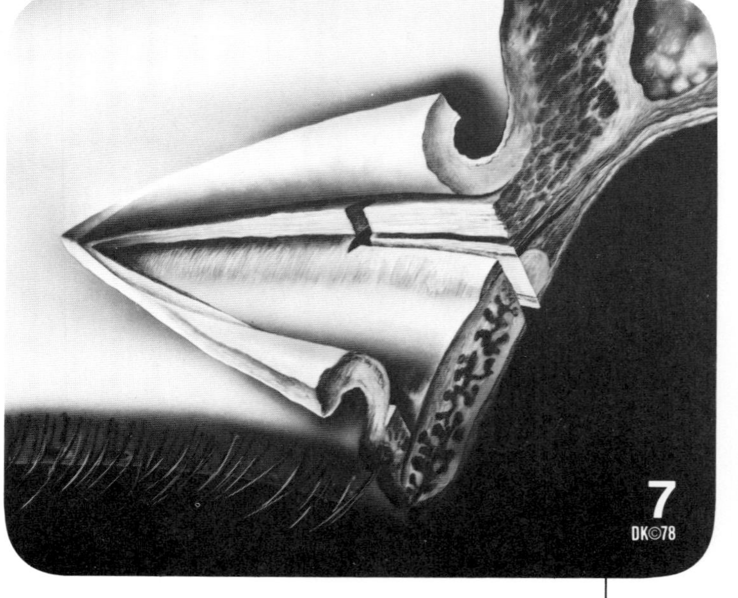
7

Donald F. Keller

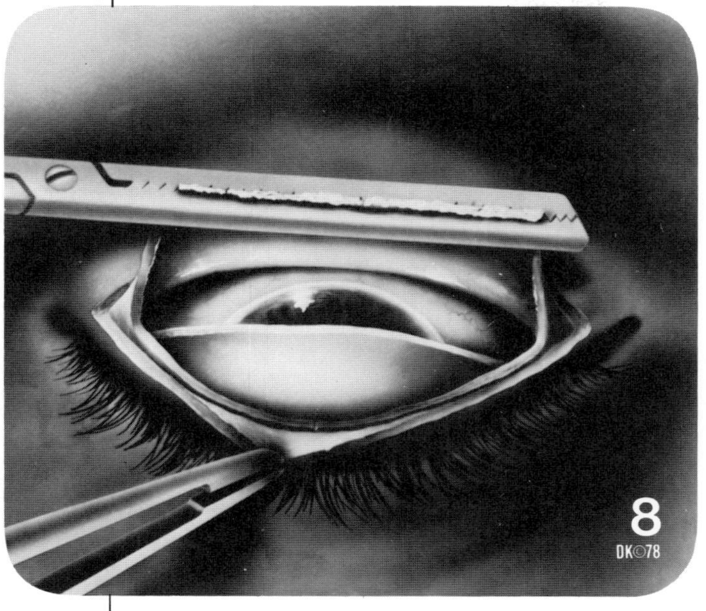

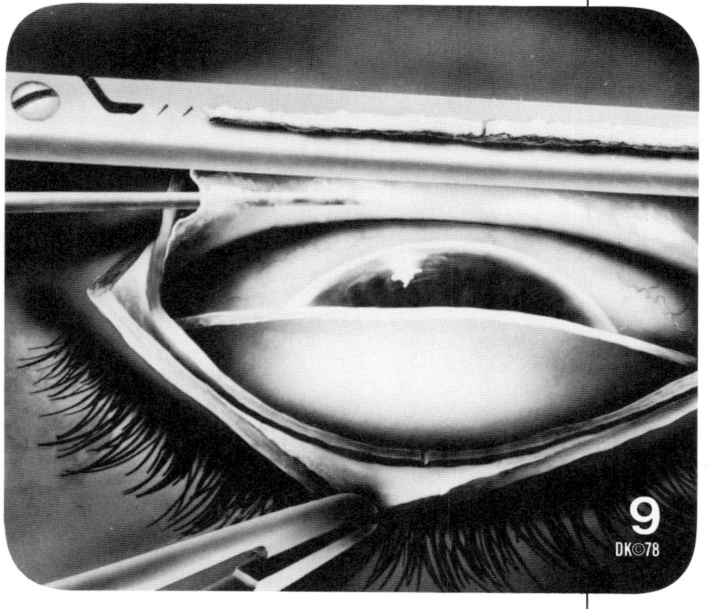

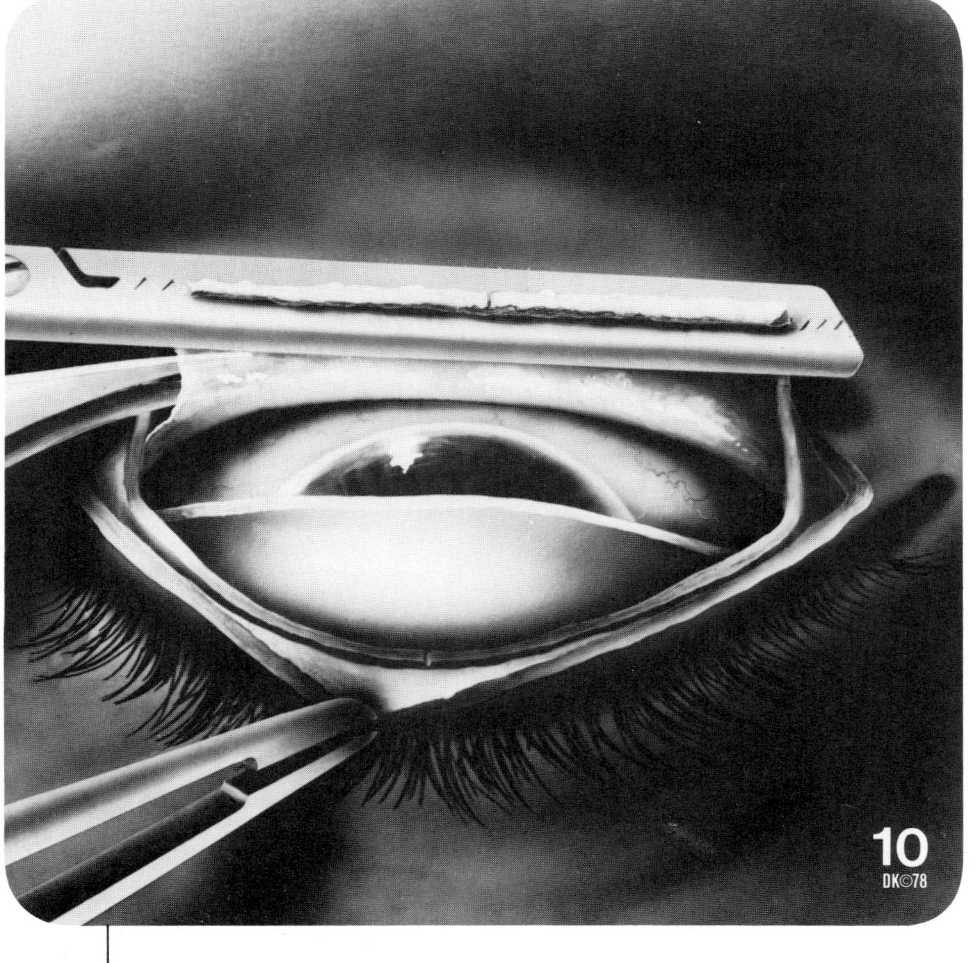

Donald F. Keller

ginal position at the upper edge of the tarsal plate with three interrupted 6-0 chromic catgut sutures [11].

After the conjunctiva is reapproximated, the surgeon must isolate levator muscle and Müller's muscle from the overlying orbital septum and orbicularis muscle, which are still held in the clamp. The location of the orbital septum is easily palpated since it originates from the superior orbital margin and inserts onto the surface of the levator aponeurosis. Orbital fat is located deep to the orbital septum. The ptosis clamp is pulled inferiorly, the upper edge of the incision is pulled anteriorly and a buttonhole incision is made 10 mm above the ptosis clamp through the orbicularis muscle and orbital septum [12]. If the septum has been perforated, the surgeon should see orbital fat herniate through the incision. Once the correct plane has been achieved, the surgeon makes a horizontal incision 25 mm long, which separates the orbicularis and orbital septum from the underlying levator muscle [13]. To confirm that the septum has been divided, the surgeon should be able to place a finger tip in the wound and palpate the orbital roof without encountering resistance. If the septum has not been cut, a tissue plane remains and diverts the surgeon's finger tip to the orbital rim.

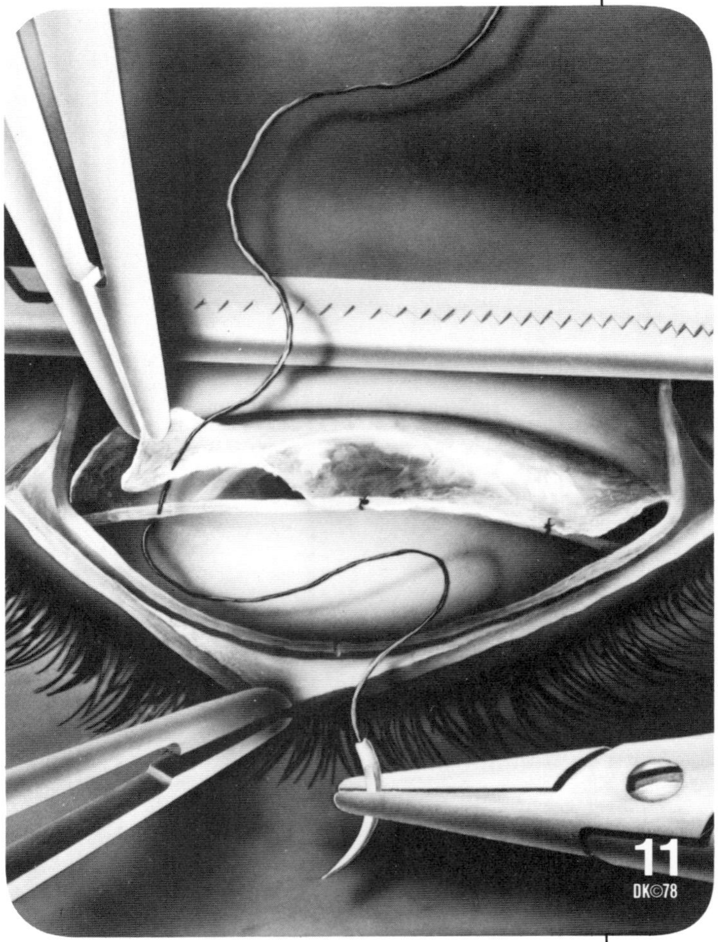

The levator muscle and Müller's muscle are now the only tissues held in the ptosis clamp. However, the aponeurosis still is not totally free, since it is attached by its medial and lateral horns. Two vertical incisions, medially and laterally, divide the horns of the levator aponeurosis [14]. As the horns are cut, care must be taken not to include the tendon of the superior oblique muscle in the medial incision and not to cut into the lacrimal gland laterally.

Donald F. Keller

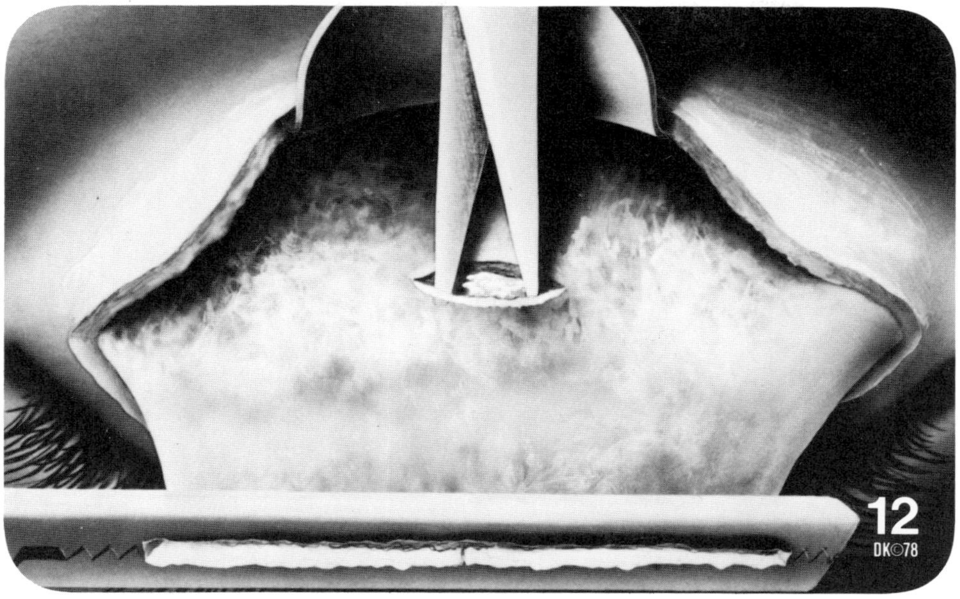

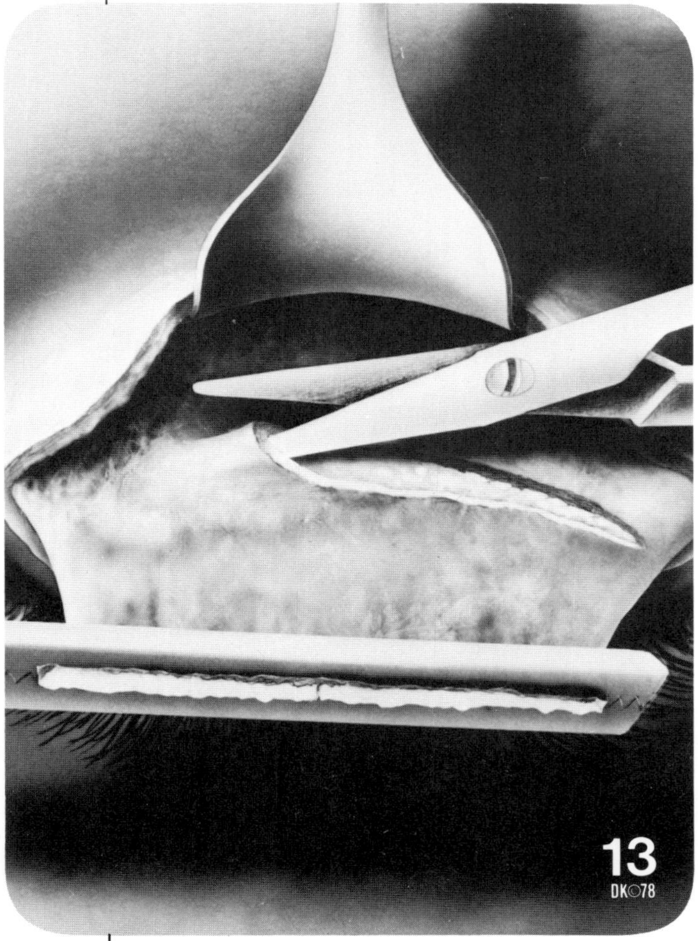

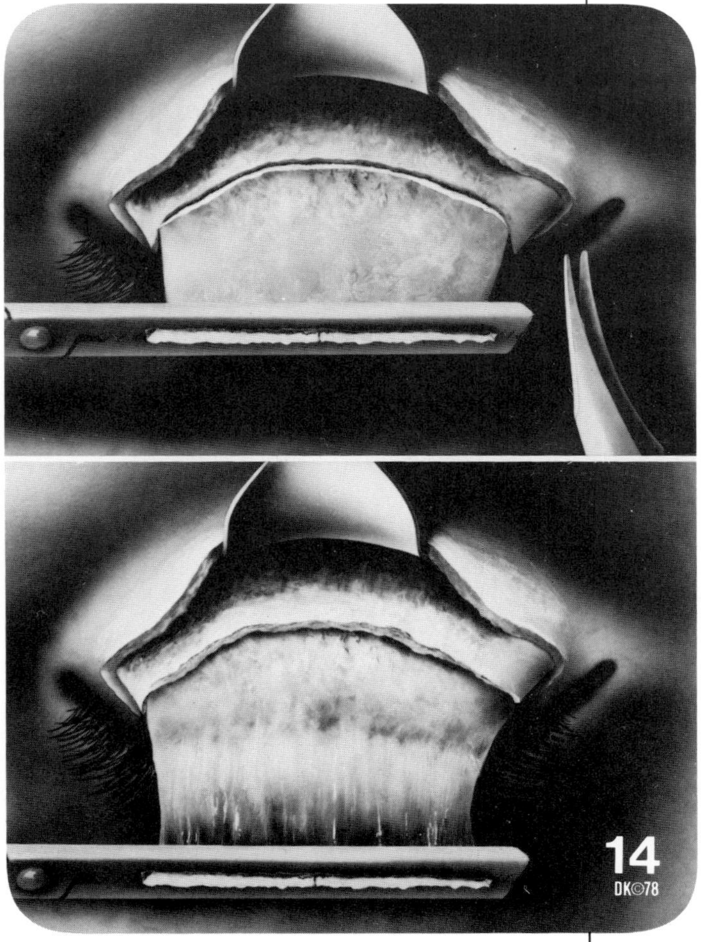

Donald A. Killer

Three double-armed 4-0 black silk sutures are placed in a lamellar fashion in the tarsal plate 15 . The bite of the suture is approximately 3 mm long, and each suture is placed approximately 5 mm apart. The levator aponeurosis is brought down the predetermined amount, and the center suture is passed through the muscle and tied with a single knot. This creates the high point of the desired lid arch and raises the lid margin to the new level created by the planned resection. The surgeon now can observe whether the lid is resting in the desired position. If alterations in the lid position are necessary, the suture is untied and repositioned.

When the surgeon is satisfied with the position of the lid arch, the medial and lateral sutures are placed through the levator muscle at the same height. All three sutures are tied loosely. The surgeon now evaluates the full lid arch to make sure that it is positioned properly. The knots are then permanently tied and cut 16 .

At this point, the levator muscle is attached firmly to the tarsal plate. The surgeon excises the excess portion of the muscles, leaving a 3-mm margin. If necessary, the surgeon may do a skin resection at the upper or lower edge of the skin incision.

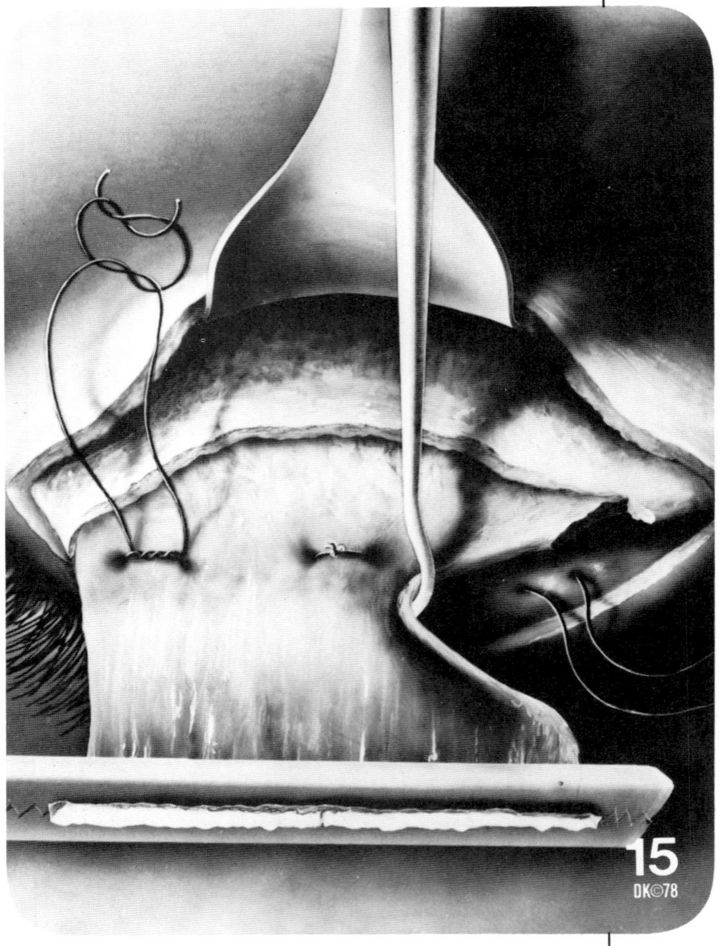

The lid fold is created with five vertically oriented 6-0 black silk sutures. The lower arm passes through the tarsoconjunctiva, tarsal plate, Müller's muscle, levator muscle, and the lower margin of the skin, 2 to 3 mm from the cut edge 17 . The superior arm of the suture is passed through the palpebral conjunctiva, Müller's muscle, and levator muscle and exits through the skin, approximately 3 mm above the cut edge.

When all five sutures are in place, they are tied snugly so that the skin edges are inverted against the levator muscle 18 .This creates a lid skin fold. A Frost suture, which is removed on the first postoperative day, is placed through the lower lid and taped to the patient's forehead. The lid is covered with a single eye patch. On the tenth postoperative day, the vertical mattress sutures are removed. We recommend the use of antibiotic ointment for lubrication two times a day until the superficial punctate keratitis due to exposure has disappeared. The lid position stabilizes in four to six weeks.

Donald A. Keller

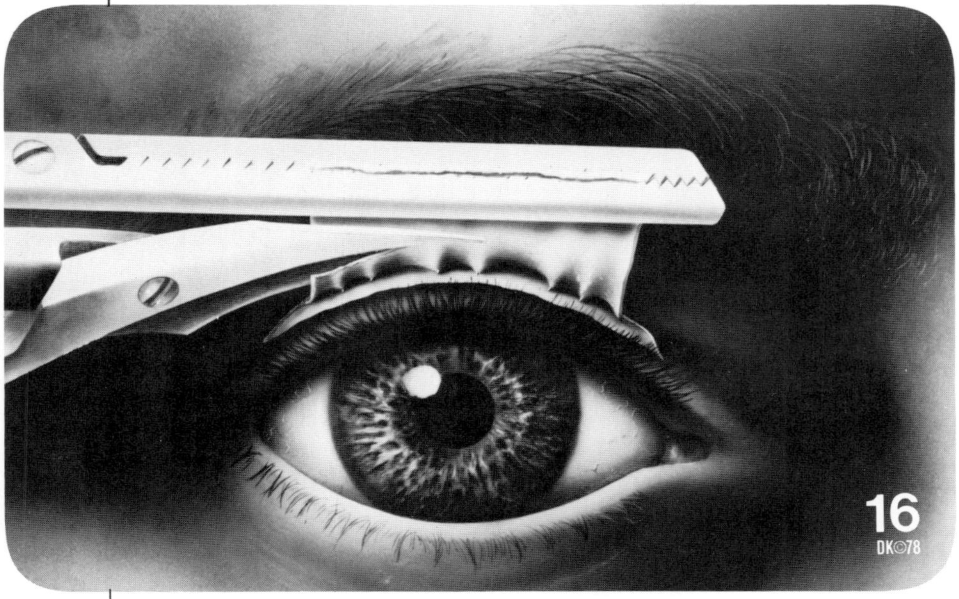

16
DK©78

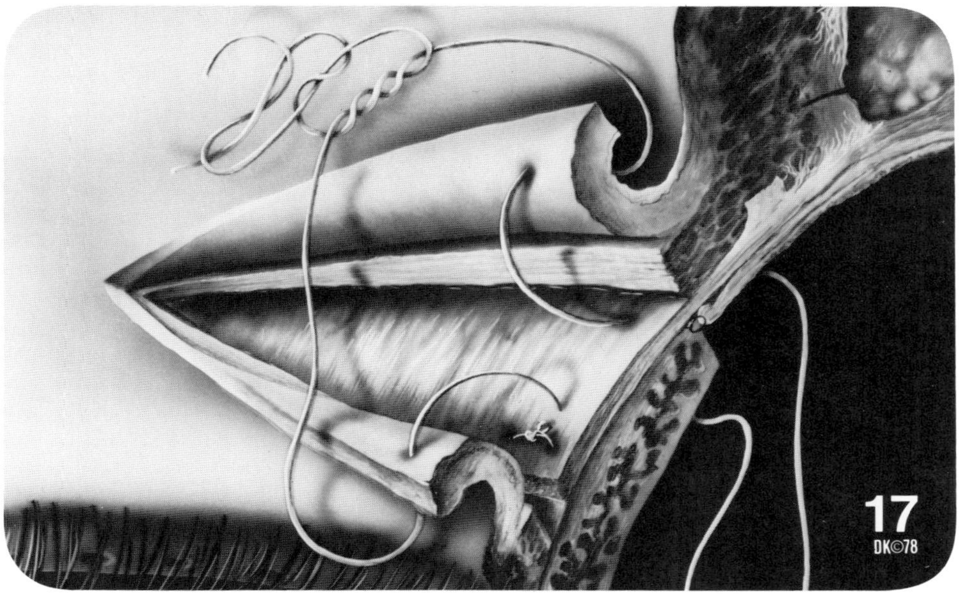

17
DK©78

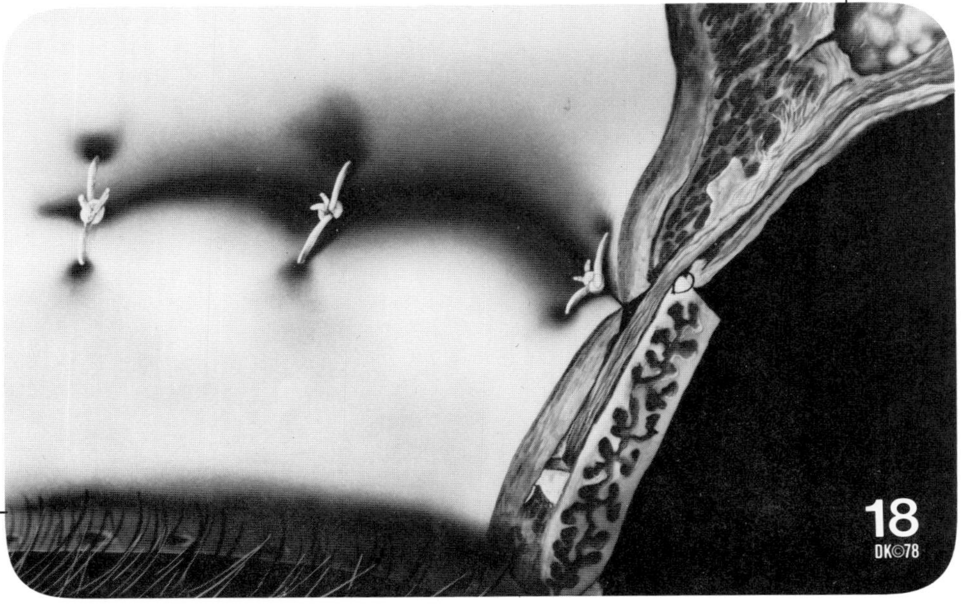

18
DK©78

Donald A. Kelker

TRANSCONJUNCTIVAL LEVATOR RESECTION

John A. Burns, M.D.

Opinion varies considerably regarding the appropriate circumstances for performing a transconjunctival levator resection. Proponents maintain that the patient undergoing this type of resection has less postoperative reaction and heals more quickly than one who has undergone external levator resection. Advocates frequently use it as their primary ptosis operation. We believe that transconjunctival levator resection is most effective in patients with mild to moderate ptosis where a possibility of overcorrection exists. This is specifically relevant to cases of acquired ptosis.

With the patient under general anesthesia, the lid is everted [1]. A traction suture is placed horizontally through the conjunctiva approximately 12 mm from the lid margin, several millimeters above the tarsal plate.

A 25-mm incision is made horizontally, 2 mm below the superior border of the tarsal plate through the tarsus to expose the levator aponeurosis [2]. A buttonhole is made through the levator aponeurosis medially and

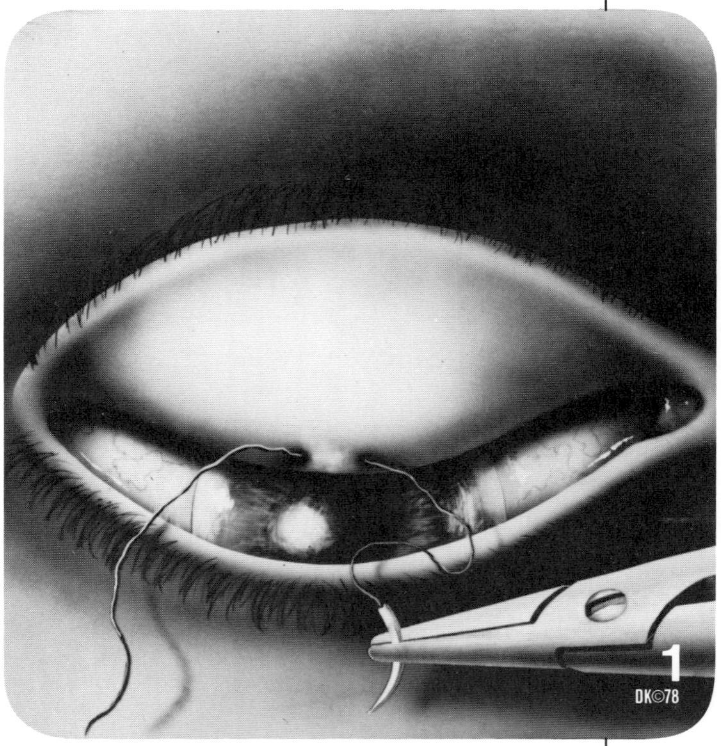

laterally, and it is separated from the orbicularis muscle by blunt dissection with Stevens scissors.

As the scissors is removed, a small, straight hemostat is inserted to grasp the levator aponeurosis. The conjunctiva is dissected from Müller's muscle superiorly to the superior conjunctival fornix [3]. The tarsal remnant is then excised [4]. The ptosis clamp is rotated inferiorly, and the levator aponeurosis is transected from its distal attachments [5].

Donald A. Keller

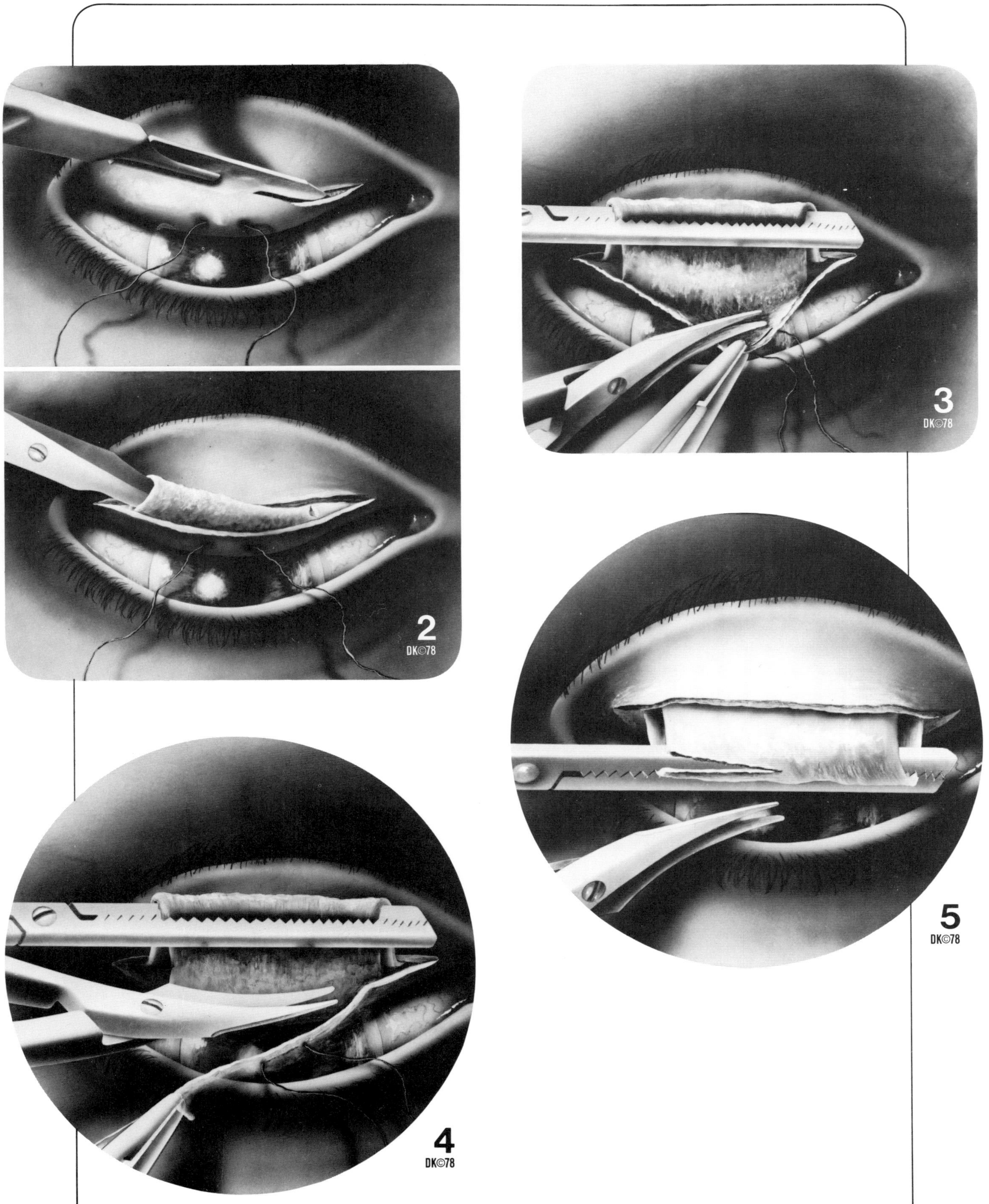

Donald A. Keller

As the levator aponeurosis is stretched, orbital septum is brought forward and exposed [6] . The plane between the levator aponeurosis and the orbital septum is opened by freeing the attachment of the orbital septum. The appearance of orbital fat between the two layers confirms the existence of the proper surgical plane. If a large resection is planned, the medial and lateral horns of the aponeurosis must be cut [7] .

Three double-armed sutures are placed through the muscle in the anteroposterior direction [8] . The placement of the sutures depends on the amount of muscle to be resected. The suture engages the upper cut edge of the palpebral conjunctiva, and the excess muscle is excised [9] . The sutures then pass through the upper end of the tarsus and

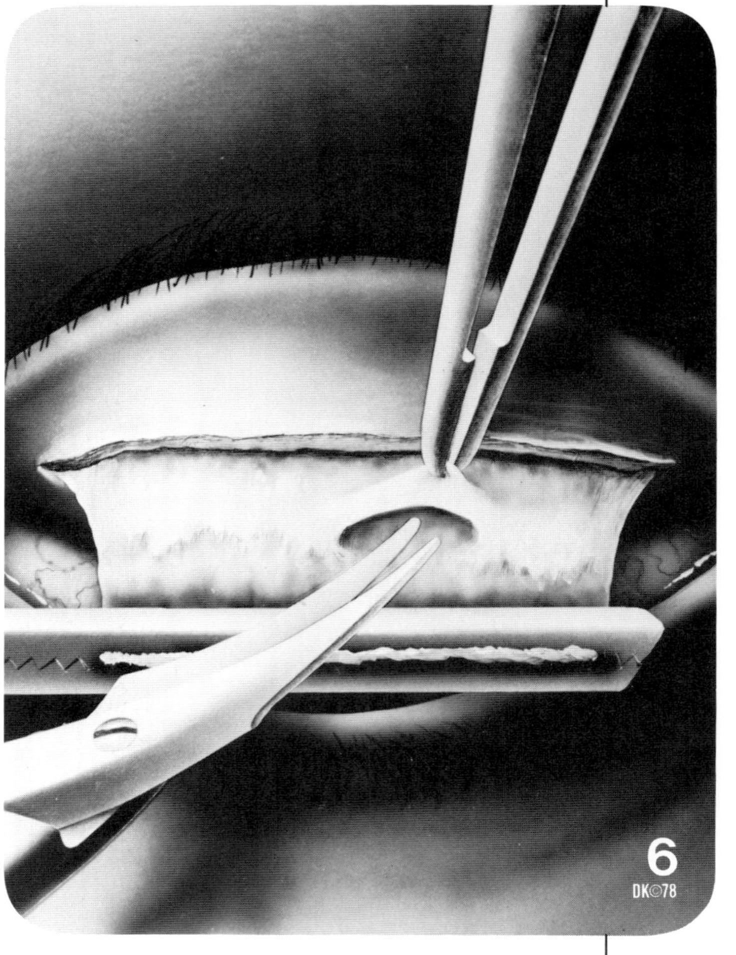

through the orbicularis muscle and skin at the level of the lid fold. They are then tied over bolsters.

After the incision is closed [10] , a Frost suture is placed in the inferior lid and is used to protect the eye for the first 24 hours after surgery. Antibiotic ointment should be applied to the eye twice a day to minimize the exposure keratitis. The lid sutures are removed on the tenth postoperative day.

Should overcorrection be recognized in the early postoperative period, the surgeon may cut the sutures and manually stretch the lid inferiorly to lower the final lid level.

Donald F. Keller

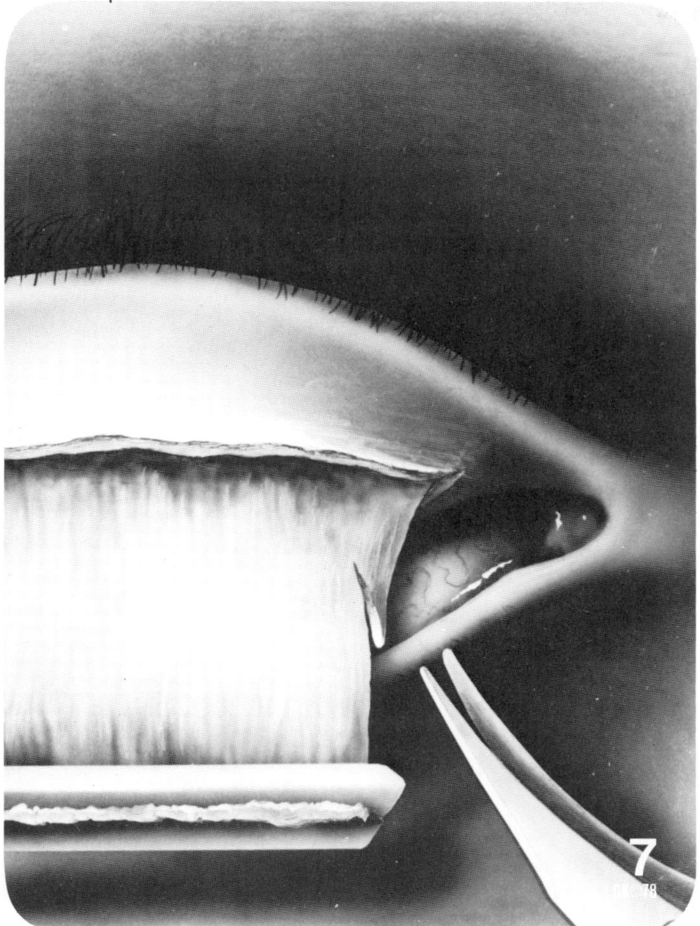

7
DK©78

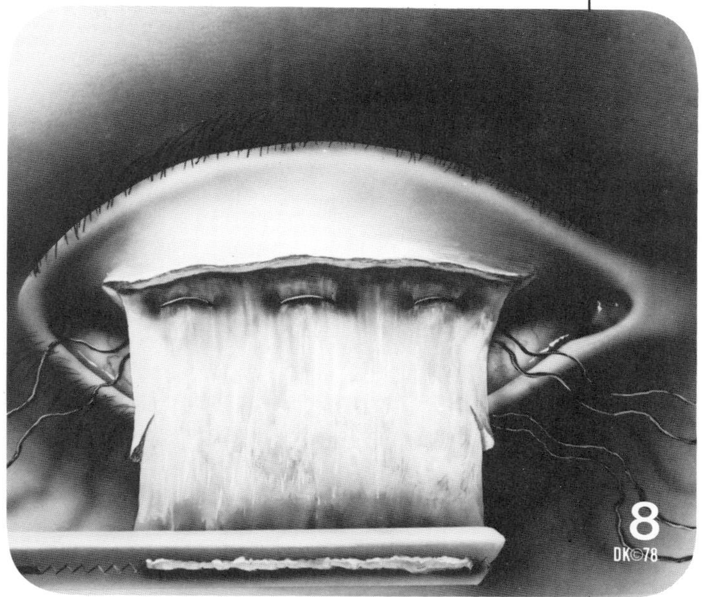

8
DK©78

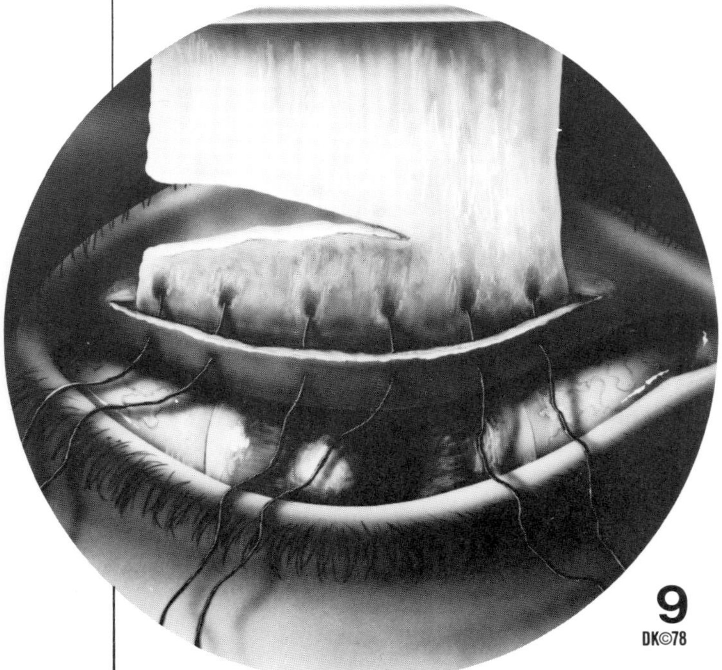

9
DK©78

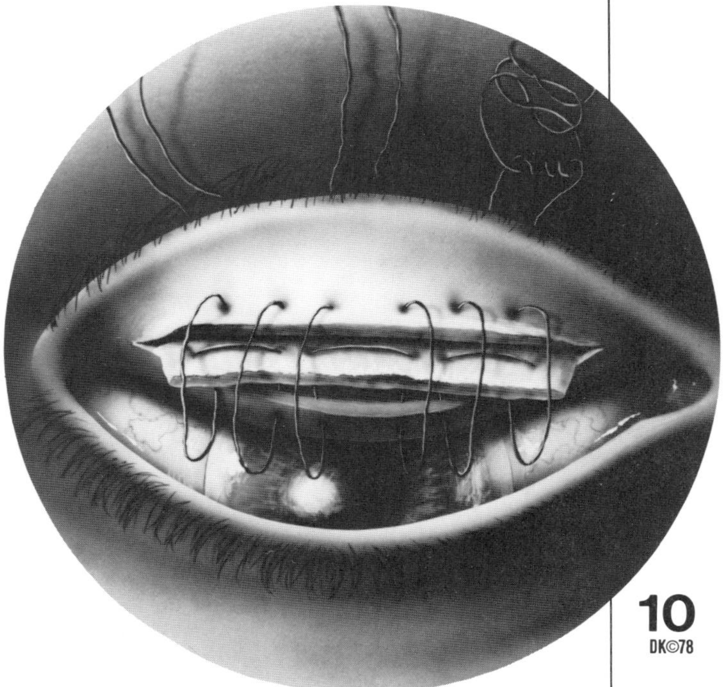

10
DK©78

Donald A. Keller

FRONTALIS SUSPENSION

John A. Burns, M.D.

A frontalis suspension creates a union between the lid and frontalis muscle. It is generally recommended for patients with very poor or no levator function, or when a levator resection has failed to achieve a sufficient lid lift.

Although a number of materials exist to create a frontalis suspension, we recommend the use of homologous or autogenous fascia lata to provide the connections between the frontalis muscle and the lid. Fascia is preferred because of its strength, uniform acceptance by lid tissue, and extremely low incidence of infection. The preparation of the fascia strips is described in the section, "Preparation of Homologous Fascia Lata Strips," in the chapter "Surgery of the Retina."

Six skin incisions, 5 mm long, are necessary for the passage of the fascial strips and are made with a scalpel. The three lid incisions are placed 2 mm above the lash line through the skin and orbicularis muscle to the tarsal plate [1]. The middle incision is centered on the lid, and the two remaining incisions are placed at the medial and lateral ends of the lid. Three incisions at the upper edge of the brow are carried down to the periosteum. The central incision is made directly in line with the central lid incision. The other brow incisions are placed 5 mm medial and lateral to their respective canthi.

A Wright needle is passed through the central brow incision, just anterior to the periosteum and over the orbital rim [2]. The needle courses beneath the orbicularis muscle, anterior to the orbital septum and tarsal plate, and exits at the central lid incision. The previously prepared fascia, cut into 30- to 35-cm strips, is placed through the eye of the Wright needle and is threaded to its midpoint. The needle is withdrawn leaving the fascia in place, and the fascia is cut [3].

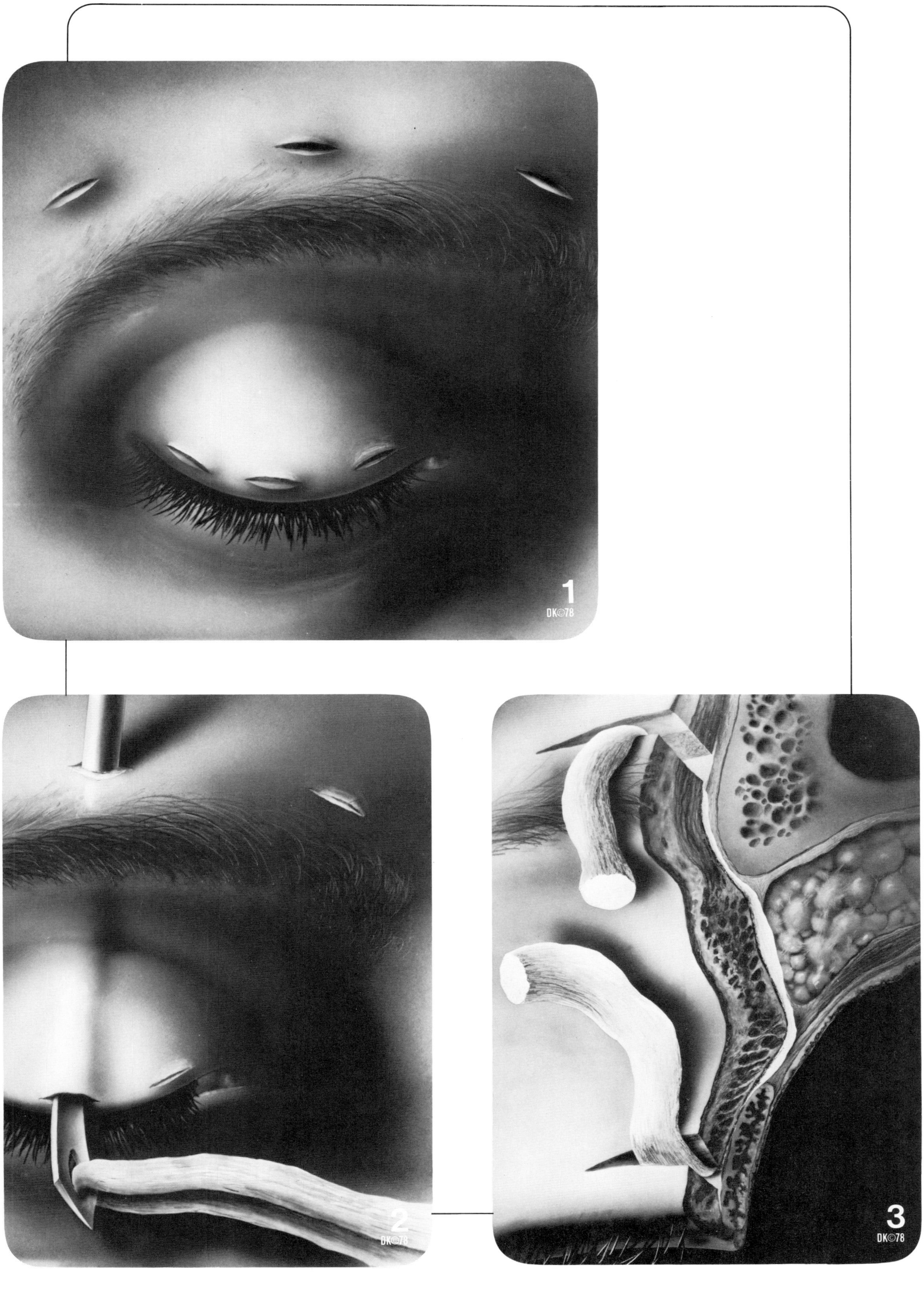
1
DK©78
2
DK©78
3
DK©78

Next, the needle is inserted through the nasal lid incision just below the orbicularis muscle and through the central incision. The fascia is placed on the needle, the needle is withdrawn, and the fascia is pulled with it through the nasal incision [4].

The needle is then passed through the medial brow incision to exit through the medial lid incision [5]. The fascia is inserted on the needle and drawn back to the brow area [6]. Finally, the needle is inserted from the medial brow above the periosteum to exit through the center brow incision. The fascia is then placed on the needle, and the end of the fascia is brought back [7]. This completes a fascial rhomboid that connects the frontalis muscle to the lid. The entire procedure is repeated on the lateral side to create a second rhomboid.

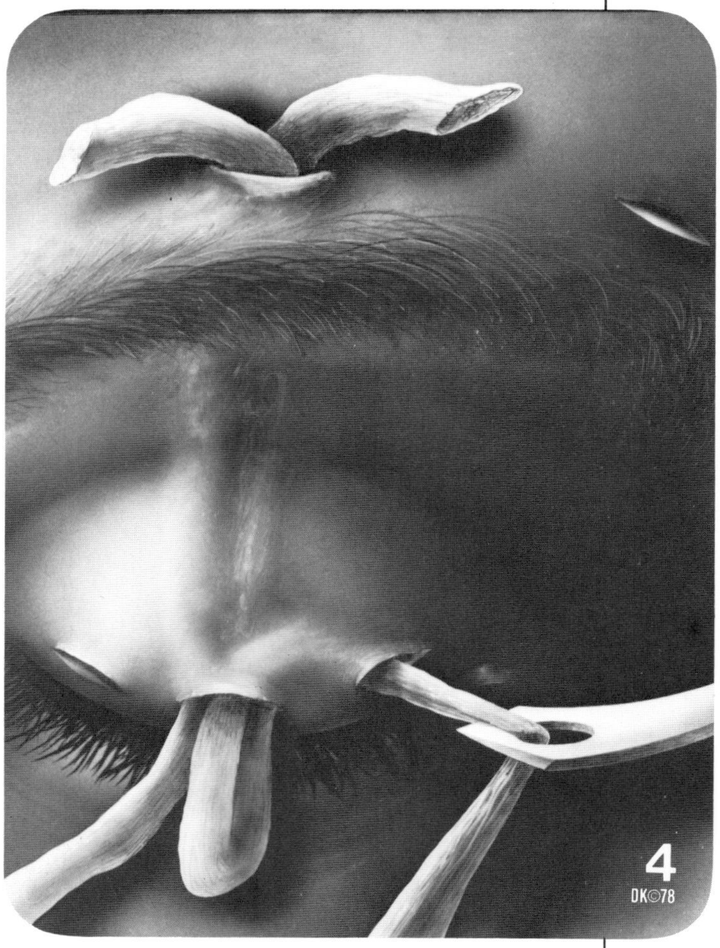

Donald F. Keller

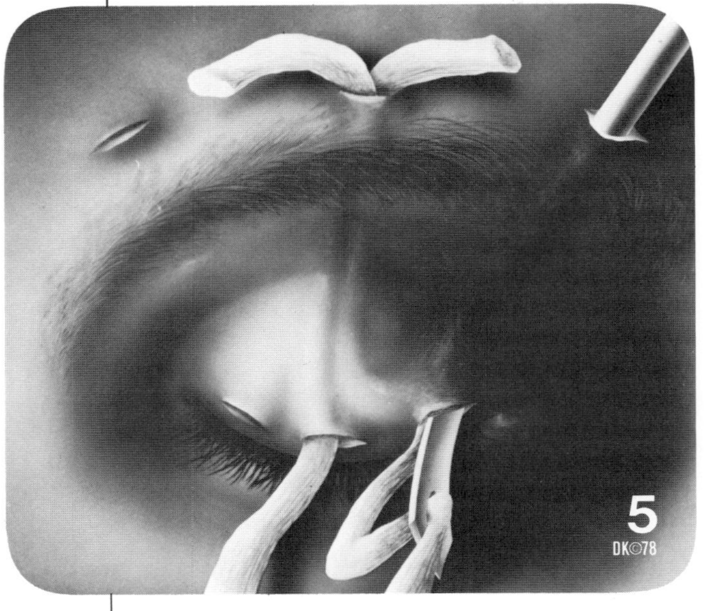

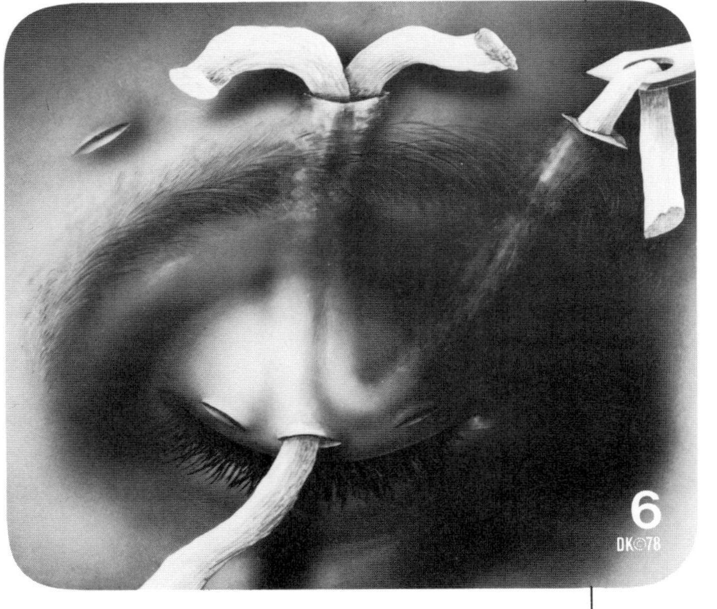

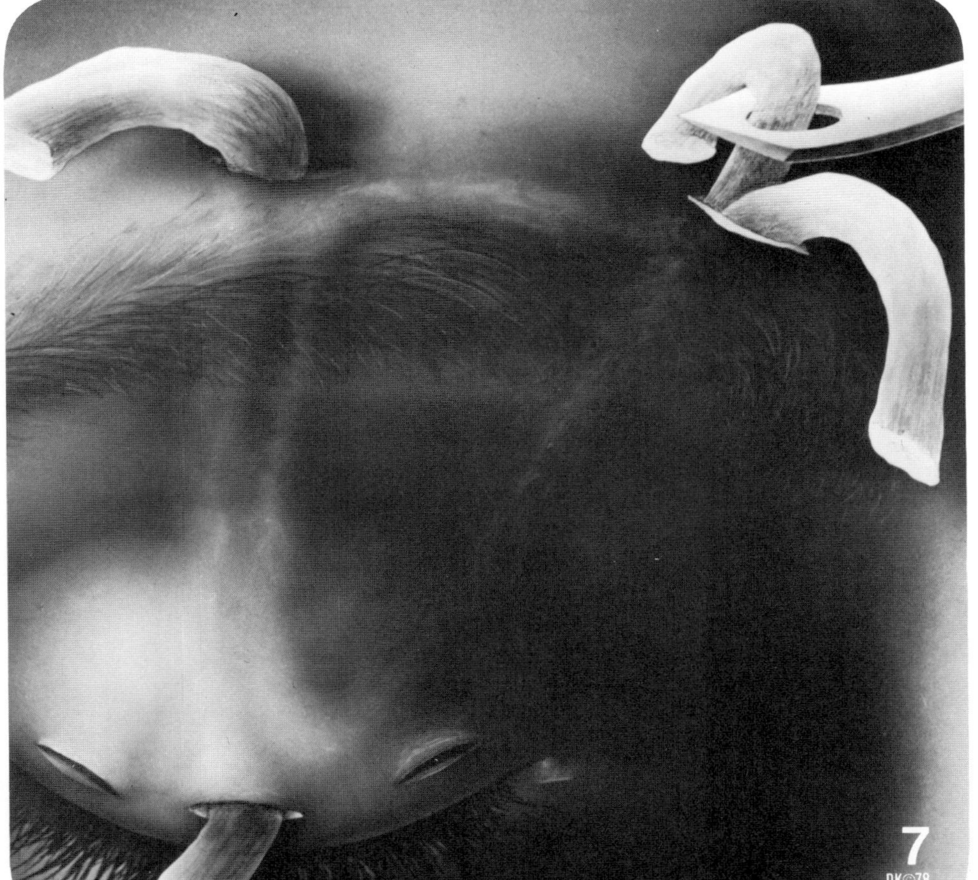

Donald A. Keller

After the two rhomboids of fascia have been formed and the two ends of fascia have been drawn to the medial and lateral sides, equal tension is placed on the strips of fascia to elevate the lid symmetrically.

Because of the slippery nature of the fascia, the surgeon cannot tie the ends together without a suture. To secure the fascia, the surgeon lays a 4-0 white silk suture across the incision site. The fascia is tied over the suture with a single overhand loop, and the suture is tied with a surgeon's knot [8]. A second overhand loop completes the square knot of fascia, and the suture is sewn through both ends of fascia to insure that the ends do not separate [9].

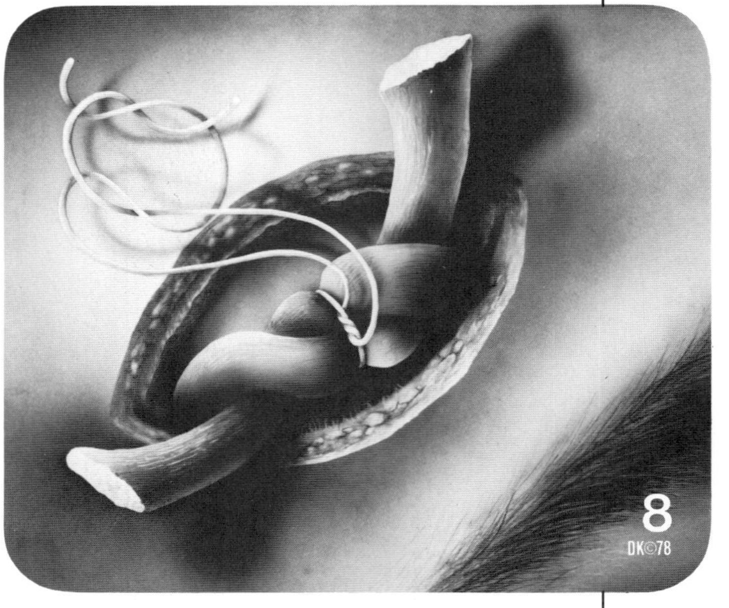

The knotted fascia must now be attached to the frontalis muscle. To achieve this, the suture that secured the fascia is passed through the frontalis muscle on the superior side of the brow incision and tied [10] [11].

Once the fascia is secured, the tails of the fascial knot are cut. The knot is pushed to the depths of the wound against the periosteum, since any fascia that extends through the incision will impair wound healing. The skin incisions are closed with 6-0 chromic catgut sutures [12]. A Frost suture holds the lids together until the following day. Because of the possibility of corneal exposure, we recommend the use of a bland ointment at bedtime postoperatively.

Donald F. Keller

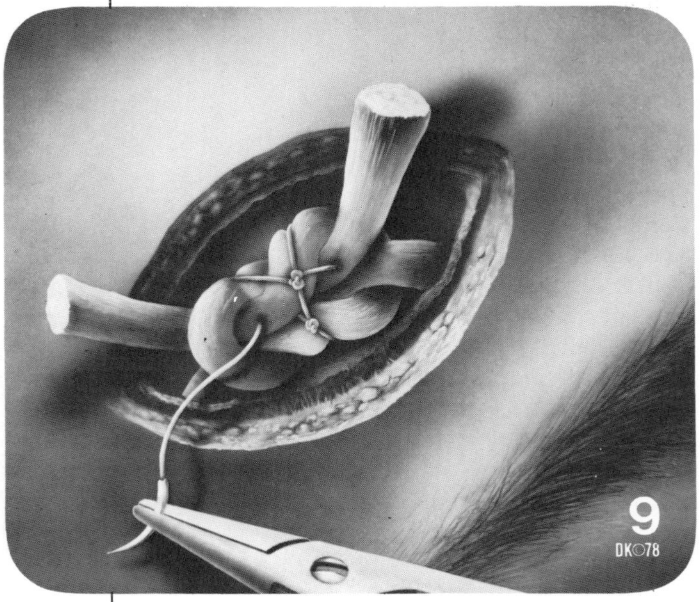

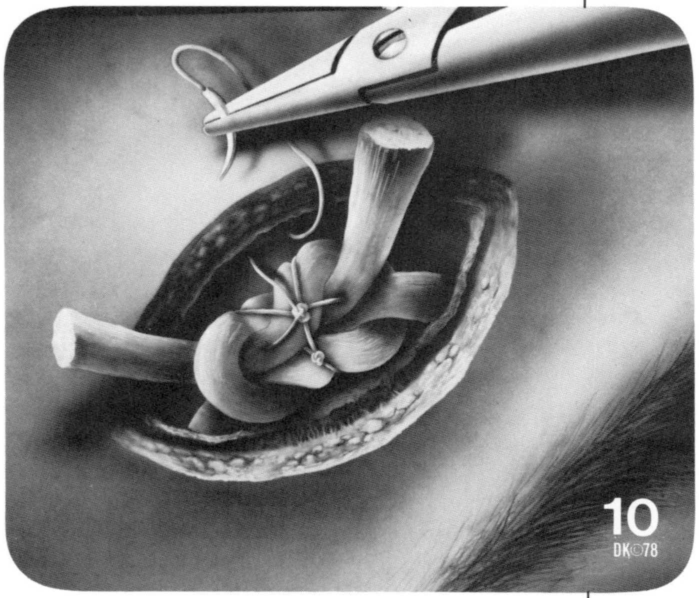

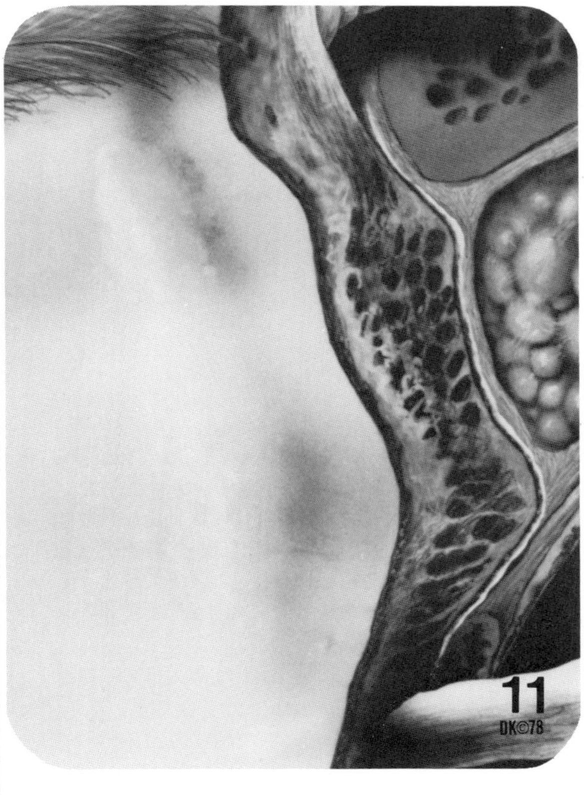

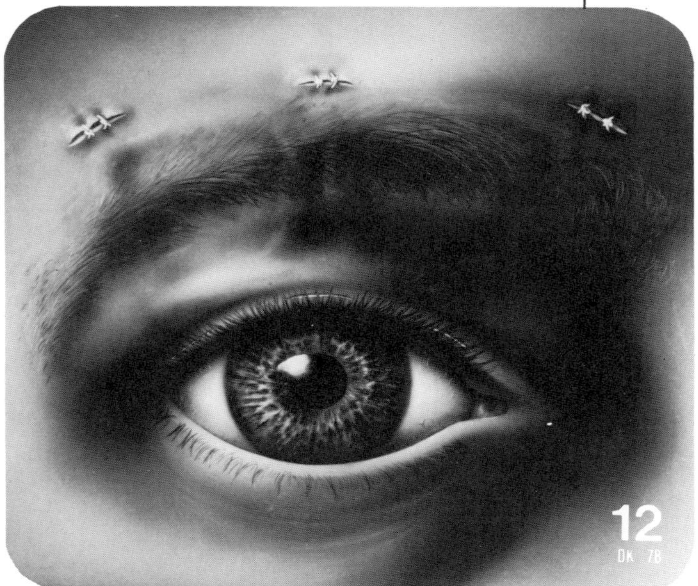

Donald A. Killer

ENTROPION

Entropion is the inward turning of the lid margin with rubbing of the lashes against the cornea and conjunctiva. Trichiasis may present a problem in the differential diagnosis. In trichiasis, the lashes are maldirected and rub against the cornea and conjunctiva, but the lid margin is in normal position. In both conditions, the patient suffers great discomfort, and chronic irritation may lead to breakdown of the corneal epithelium and may be visually threatening as well.

Four types of entropion exist: senile, cicatricial, congenital, and true spastic. Senile, the most common type, is ordinarily caused by laxity of the lid tissue and involves only the lower lid. Cicatricial entropion, which may involve upper or lower lid, may result from infection or chemical injury that scars the tarsus and conjunctiva, leading to secondary contracture. Congenital entropion is rare and is usually secondary to microphthalmus. True spastic entropion is a result of ocular irritation, frequently encountered postoperatively. It is transient and self-limited and does not require surgical correction.

One well-accepted cause is laxity and weakness of the inferior aponeurosis, which permits the inferior border of the tarsus to move anteriorly; the preseptal muscle then overrides the tarsus and forces the lid margin to turn in. Atrophy of orbital fat in the aged and the ensuing relative enophthalmos contribute to the poor apposition of the lower lid to the globe, and the lid rotates inward. In addition, horizontal laxity of the lid, results in elongation.

The choice of surgical procedures depends on the degree of horizontal elongation and the extent of inferior aponeurosis weakness. Inferior aponeurosis weakness can be diagnosed by loss of excursion of the lower lid on downward gaze. The aims in general are to strengthen tissues that are weak or to shorten those that are lax.

The Ziegler cautery method is an office procedure which can be used in patients with slight horizontal laxity and minimal inferior aponeurosis weakness. The double triangle repair of entropion may be indicated for those patients with senile entropion who do not have marked lid laxity or weakness of the lower lid retractors. In patients with moderate to severe senile entropion with marked horizontal laxity of the lid, a full-thickness lid resection at the lateral canthus is indicated. Moderate to severe senile entropion with little horizontal elongation but evidence of inferior aponeurosis weakness is an indication for tucking of the inferior aponeurosis.

ZIEGLER CAUTERY

Robert B. O'Dair, M.D.

Many techniques have been described in which a thermal burn is used to correct entropion of the lower eyelid by creating an adherent scar between skin, orbicularis muscle, and tarsus. The barrier created prevents the orbicularis muscle from riding upward and turning the lid in. Since Ziegler cautery is rapid and easy to perform, it may be useful in elderly patients with mild entropion who wish to avoid more extensive surgical procedures. The major disadvantage of this procedure relates to the difficulty in controlling the burn. Occasionally, an overcorrection may occur if excess cautery is applied.

Anesthesia is obtained by infiltration. Two rows of penetrating electrocautery are applied to the lower lid along the length of the tarsus in parallel lines 4 and 7 mm from the lid margin [1]. The lower row is placed below the tarsal margin. Usually, five or six equally spaced burns in each row are sufficient. The upper row achieves adherence between skin, orbicularis muscle, and tarsus, and the lower row between skin, orbicularis muscle, and the deeper tissues.

The patient should be warned about the charring from the burn reaction, which may be alarming initially. Cool compresses for the first week relieve discomfort. The skin lesions heal in two or three weeks, leaving almost imperceptible scars.

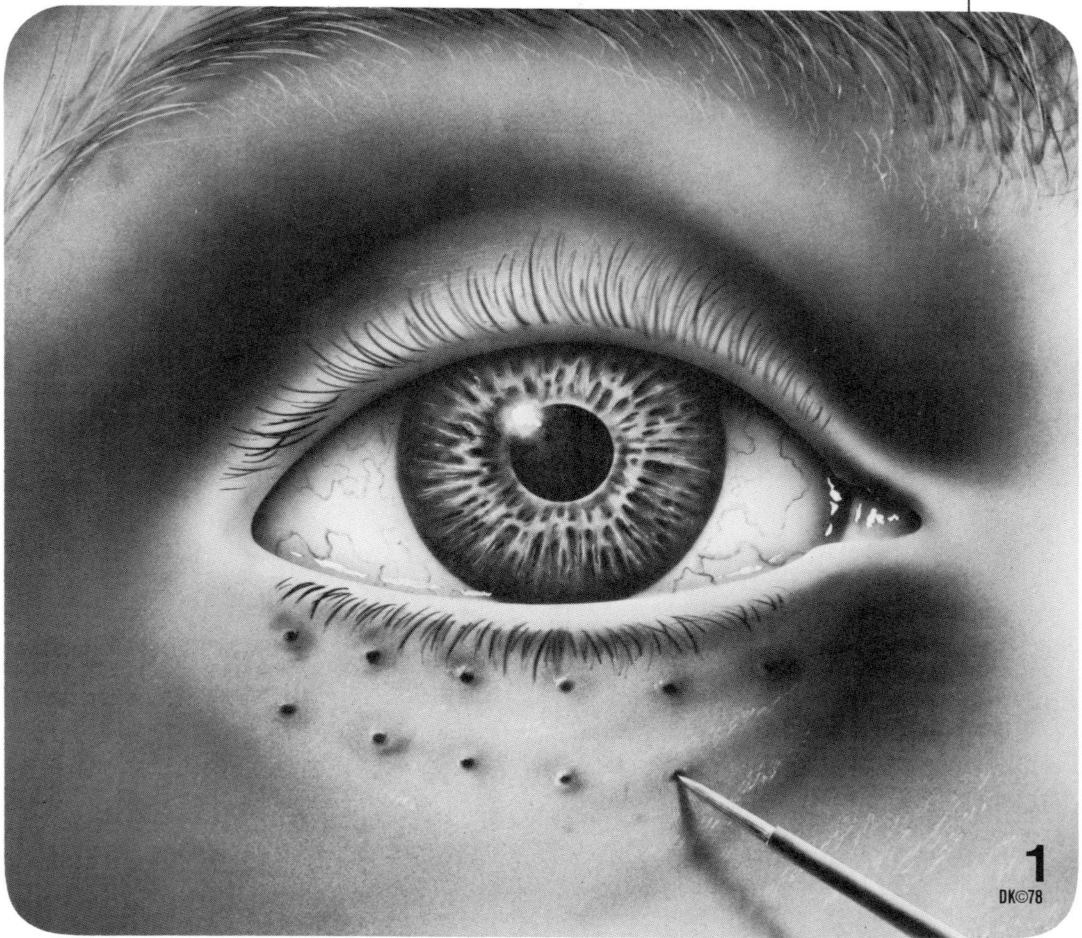

Donald A. Killer

DOUBLE TRIANGLE REPAIR OF ENTROPION

Robert B. O'Dair, M.D.

The Fox double triangle repair has enjoyed consistent success throughout the years for correction of senile entropion. Without changing the horizontal dimension of the lid margin, the procedure accomplishes shortening of the lower lid, particularly the lower tarsus, and tightens horizontal support of the lower lid by skin and orbicularis muscle.

Anesthesia is obtained by infiltration. A large chalazion clamp, applied to the center of the everted lower lid, extends below the lower margin of the tarsus [1]. The planned apex of the inner triangle is at the lid margin and includes the gray line. The base of the triangle, at the tarsal border, measures 6 to 8 mm. The incisions are made with a Bard-Parker No. 15 blade and include only tarsus, not underlying orbicularis muscle. The apex of the tarsal triangle is grasped with forceps, and the triangle is dissected from the underlying orbicularis muscle with Westcott scissors [2].

A base-up triangle is made on the skin surface, 2 mm temporal to the lateral canthus. The base of the triangle is horizontal and at the same level as the canthus. All sides of the triangle measure 10 to 12 mm [3]. This triangle of skin and orbicularis muscle is excised [4].

The tarsal triangle is closed with four or five interrupted 5-0 chromic catgut sutures. The sutures are placed so that the knots are buried on the orbicularis side of the wound. Five or six interrupted sutures of 6-0 black silk close the skin triangle. The redundant skin fold created superiorly is excised and sutured [5]. The redundant fold of conjunctiva is also excised [6].

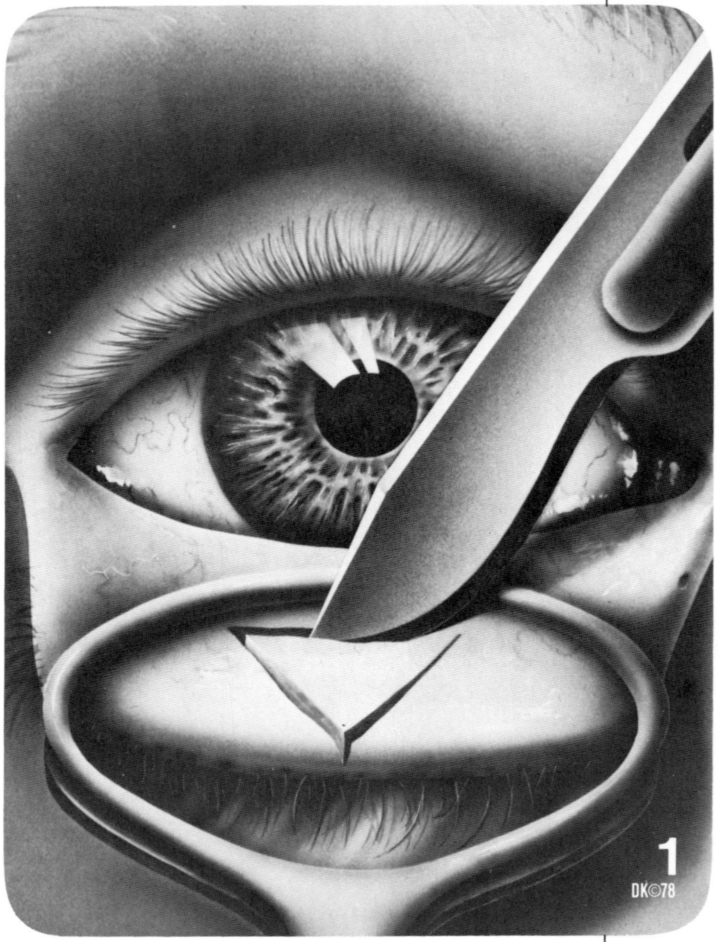

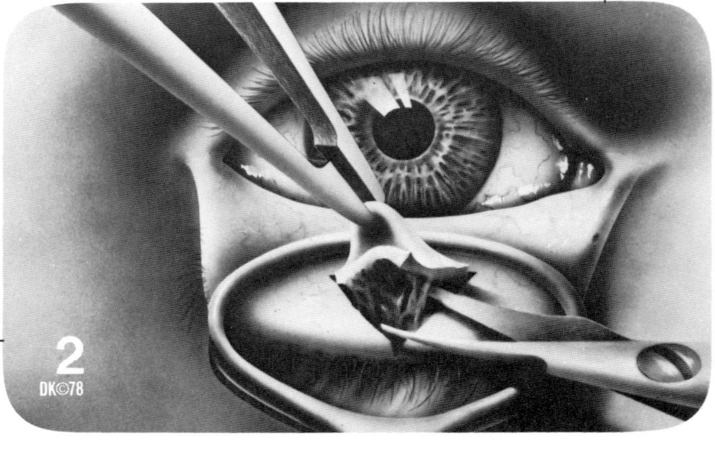

Donald H. Keller

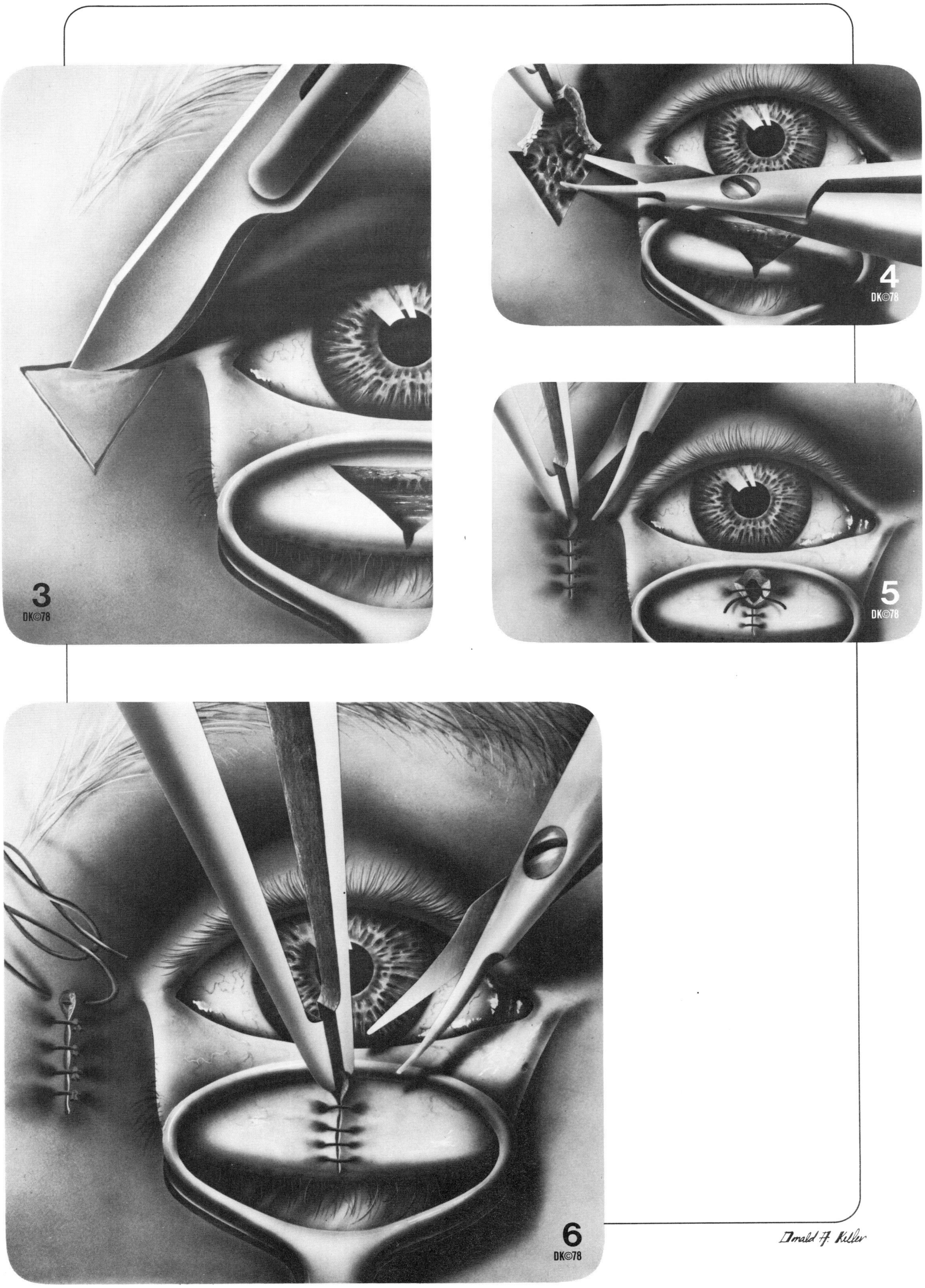

Donald A. Keller

HORIZONTAL LID SHORTENING

Robert B. O'Dair, M.D.

Horizontal shortening of the lid with plication of the orbicularis muscle is particularly well suited to those patients with entropion who show marked horizontal elongation of the lower lid. This procedure, which is modified from the original description by Bick, has been effective in approximately 75 percent of patients with senile entropion.

Infiltrative anesthesia is accomplished by injecting 1 percent lidocaine with epinephrine into the lower lid and lateral canthus. The planned line of incision at the lateral canthus extends the curve of the upper eyelid [1]. The lid is grasped with a skin hook near the canthus. The interior blade of a Stevens scissors is placed deep within the cul-de-sac at the canthus, and the external blade is on the skin surface [2]. The lid is completely severed from its attachment to the lateral canthal tendon. Bleeding usually is minimal and can be controlled with pressure.

The lower lid is drawn laterally to determine the amount of horizontal laxity, usually 3 to 6 mm. If too much lid is excised, the punctum will be directed too far laterally, outside the lacrimal lake, and tear drainage may be impaired. In addition, excessive shortening of the lid may cause a cosmetic blemish. Too little shortening results in undercorrection and recurrence. A 2-mm razor blade incision is made at the point where the lid crosses the outer canthus. This helps insure a clean edge for subsequent re-formation of the lateral canthus [3]. The scissors completes excision of the full thickness of the eyelid. The lower quarter of the lid excision extends laterally on an oblique angle to avoid creating a redundant skin fold at the lower margin [4].

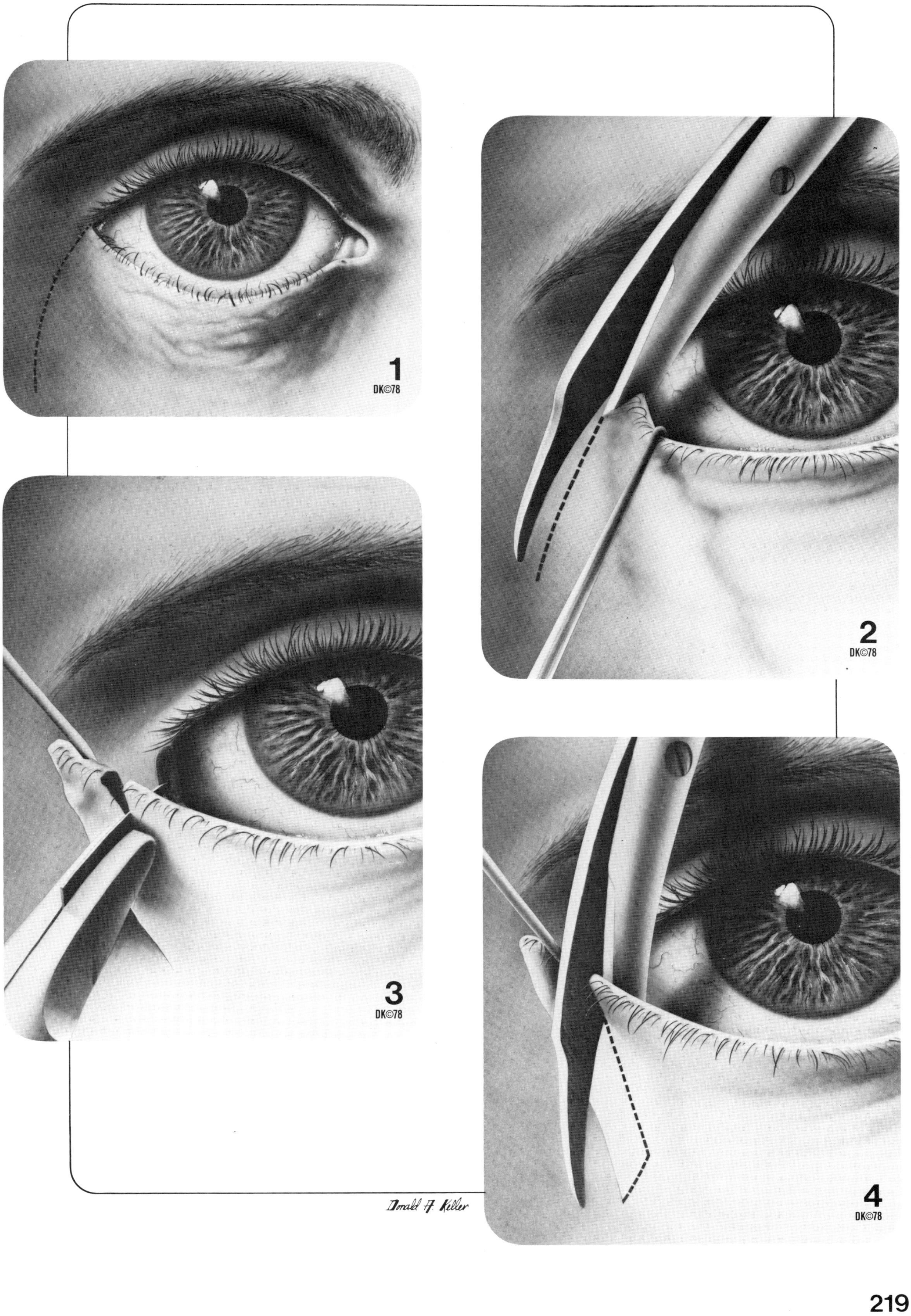
1
DK©78
2
DK©78
3
DK©78
4
DK©78
Donald A. Keller

A 4-0 black silk suture re-forms the lateral canthus [5]. It is placed first through the medial margin of the wound, starting 2 mm below the lash line. This bite includes skin, orbicularis muscle, and tarsal plate (OM) and (TP). The needle is then passed through the lateral margin of the wound to include a firm bite of the lateral canthal tendon (LCT); it exits through muscle and skin. In passing this suture through the lateral part of the wound, the surgeon can usually tell by feel that the relatively immobile canthal tendon is included in the bite. The suture is drawn taut temporarily with a single loop of a surgeon's knot to test approximation and re-formation of the lateral canthus. When the surgeon is satisfied with placement of this suture and the angle of the lateral canthus, the suture is loosened, and the muscle layer closed with interrupted sutures of 5-0 chromic catgut [5] [6]. These sutures reapproximate the orbicularis muscle with long subcutaneous bites through the muscle and appose the lower portion of the lid against the globe. Interrupted sutures of 6-0 silk close the skin [5] [6]. Exact approximation of the lateral canthus can be accomplished with one additional suture of 6-0 silk through the gray line [7]. Good surgical technique leaves the lid everted with snug apposition to the globe.

Usually no dressing is necessary. The 6-0 silk sutures may be removed on the fifth postoperative day, and the 4-0 silk suture usually remains for seven to ten days.

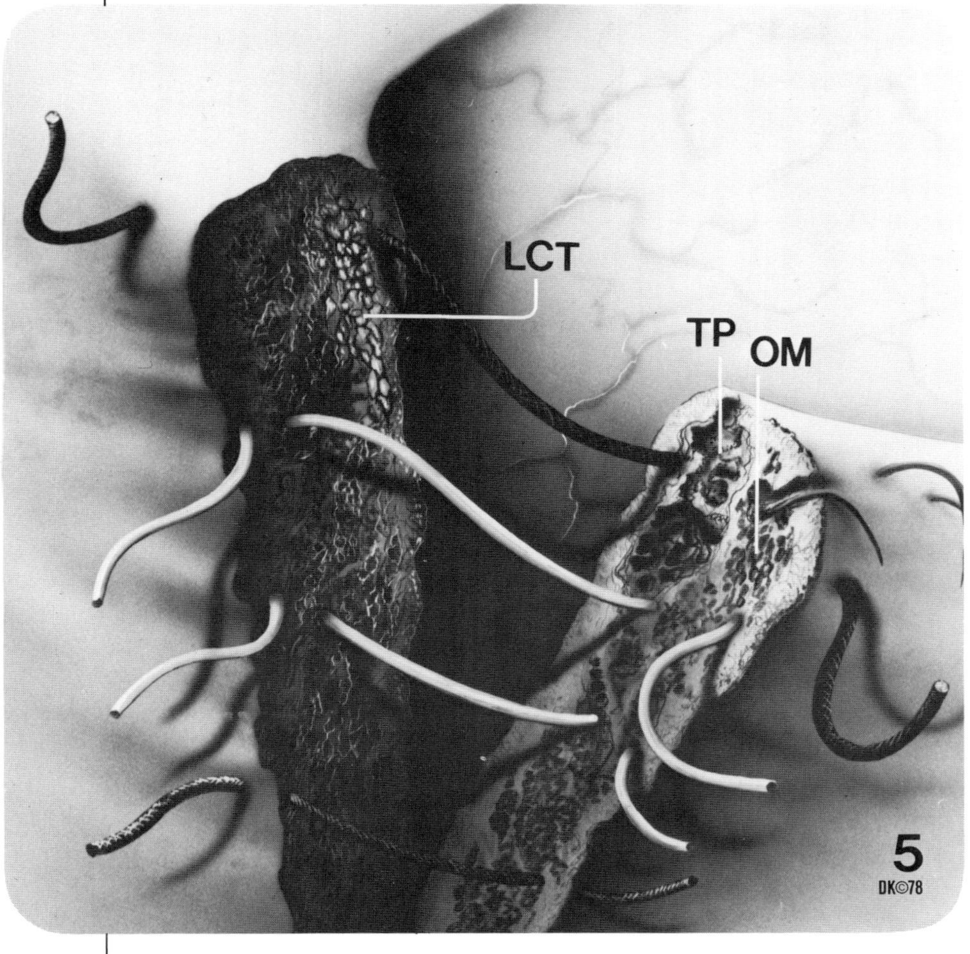

5
DK©78

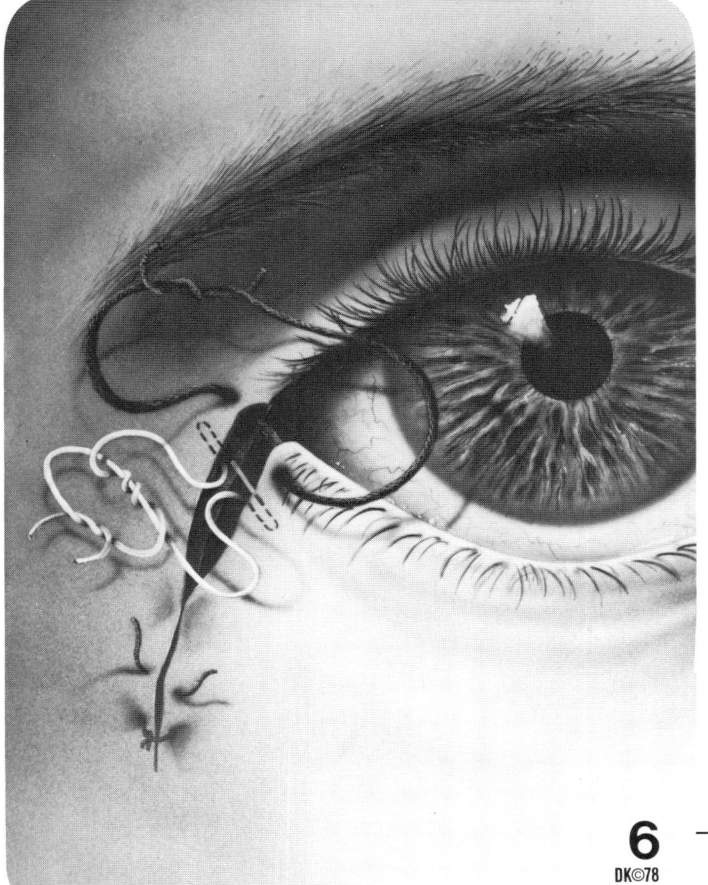

6
DK©78

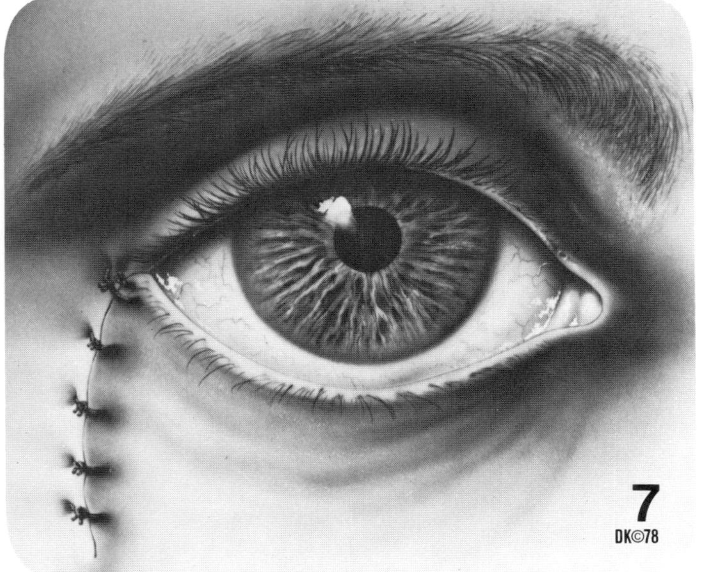

7
DK©78

Donald H. Keller

TUCKING OF THE INFERIOR APONEUROSIS

Robert B. O'Dair, M.D.

Tucking of the inferior aponeurosis is the entropion procedure particularly well suited to those patients without marked horizontal laxity who demonstrate a loss of downward movement of the lid on downgaze.

After anesthetic infiltration of the lower lid, skin incision is made 5 mm below and parallel to the lid margin along the lateral two thirds of the lid to expose the underlying orbicularis muscle [1]. The orbicularis muscle is divided bluntly and dissected upward, revealing the lower border of the tarsus and the filmy attachment of the orbital septum, T and S [2].

The orbital septum is dissected free from its attachment to the lower tarsal border for a distance of 10 mm horizontally by wiping a cotton-tipped applicator in a downward direction to expose the inferior aponeurosis [3]. Redundant skin and orbicularis muscle along the lower margin of the incision are excised [4]. To avoid undesirable shortening of the lid, usually not more than a 3- to 5-mm strip of orbicularis muscle and a lesser amount of skin are excised.

A 4-0 black silk suture is passed through the inferior skin border, and a 2-mm bite is made through the inferior aponeurosis, IA [5] [6]. Care must be taken not to penetrate the conjunctiva, arrow [5]. At this point, the inner surface of the lid is inspected to determine that the needle is visible through the conjunctiva. The suture is passed through the inferior border of the tarsus, T [5] [6], and finally through the skin.

The suture is tied temporarily with a surgeon's knot, and the lid is inspected. Ideally at this point, the patient has 3 mm of downward movement of the lid on downgaze. If this has been achieved, the suture is loosened, and four additional sutures are placed in a similar manner, approximately 3 mm apart [6]. If ectropion is present, the suture is removed, and a bite of the inferior aponeurosis is taken closer to the inferior tarsal border. If there is an undercorrection, the suture through the inferior aponeurosis is replaced further from the lower border of the tarsus.

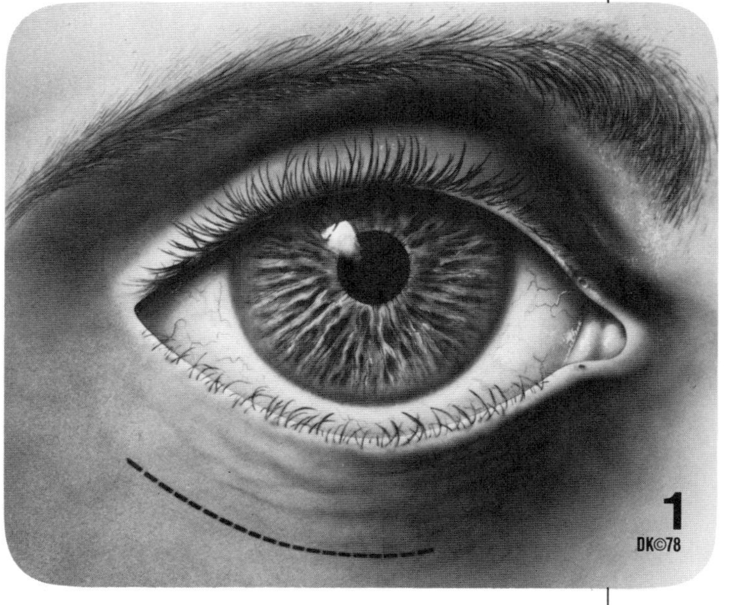

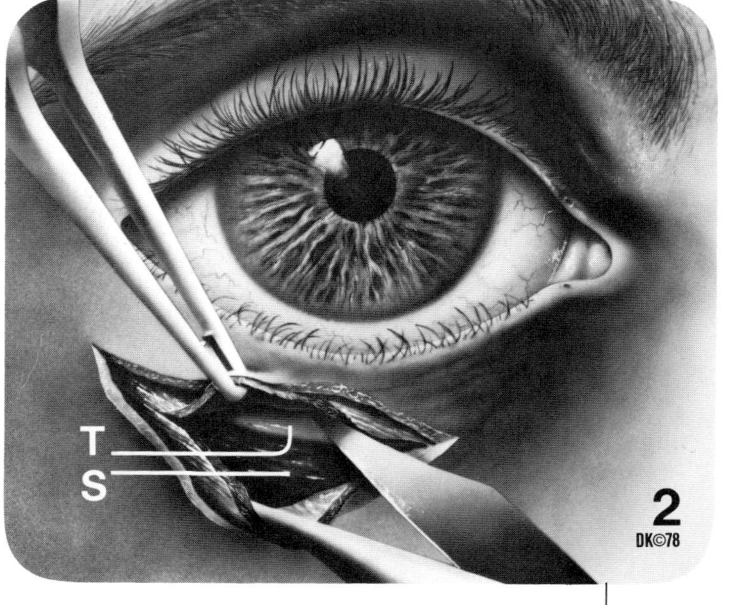

Usually no dressing is necessary, and cool compresses in the early postoperative course minimize edema. Sutures are removed in six to eight days. If overcorrection becomes apparent, sutures may be removed somewhat earlier.

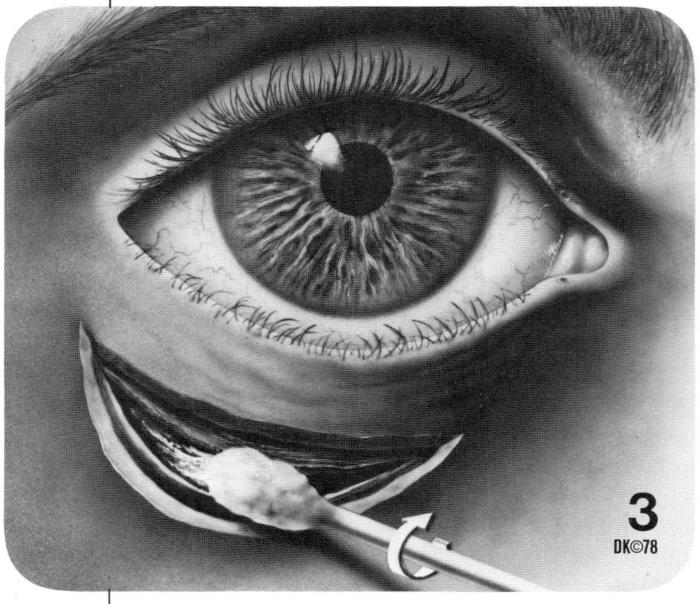
3
DK©78

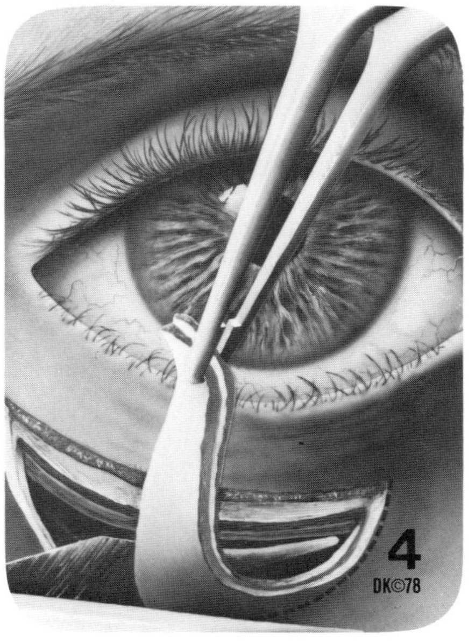
4
DK©78

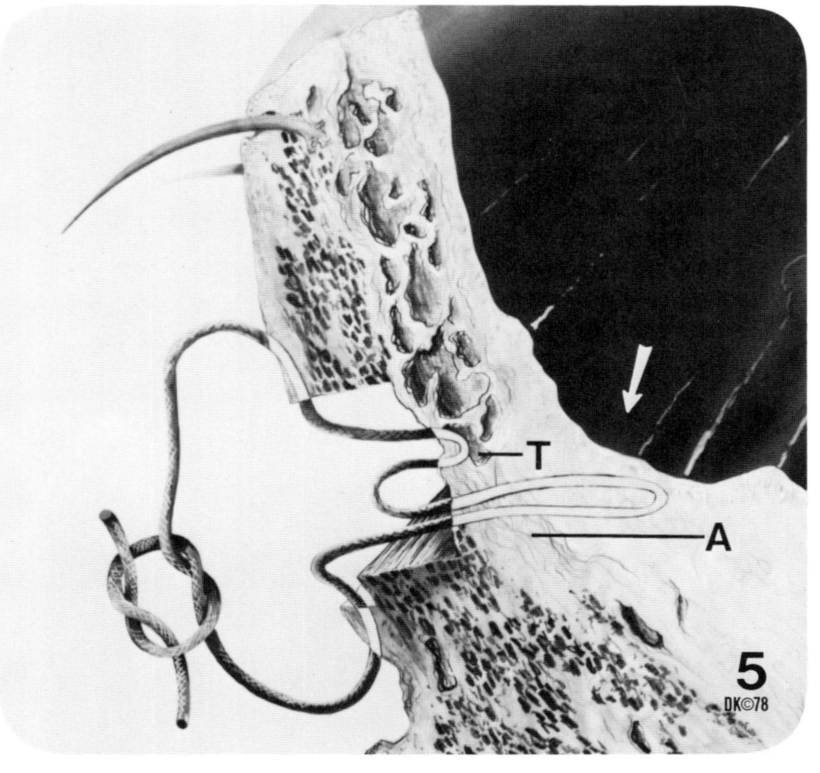
T
A
5
DK©78

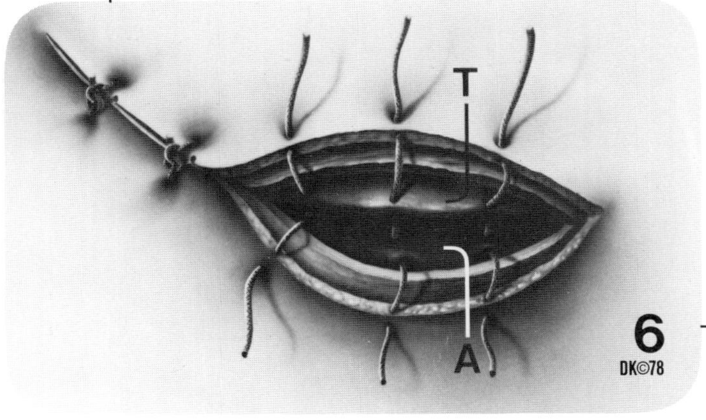
T
A
6
DK©78

TRANSVERSE BLEPHAROTOMY WITH LID ROTATION

Robert B. O'Dair, M.D.

Cicatricial entropion may involve the upper or the lower lid. The common causes are chemical burns, trauma, infections, such as trachoma, and inflammation seen with ocular pemphigoid. For slight cicatricial entropion of the lower lid, tucking of the inferior aponeurosis may be adequate. For moderate to severe entropion, the Weis procedure to attach palpebral conjunctiva to lid skin is the most reliable.

The proposed line of incision [1] begins slightly lateral to the punctum and extends parallel to the lid margin, just short of the lateral canthus. To guard against inadvertent corneal damage, a cornea protector is placed prior to attaching a large chalazion clamp. This clamp stabilizes the lid and allows more accurate incision [2]. A razor blade incision is made 3 mm below the lower lid margin to expose the underlying orbicularis muscle. The clamp is reversed and a similar incision is made on the conjunctival surface through the tarsus [3]. A Stevens scissors creates a small buttonhole to join the two incisions, and the orbicularis is cut along the entire extent of the wound, thereby creating a transverse blepharotomy [4].

Four double-armed 4-0 black silk sutures are passed through the conjunctiva and tarsus, T [5] at the lower edge of the wound, and then anteriorly and subcutaneously through the upper section of the wound to emerge at the lash line [5] [6].

These evenly placed sutures are tied securely over cotton pledgets [5] [6]. The tension created along the anterior portion of the wound is usually sufficient to evert the lid margin. The sutures remain in place for one week but can be removed earlier if overcorrection becomes apparent. Interrupted sutures of 6-0 black silk close the skin incision [5] [6]. These may be removed on the fifth postoperative day.

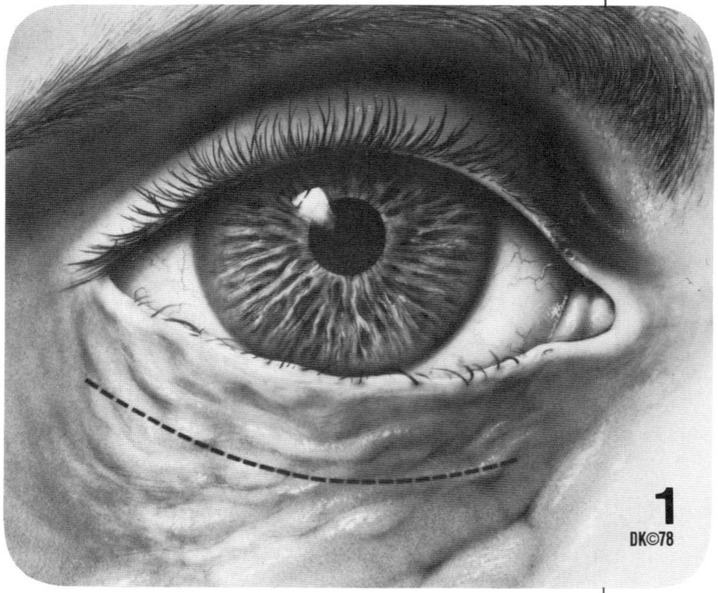

1
DK©78

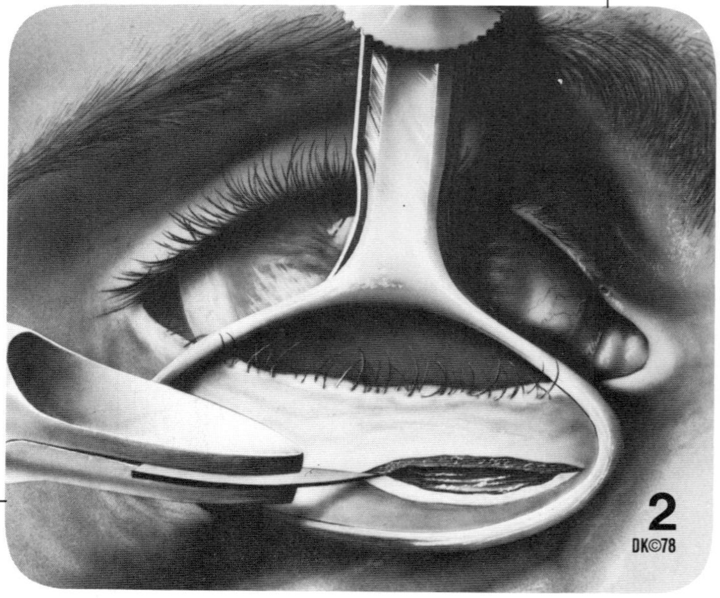

2
DK©78

Donald A. Killer

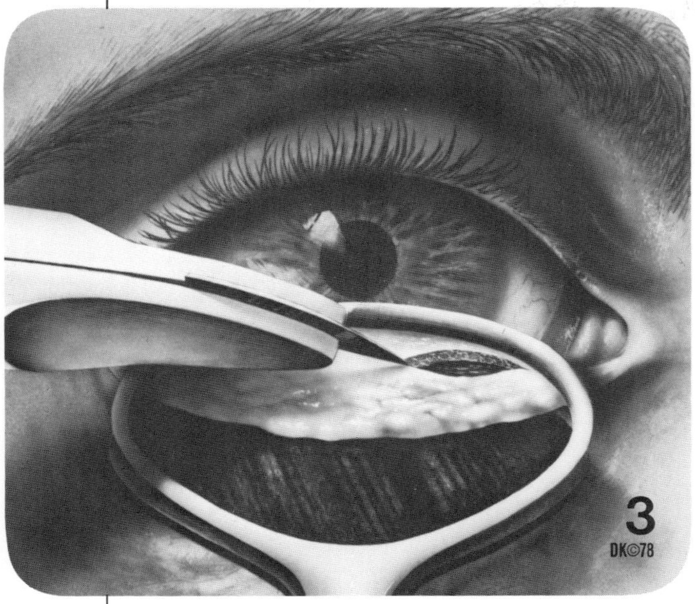
3
DK©78

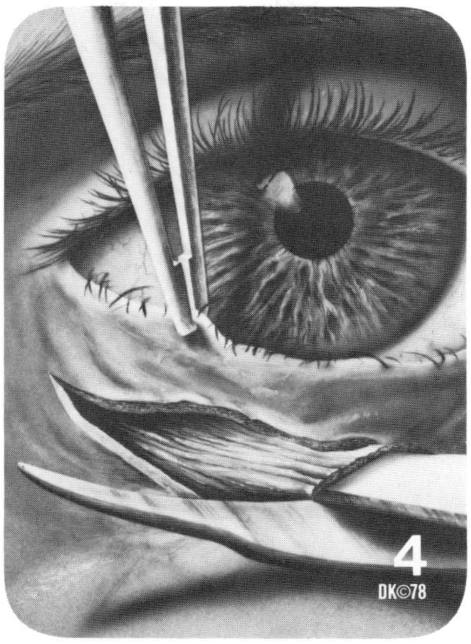
4
DK©78

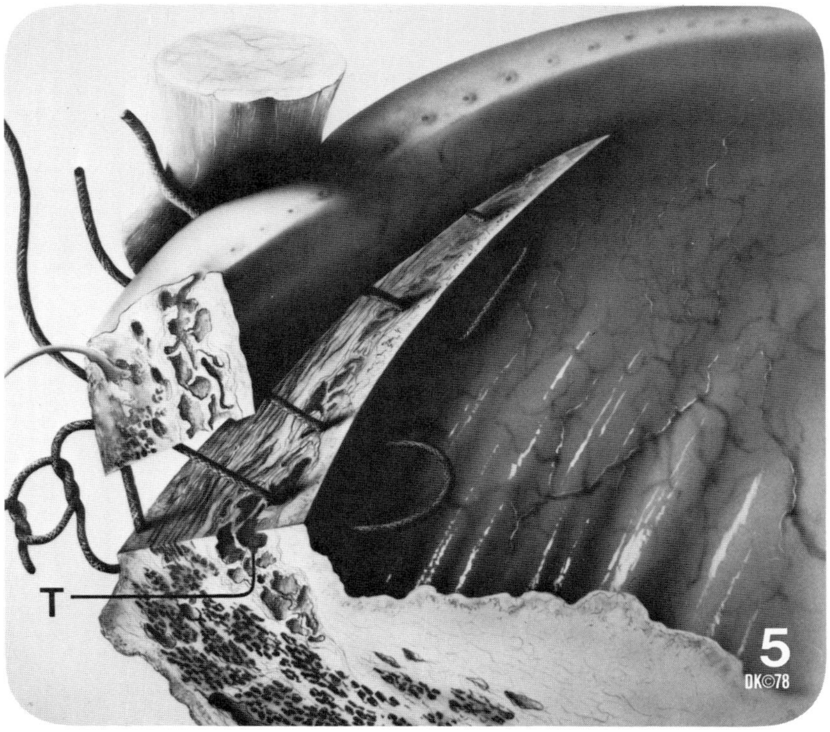
T
5
DK©78

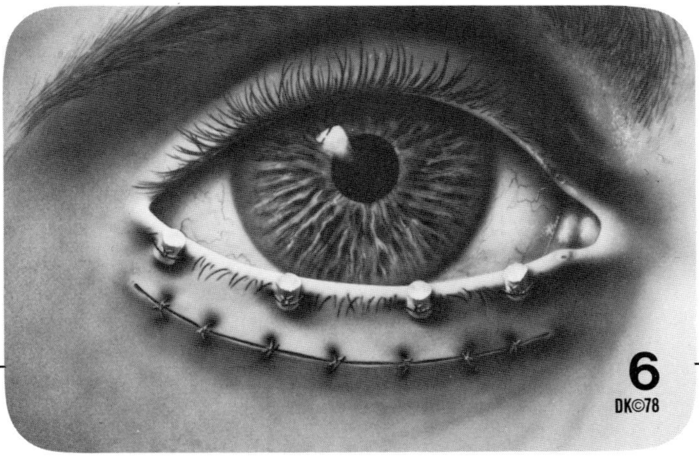
6
DK©78

ECTROPION

Ectropion is an outward turning of the eyelid. Most common is the senile type, which involves the lower lid. Cicatricial ectropion may be secondary to shortening of the skin-orbicularis layer after trauma or infection. Mechanical ectropion is usually caused by the external traction of a lid tumor. Congenital ectropion is rare and frequently associated with other congenital facial abnormalities.

The basic cause of senile ectropion is relaxation of the lower lid, accompanied by horizontal elongation and loss of muscle tone. The process is first noted medially with eversion of the punctum. Epiphora is often the first symptom, and the constant wiping of overflow tears by the patient tends to be aggravating. Further eversion with keratinization of the conjunctiva ensues. The final result is laxity of the entire lid, with or without elongation of the medial canthal tendon. Treatment depends on the stage of the pathologic process and the most predominant tissue defect. The following three procedures may be used alone or in combination to manage senile ectropion.

EXCISION OF MEDIAL SPINDLE OF CONJUNCTIVA

Robert B. O'Dair, M.D.

This procedure is used to treat mild punctal eversion. In more severe cases of punctal eversion, it may be combined with full-thickness excision of the lid at the lateral canthus.

Anesthesia of the lower lid is achieved by infiltration. The area of conjunctiva to be excised is a spindle about 6 mm long, centered horizontally below the punctum [1]. The assistant holds a lacrimal probe in the lower canaliculus to mark its location and to prevent inadvertent damage to this structure. A No. 11 Bard-Parker blade creates the superior curved incision beginning 3 mm below the punctum to avoid damage to the ampulla. The incision outlines the spindle of tissue to be excised, which extends in depth to the orbicularis muscle [2]. One end of the spindle is grasped with a Castroviejo forceps, and the spindle is excised with Westcott scissors [3]. Closure with three interrupted sutures of 6-0 black silk corrects the punctal eversion [4].

Postoperatively, warm compresses diminish the surgical reaction and make the patient more comfortable. The sutures are removed one week after surgery.

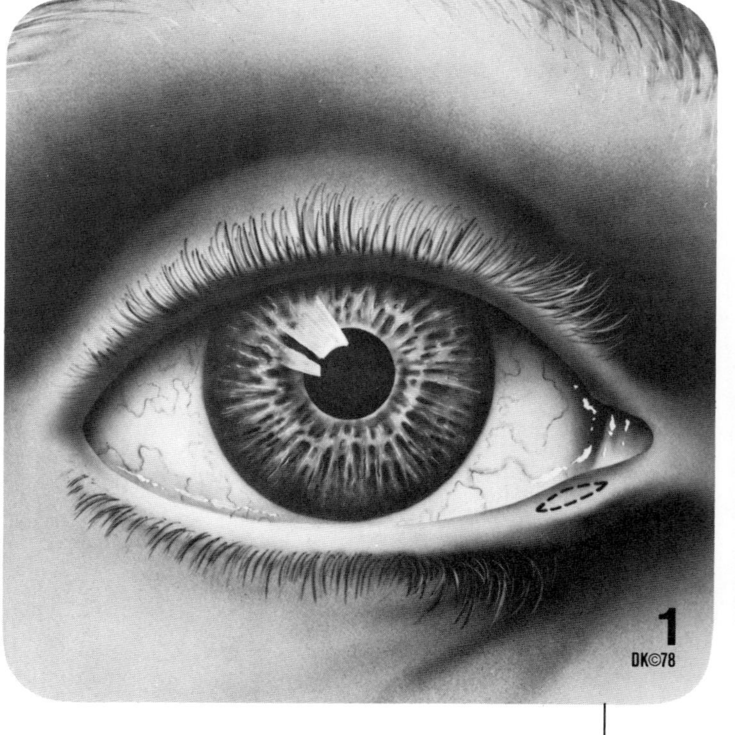

Donald F. Keller

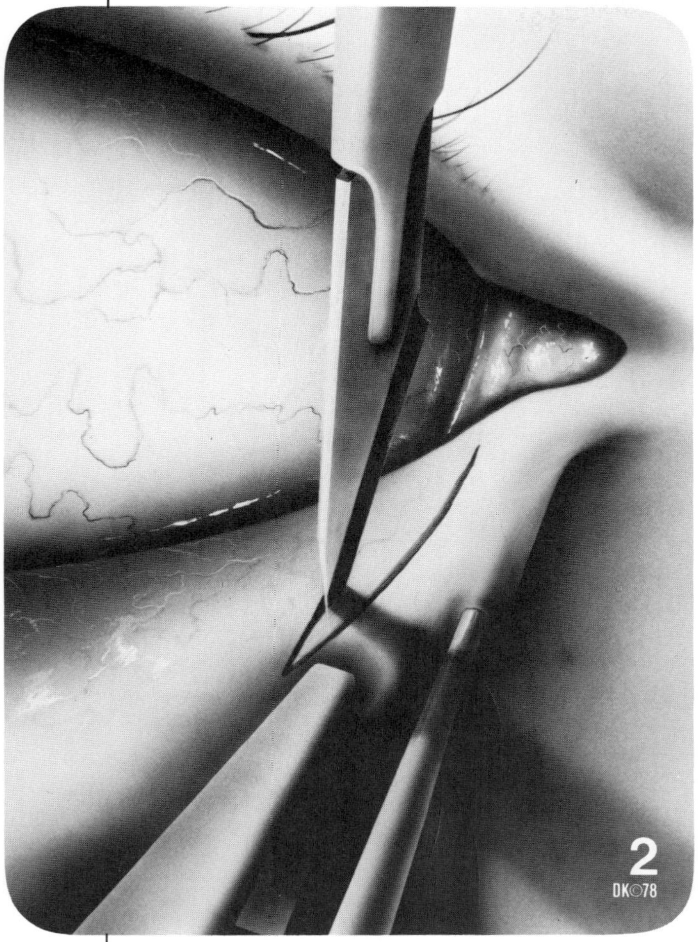

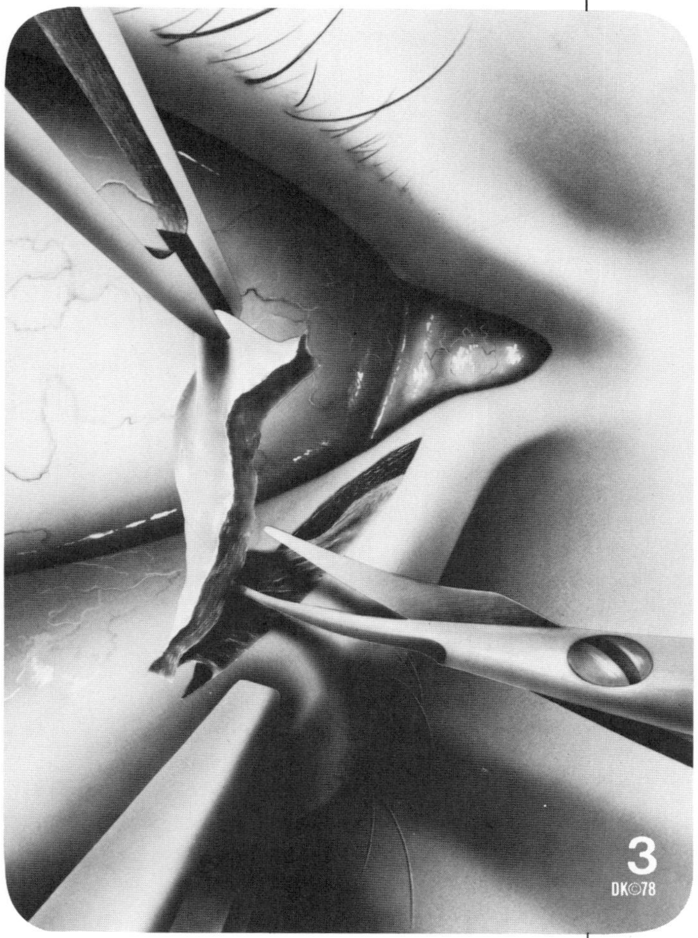

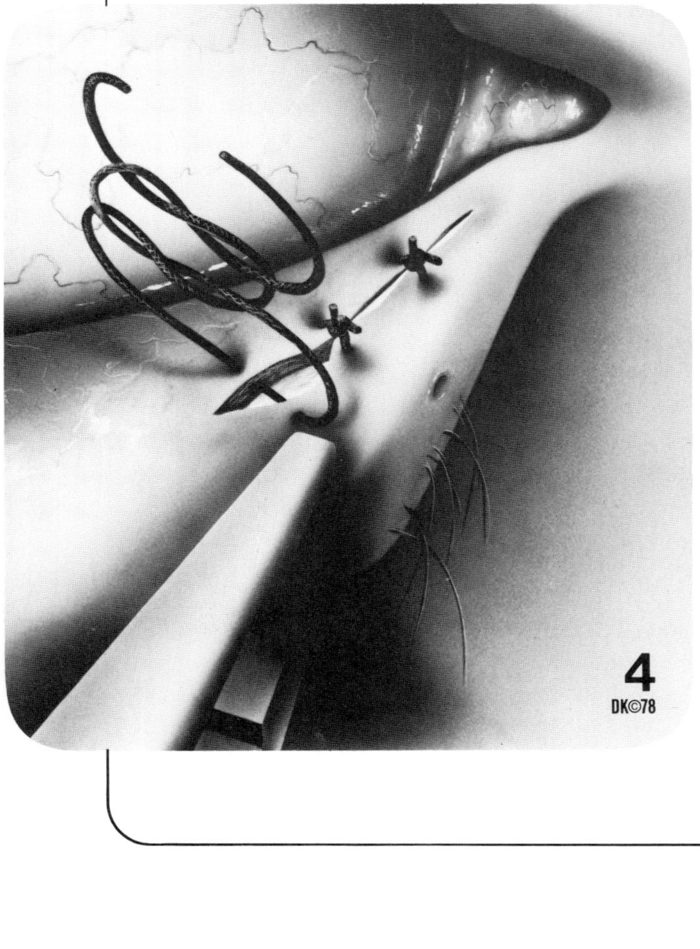

Donald A. Keller

TUCKING OF THE MEDIAL CANTHAL TENDON

Robert B. O'Dair, M.D.

Tucking of the medial canthal tendon is helpful in treating moderate senile ectropion when the defect is laxity and elongation of the medial canthal tendon. In severe cases, this procedure may be combined with shortening of the lid at the lateral canthus.

After administration of local anesthesia by infiltration, a probe is placed in the lower canaliculus to mark its location. An incision through the skin to orbicularis begins slightly medial to the punctum, parallel to and 2 mm below the lid margin. It extends approximately 6 mm and follows the curve of the lid to the point overlying the insertion of the medial canthal tendon [1]. The skin is dissected inferiorly away from the underlying orbicularis muscle for approximately 3 mm and the upper skin flap superiorly to the lid margin to expose the medial canthal tendon. Care is taken to avoid injury to the canaliculus.

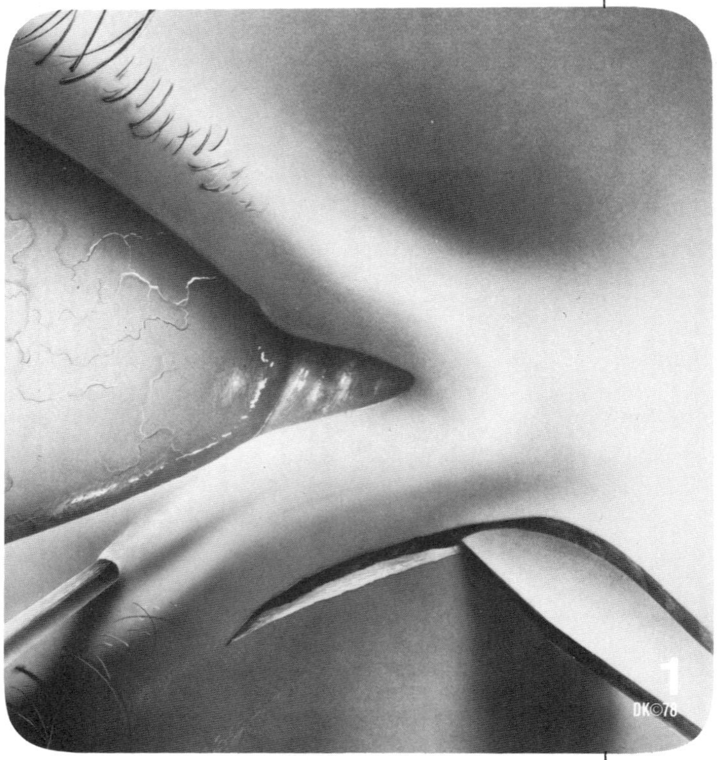

Since the angular vessels cross the medial canthal tendon 2 to 3 mm from its attachment to bone, the surgeon retracts the vessels with a muscle hook. If the angular vessels are cut inadvertently, the bleeding is easily controlled with cautery.

With a suture of 6-0 white silk, the surgeon takes a firm bite of the tendon at its insertion [2]. A Thorpe forceps is used to grasp the tendon laterally and draw it toward its insertion to estimate the amount of its laxity. When the lid is sufficiently tightened, a second bite of the tendon is taken to shorten it, and the square-knot tie is completed [3]. This may result in a temporary distortion of the canaliculus, yet ultimately does not interfere with lacrimal drainage.

Meticulous closure of the skin with 6-0 black silk assures covering of the plicated tendon [4].

Warm compresses reduce postoperative inflammation. The 6-0 white silk suture remains, while the skin sutures of 6-0 black silk may be removed one week after operation.

Donald F. Keller

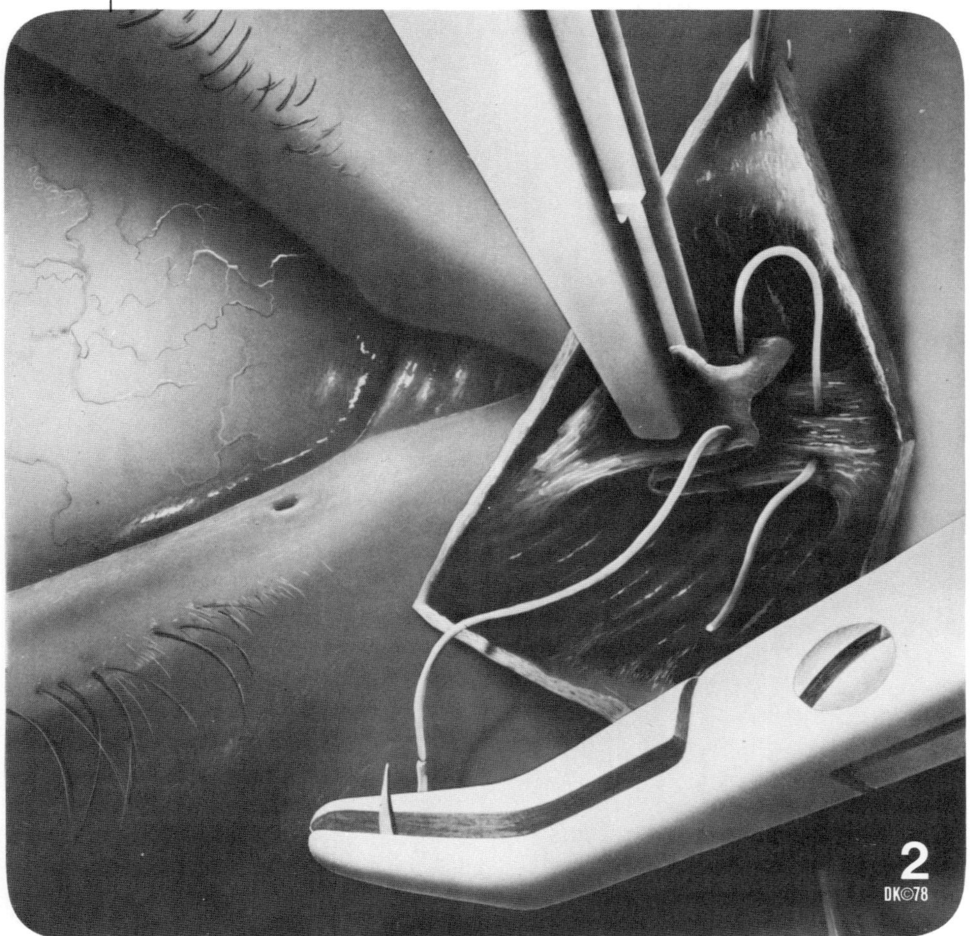

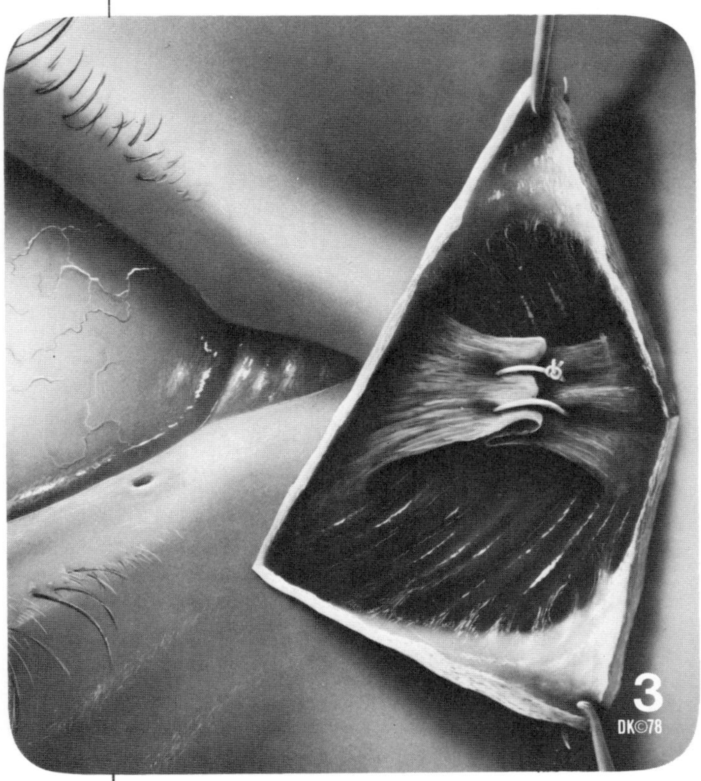

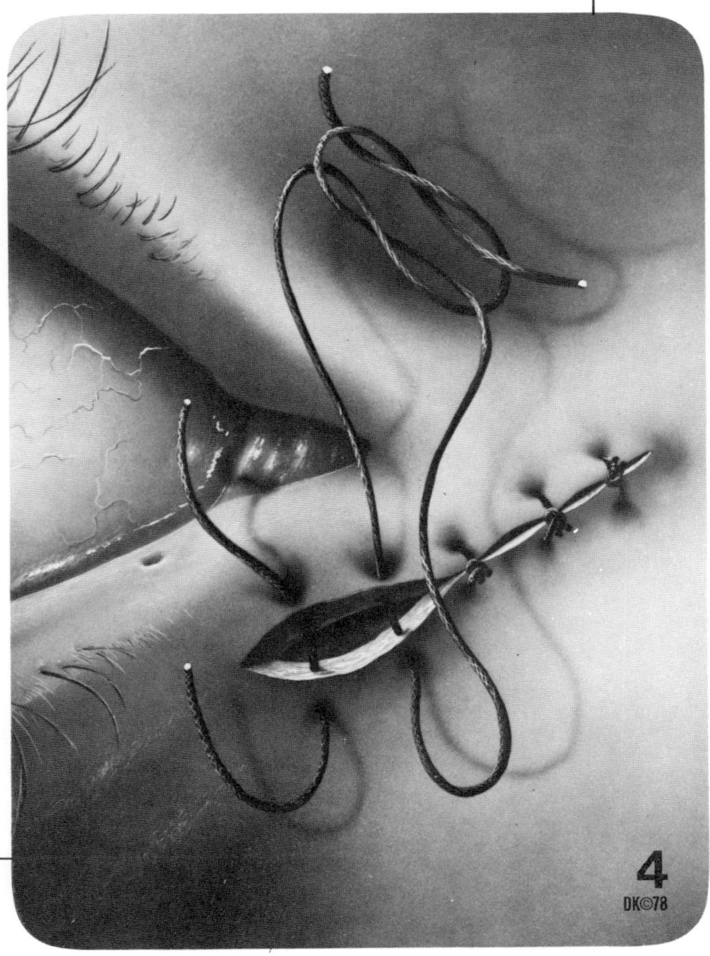

Donald A. Keller

HORIZONTAL LID SHORTENING

Robert B. O'Dair, M.D.

Full-thickness wedge excision at the lateral canthus is useful to shorten the lower lid horizontally in moderate to severe senile ectropion, when the laxity involves the entire lid. It may be used in combination with conjunctival spindle excision or shortening of the medial canthal tendon.

The preliminary steps of this procedure are identical to those of horizontal lid shortening with plication of the orbicularis muscle to correct marked senile entropion. The differences between the two procedures are the shape of the wedge excised—triangular in this procedure and trapezoidal in the entropion procedure—and simple end-to-end reapproximation of the orbicularis muscle without plication in this procedure.

After local infiltration, the lid is grasped with a skin hook near the lateral canthus. The lid is detached at the canthus with Stevens scissors, one blade of which is placed deep within the cul-de-sac, in a line corresponding to an extension of the upper lid curve [1]. Bleeding may be controlled by pressure.

The surgeon draws the lid laterally to estimate the proper amount of shortening, usually 3 to 6 mm. The point at which the lid crosses the canthus is marked with a 2-mm vertical razor blade incision through the lid margin [2]. The scissors completes excision of the full-thickness base-up triangle of the eyelid [3].

The canthus is re-formed with a suture of 4-0 black silk that passes from the skin edge of the severed lid to take a firm bite of orbicularis muscle and tarsus and then exits from the wound. It is then passed through the lateral canthal tendon, muscle, and skin on the opposing wound edge [4]. The suture is tightened temporarily to test approximation and re-formation of the lateral canthus. After the accuracy of approximation is assured, the knot is loosened; the muscle is closed with interrupted sutures of 5-0 chromic catgut and the skin with interrupted sutures of 6-0 black silk [5] [6]. One additional suture of 6-0 black silk at the lid margin assures precise re-formation of the gray line.

Usually no dressing is necessary. The 6-0 sutures can be removed on the fifth post-operative day and the 4-0 black silk after ten days.

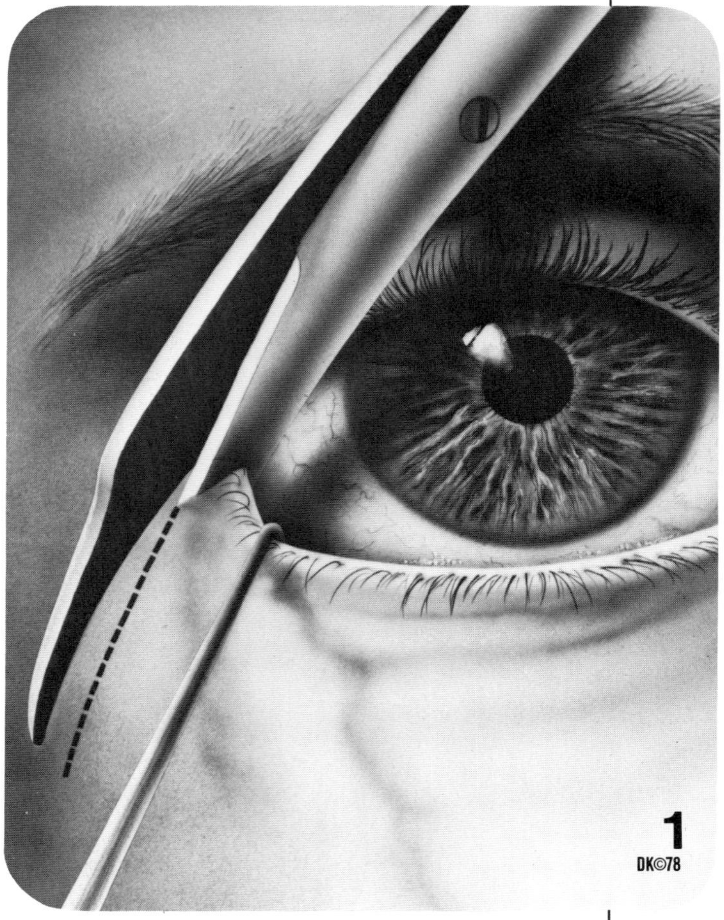

1

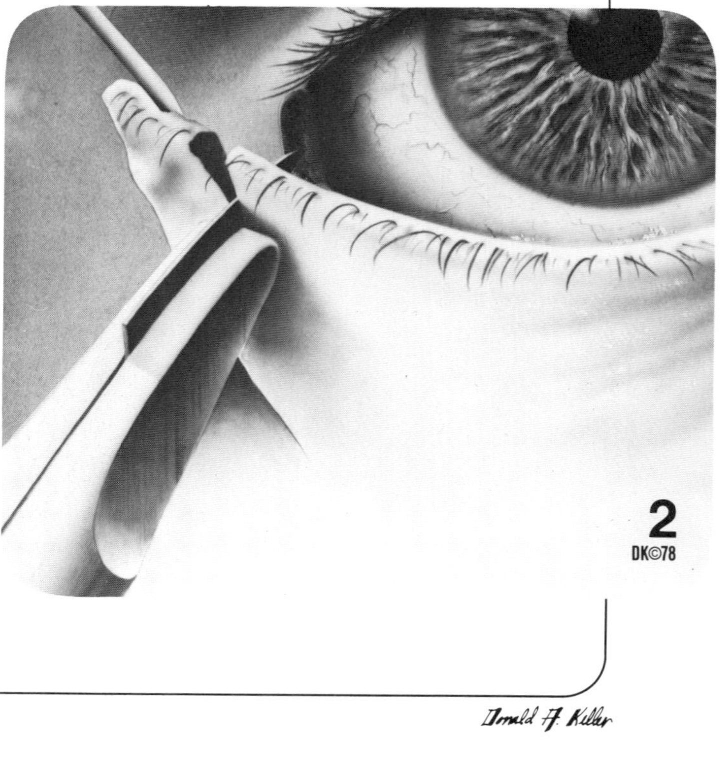

2

Donald F. Keller

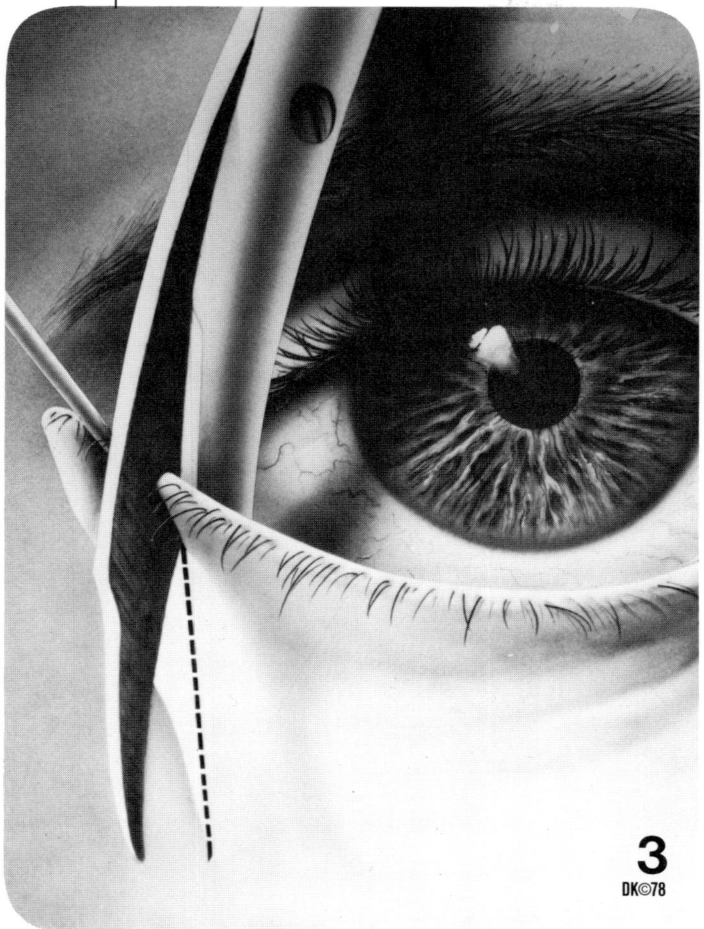

3
DK©78

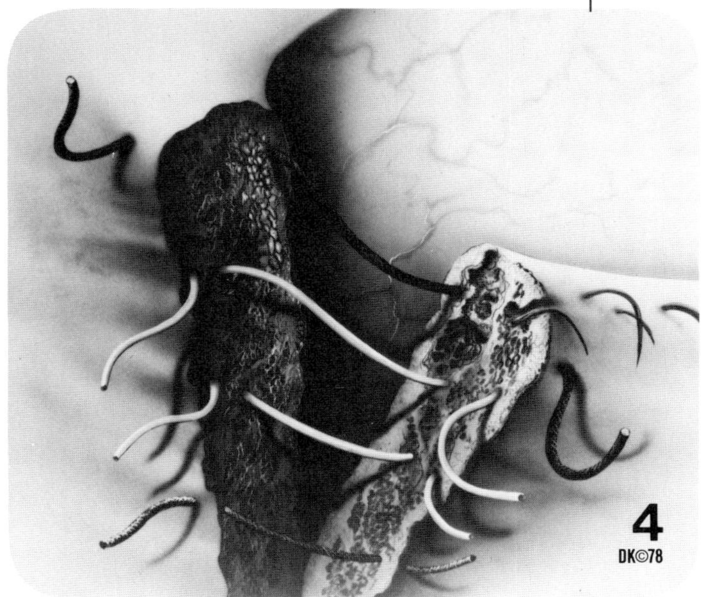

4
DK©78

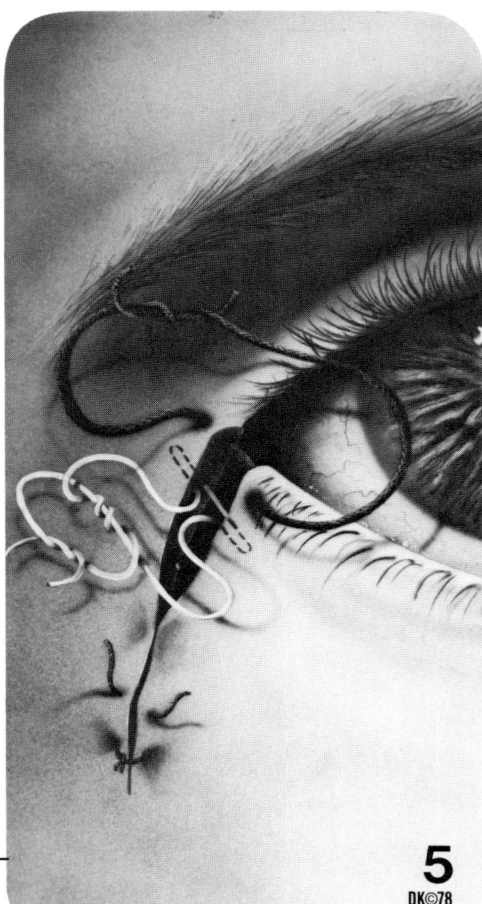

5
DK©78

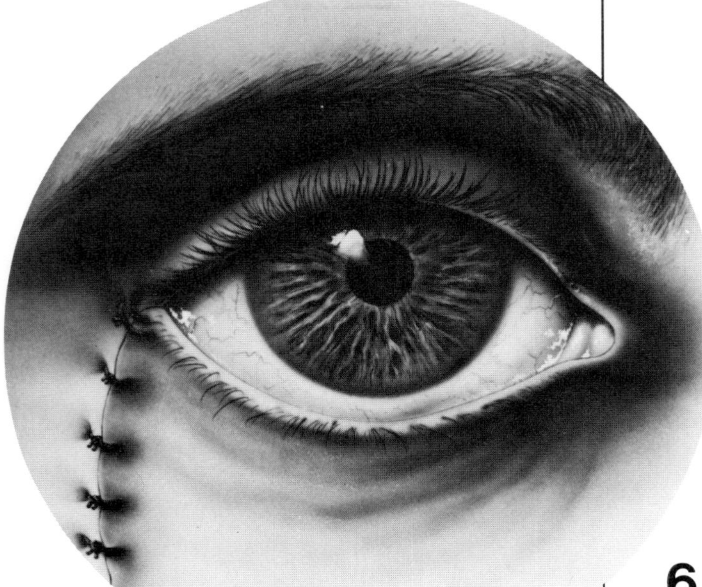

6
DK©78

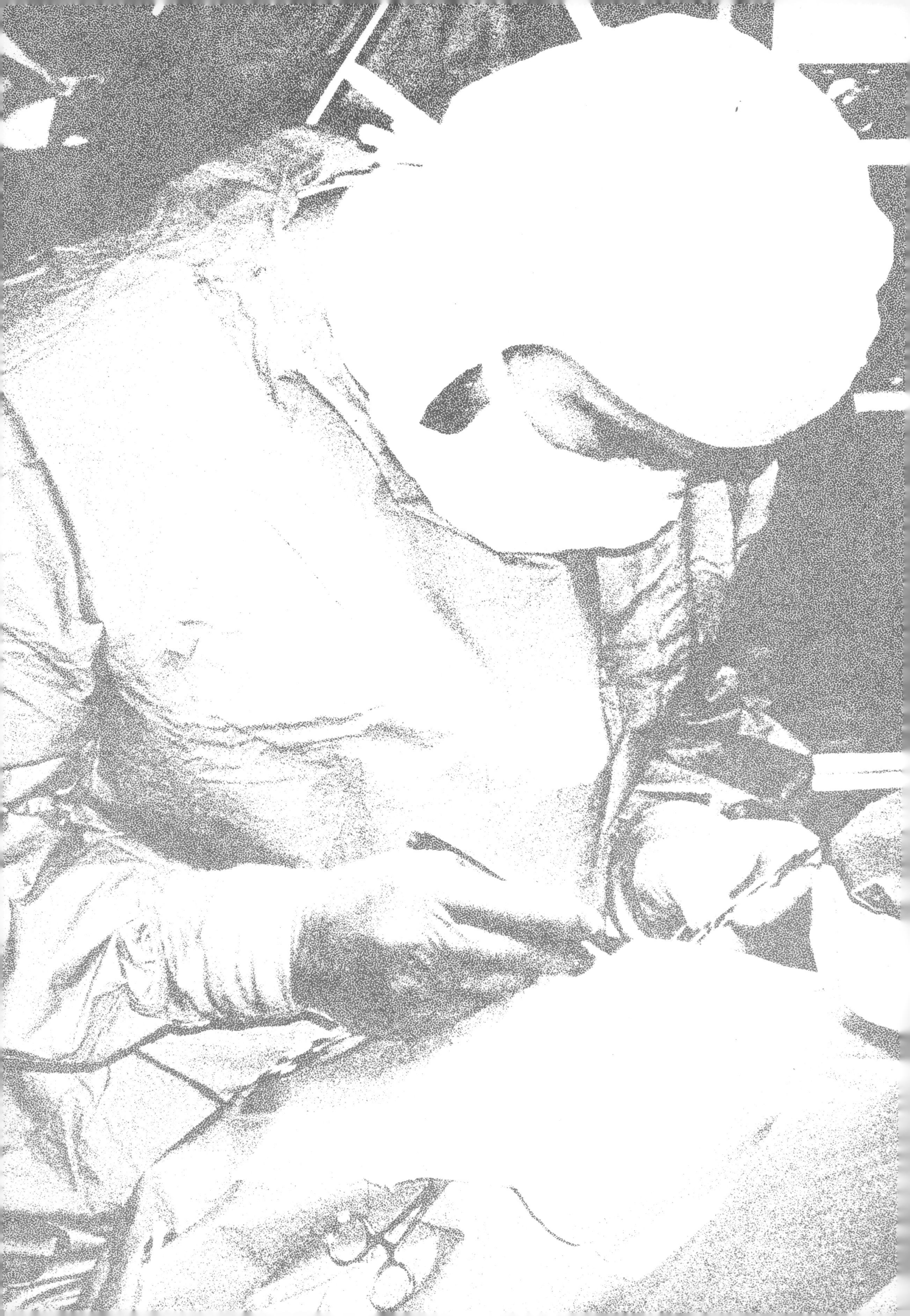

8
LACRIMAL APPARATUS
SURGERY

ANATOMY OF THE LACRIMAL EXCRETORY SYSTEM

John A. Burns, M.D.

A comprehensive knowledge of the lacrimal excretory system is extremely important in preoperative and intraoperative management of patients with either lacrimal obstruction or trauma to this region.

A lacrimal papilla, PA [1], appears on the medial aspect of the upper and lower lid margins, slightly elevated from the surface. The inferior punctum is 7 mm from the medial canthus, while the superior punctum is 6 mm from the medial canthus. In the center of the papilla is the punctum, PU [2], easily recognizable by the glistening white ring of fibroelastic tissue that surrounds the opening. The punctal opening, about 0.3 mm in diameter, faces slightly posteriorly and leads to the vertical canaliculus (VC) and then the horizontal canaliculus (HC). Immediately within the canaliculus, the system dilates to approximately 0.5 mm and extends vertically 2 mm. The medial portion of the canalicular system, the horizontal canaliculus, is approximately 8 mm long. In actuality, the lower lid canaliculus is inclined upward to the lateral wall of the lacrimal sac at approximately a 15-degree angle. The upper canalicular system is similar, with the exception that the papilla is located approximately 1 mm more medially than in the lower lid, and the angle is inclined downward at approximately 25 degrees. In 90 percent of the population, the upper and lower canaliculi join just lateral to the lacrimal sac to form the common canaliculus (CC) at a point called the ampulla (AMP). The common canaliculus enters into the lateral wall of the lacrimal sac just above and posterior to its center at the common internal punctum (CP). In the absence of a common canaliculus, there are two openings into the lacrimal sac.

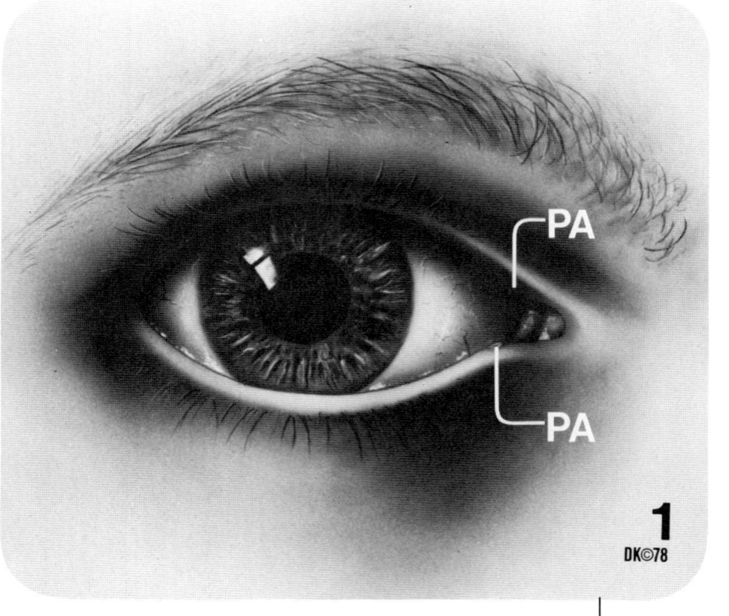

A view of the lacrimal sac from the inside shows a slight depression below the entrance of the common punctum, which is called the sinus of Maier (SM). A small flap of mucosa, the valve of Rosenmüller (VR), overhangs the sinus of Maier and the entrance of the common canaliculus, which is the common internal punctum (CP). The lacrimal sac is in the lacrimal fossa, LF [3], which is formed by the junction of the medial orbital and infraorbital rims. The orbital septum, SEP (broken line) passes posterior to the sac. The lacrimal sac, therefore, technically lies outside the orbital septum. The anterior wall of the lacrimal fossa is formed by the anterior lacrimal crest (ALC), which is a medial extension of the frontal process of the maxillary bone (MB). It is most easily found by following the infraorbital rim (IR) medially. The posterior aspect, the posterior lacrimal crest, PLC [4], is part of the lacrimal bone (LB) and is a direct downward projection of the medial orbital rim (MR). The junction of the maxillary and lacrimal bones forms the medial wall of the lacrimal fossa.

Horner's muscle (HM) inserts onto the posterior lacrimal crest immediately anterior to the attachment to the orbital septum. The

Donald F. Keller

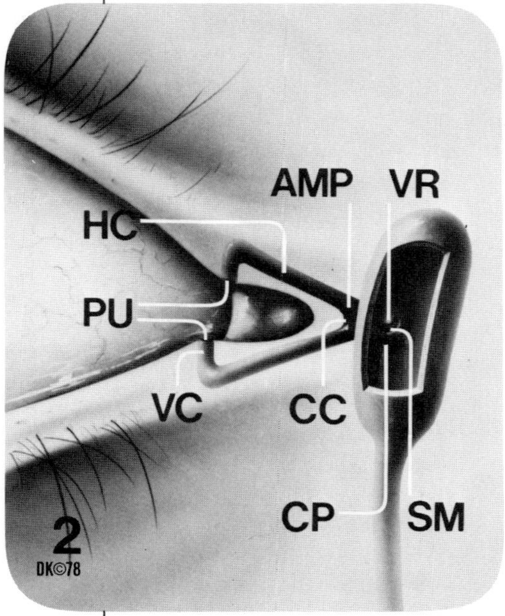

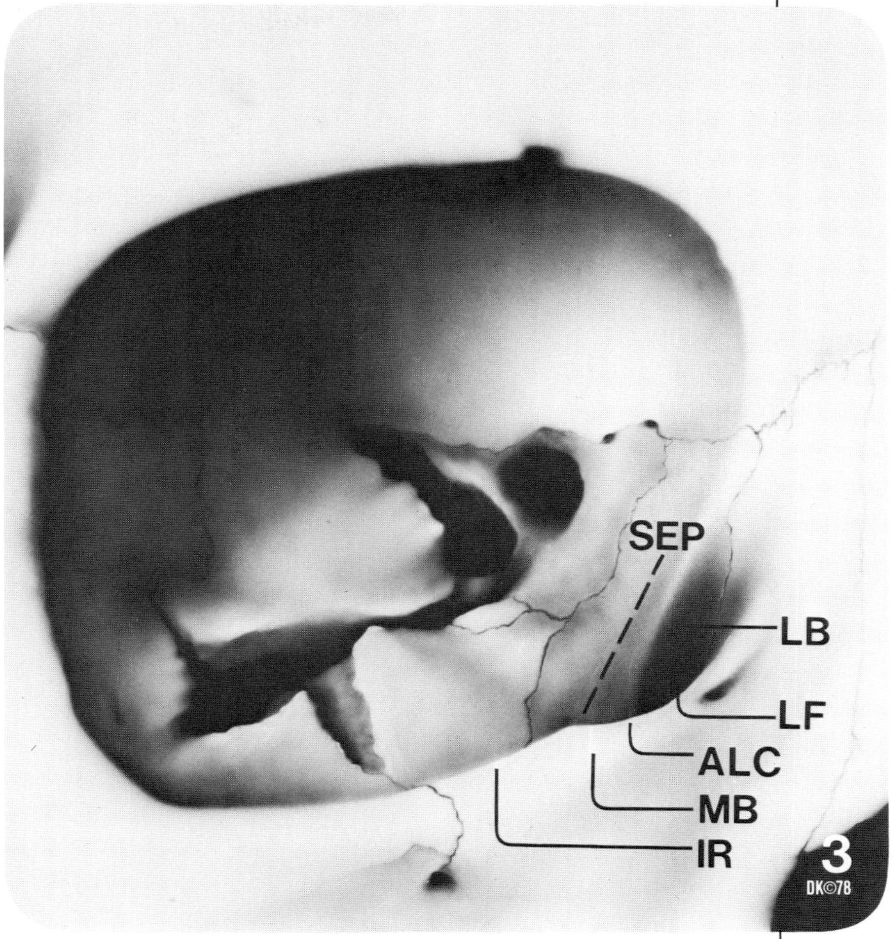

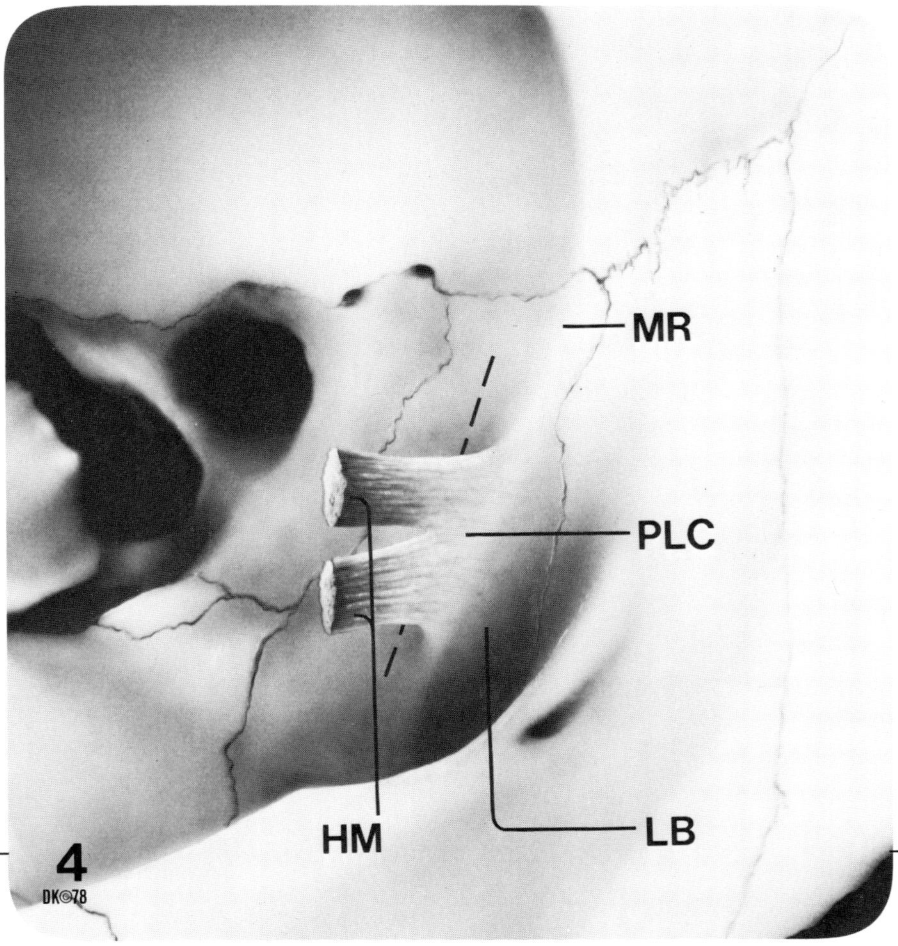

Donald A. Keller

periosteum, PER [5], surrounds the lacrimal sac (LS), creating a sac within a sac. Anterior to the sac, the pretarsal muscles (PTM) extend as the medial canthal tendon (MCT). The medial canthal tendon divides the sac into two portions—the dome, which is called the fundus (F) and the lower portion, which is called the body (B). The enveloping periosteum, pretarsal muscles, and Horner's muscle comprise the diaphragm of the lacrimal sac, necessary for normal functioning of the lacrimal pump.

The nasolacrimal duct, NLD [5] [6], passes into the nose through the bony opening formed by the lacrimal, maxillary, and inferior turbinate bones, LB, MB, and ITB [6]. The duct is divided into the interosseous and meatal portions. The interosseous portion is 12 mm long, and the meatal portion is 5 mm long. The nasolacrimal duct angles posteriorly approximately 15 degrees [7], as well as 10 degrees medially [6]. The bony opening of the duct is in the inferior meatus, IM [6] [7], at the junction of the anterior one third and posterior two thirds of the inferior turbinate bone, ITB [7]. The opening into the nasal cavity is created by an extension of the nasolacrimal duct which is covered by nasal mucosa. In the adult, this opening is approximately 35 mm posterior to the naris [7].

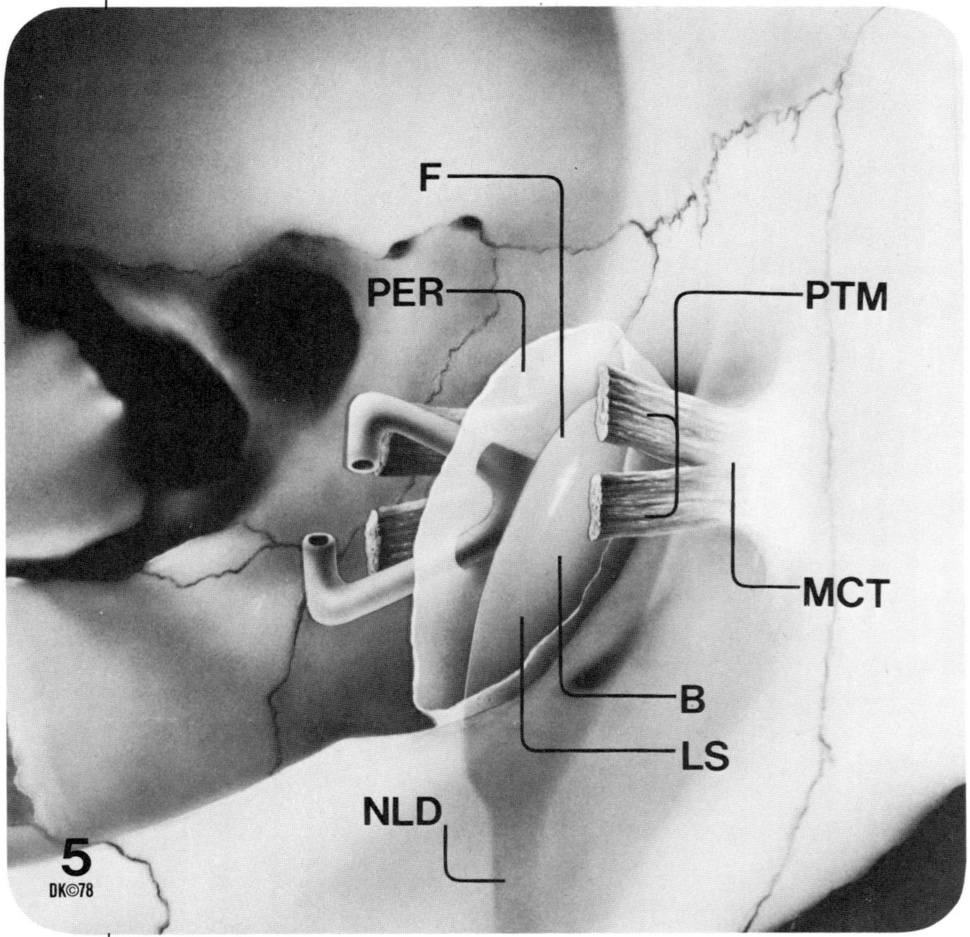

5
DK©78

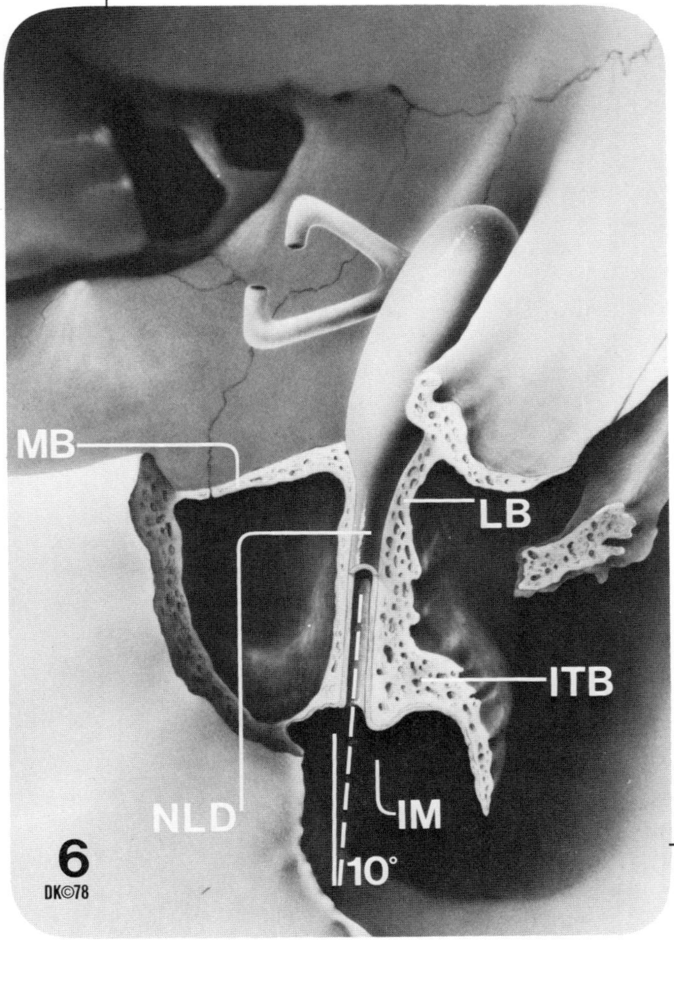

6
DK©78

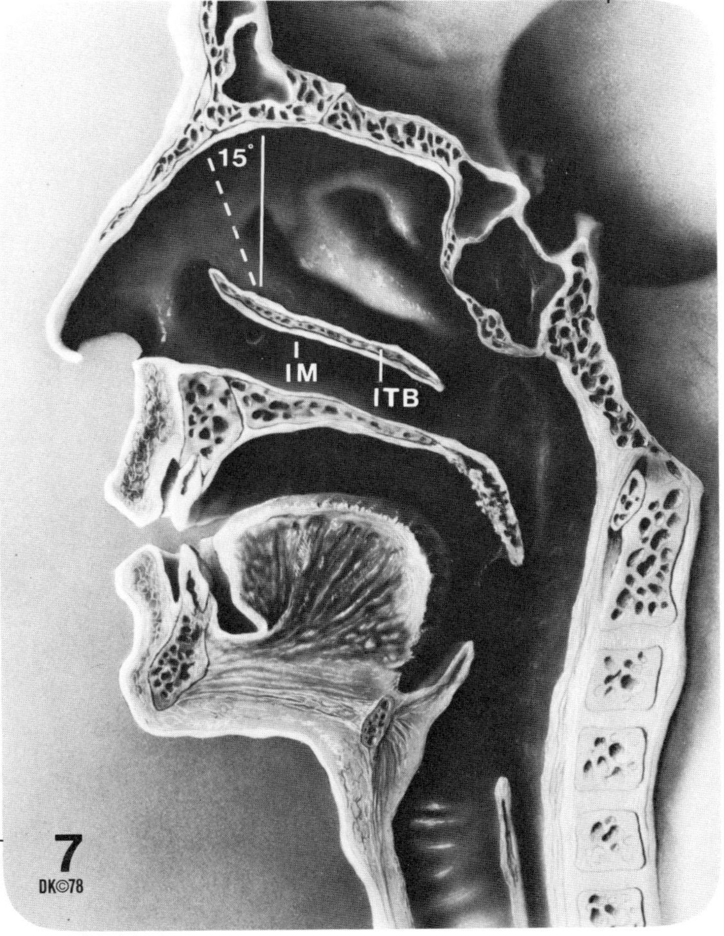

7
DK©78

Donald A. Keller

DIAGNOSTIC TESTS OF THE LACRIMAL SYSTEM

Although a complete discussion of all important diagnostic tests of the lacrimal system is beyond the scope of this surgical atlas, certain tests are included because they are surgical in nature. These tests include tear duct irrigation and probing and the primary and secondary dye tests to determine the cause of epiphora. They allow the clinician to identify an obstruction in the lacrimal system and its location and to determine if the lacrimal pump is functioning normally. Epiphora occurs most commonly as a secondary manifestation of chronic and acute dacryocystitis.

These diagnostic tests are normally outpatient procedures. To perform these tests adequately, it is essential that certain equipment and instruments be available. An examining chair with a back that tilts and good focal illumination of the patient's eye and face are essential. The surgeon needs an ordinary operating loupe to magnify the surgical field for the ocular portion of these tests and an ENT headlight, preferably with a built-in light source, for the nasal portion. The necessary instruments include an adult and a pediatric nasal speculum; blunt and sharp punctal dilators; Bowman lacrimal probes, sizes 00 and 0, 1 and 2, and 3 and 4; a 3-ml syringe with a lacrimal cannula; bayonet forceps; and several Quickert No. 1 straight lacrimal probes. Additionally, sterile saline and cotton balls, a topical anesthetic such as proparacaine hydrochloride, and a nasal decongestant agent such as phenylephrine hydrochloride 0.5 percent are necessary.

LACRIMAL IRRIGATION

John A. Burns, M.D.

Lacrimal irrigation is the initial test to determine the patency and function of the lacrimal excretory system. The test is rapid to perform, and in a majority of patients, the examiner can identify the cause of epiphora and the site of obstruction.

Prior to the irrigation, the upper and lower canaliculi are inspected for patency and anatomic location. In some cases of epiphora the problem is related to punctal abnormalities and the anatomic relationship between the lid and the globe.

The irrigation is best performed with the patient in a semisupine position. The cornea is anesthetized. To reduce the possibility of creating a false passage through the base of the ampulla, the examiner first dilates the punctum, using a sharp punctal dilator. The index finger draws the lid laterally, placing it under maximum horizontal stretch to straighten the lower canaliculus [1].

The examiner inserts a straight lacrimal cannula on a 3-ml, saline-filled syringe vertically into the canaliculus for a distance of 2 mm. The examiner rotates the handle of the cannula to 15 degrees below the horizontal plane [2]. The cannula is then inserted an additional 10 mm to touch the medial wall of the sac [3].

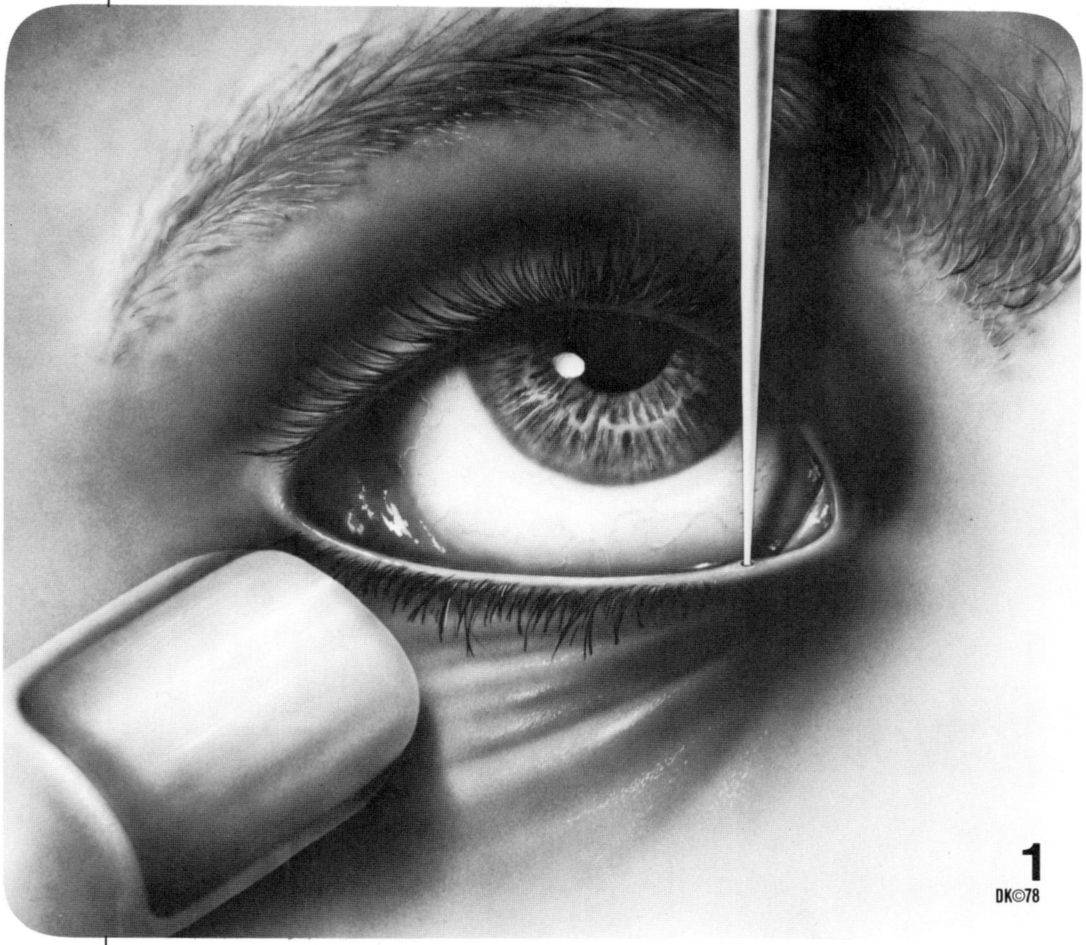

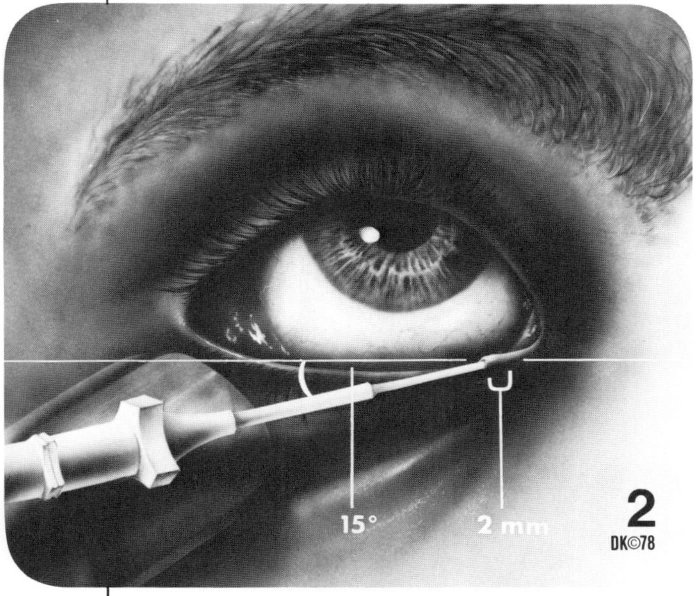

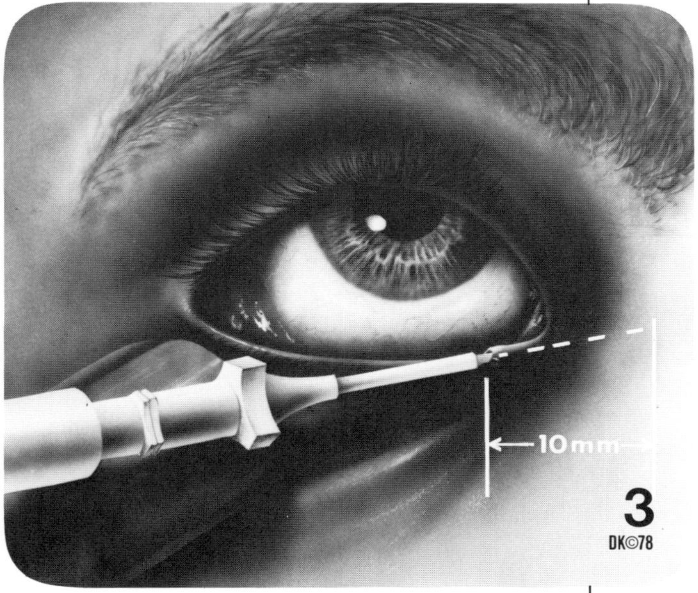

Donald F Keller

A hard stop [4] is the firm feeling as the lacrimal cannula touches the medial wall of the lacrimal sac and the underlying lacrimal bone. A soft stop—a spongy feeling as the cannula presses the common punctum and lateral wall of the sac against the medial wall [5] —usually indicates an obstruction at the lower canaliculus or common punctum. Any resistance to passage of the cannula through the lower canaliculus should be noted as a possible area of stenosis or atresia.

Before beginning the irrigation, the examiner places one finger over the lacrimal fossa to palpate the lacrimal sac during the test. If the lacrimal sac is normal, little or no bulging of the sac occurs on irrigation, and saline flows freely into the nose. If the lower canaliculus is obstructed, saline regurgitates from it. If the site of obstruction is the common punctum or common canaliculus, saline flows from both the upper and lower canaliculi. Both of these results follow a soft stop. If the obstruction is in the lacrimal sac or nasolacrimal duct, the sac bulges on irrigation, and the saline may regurgitate from either canaliculus. If the sac is infected, the regurgitated fluid may be purulent.

The examiner estimates the size of the sac on a rating scale of 1 to 4: 1) no bulge; 2) bulge below the medial canthal tendon; 3) bulge above and below the medial canthal tendon; and 4) dilation visible without irrigation.

In certain conditions, a functional obstruction may not be severe enough to interfere with irrigation. Rarely does lacrimal irrigation cure obstruction in an adult patient.

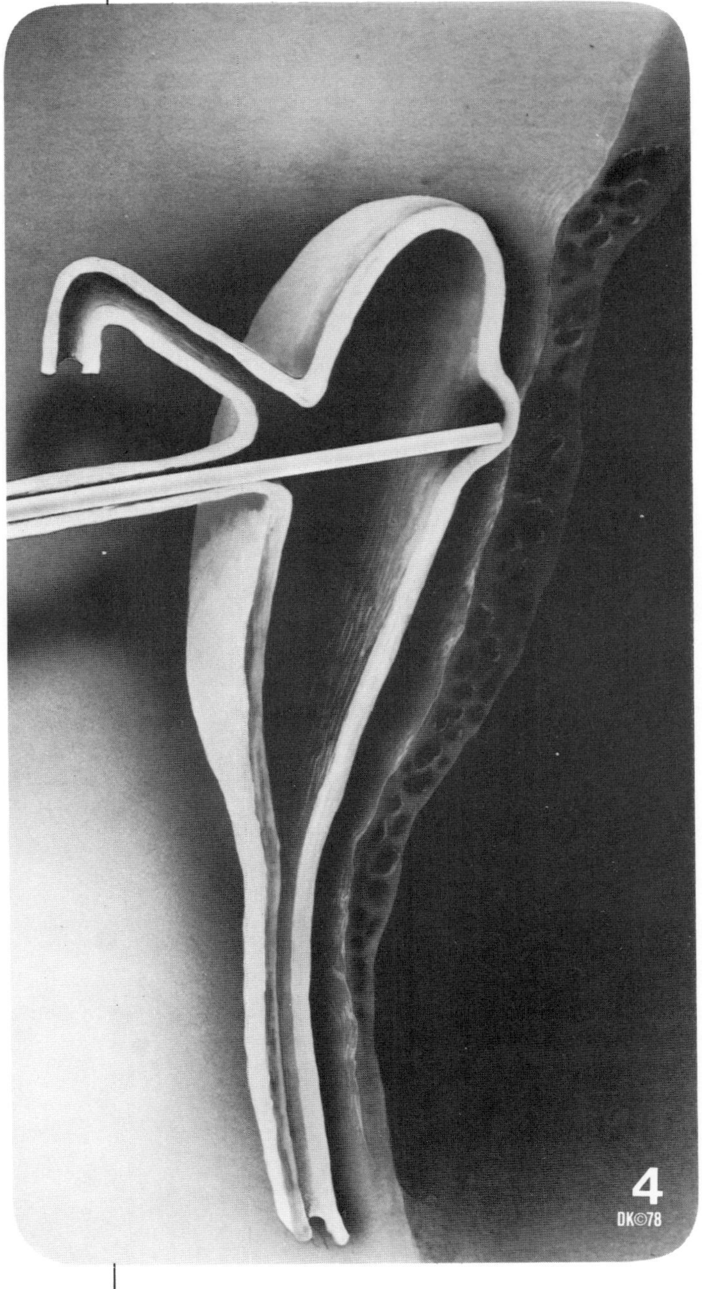

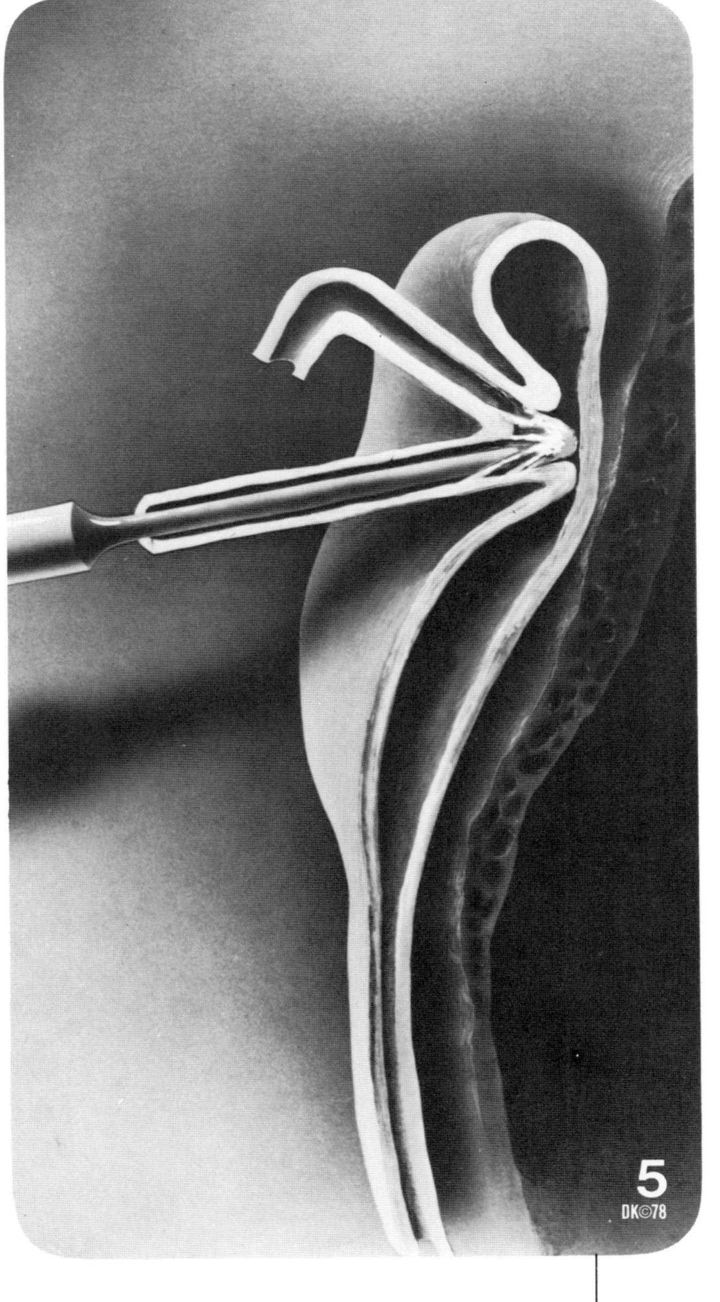

Donald F. Keller

TEAR DUCT PROBING

John A. Burns, M.D.

Tear duct probing is intended to confirm or identify the site of partial or complete obstruction in the lacrimal excretory system previously suggested by lacrimal irrigation. Probing may be therapeutic by breaking the obstruction, but this occurs rarely in the adult patient.

After the lower punctum is dilated, drops of 0.5 percent phenylephrine hydrochloride are instilled into the nose to shrink the nasal mucosa. Constriction of the nasal mucosa is as important to thorough nasal examination as pupillary dilatation is to complete fundus examination. Probing may cause moderate, transient discomfort to the patient. I have found that it is better to request that the patient tolerate the discomfort, which subsides in a matter of seconds after the probe is positioned, than to attempt to anesthetize both the facial and nasal portions of the lacrimal excretory system.

With the lid under lateral tension, the lacrimal probe is passed slowly (to note any area of stenosis or scar formation or the presence of lacrimal stones) at the angle of the normal canaliculus, in the same manner as the cannula is passed for irrigation. The probe comes to either a hard or a soft stop [1] [2] . The examiner releases the lid tension and rotates the handle of the probe vertically, where its tip is perfectly aligned to pass from the isthmus of the sac into the nasolacrimal duct [3] . Frequently, as the tip

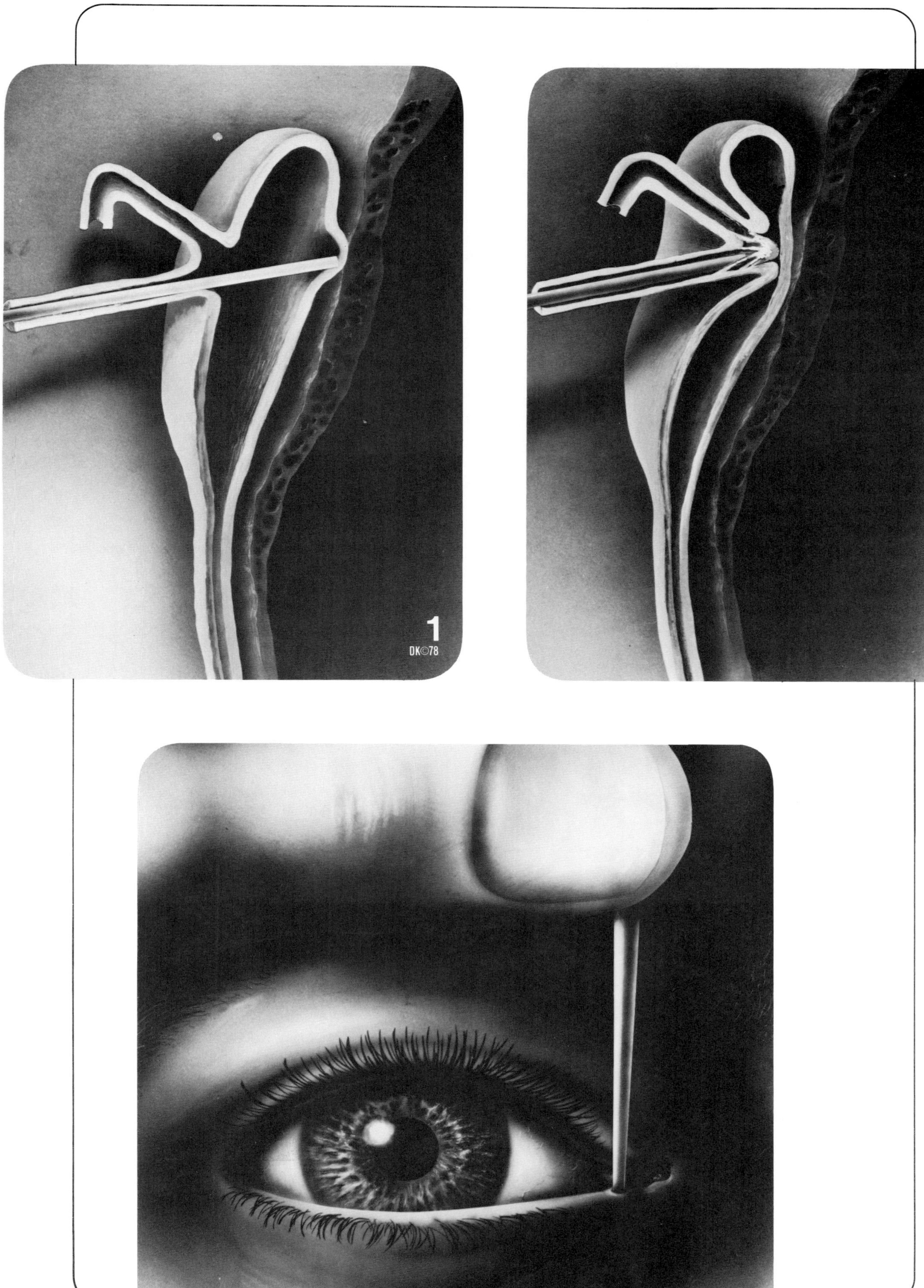
1
DK©78
2
DK©78
3
DK©78

of the probe engages the sac opening into the nasolacrimal duct, gentle pressure is necessary to start the passage, even in a normal patient.

When the tip of the probe has been inserted approximately 15 mm, it is in proper position at the isthmus. Passage of the probe an additional 20 mm downward positions the tip under the inferior turbinate in the inferior meatus and against the floor of the nose **4**. By noting the number of millimeters the probe is advanced, the examiner can estimate when the probe is under the inferior turbinate.

The examiner changes from the operating loupe to an ENT headlight to examine the nose. If the patient's nasolacrimal duct is normal, the probe appears in the inferior meatus, approximately 35 mm posterior to the naris **5**. The location of the mucosal opening varies considerably, from the top of the inferior meatus to any point on the lateral wall. The most common location is 5 mm below the dome of the inferior meatus on the lateral nasal wall. Periodically, probings in patients with epiphora and probable nasolacrimal duct obstruction may create false passages that allow the probe to pass into the nose at a point somewhere between the anterior end of the middle turbinate and the top of the inferior turbinate. After the probe has been withdrawn, the diagnostician may frequently find that irrigation through the false passage is possible. Unfortunately, these passages close in a matter of hours and are of no lasting functional benefit.

If probing yields normal findings and epiphora continues, primary and secondary dye testing is indicated.

PEDIATRIC TEAR DUCT PROBING

As many as 30 percent of infants may have closed nasolacrimal ducts at birth, although the great majority of ducts open spontaneously during the first three months of life. If the child is examined before the fourth month of life, conservative medical management, such as instillation of antibiotic solutions and massage of the lacrimal fossa, is recommended. If epiphora and/or chronic infection persist after six months of age, tear duct probing is indicated, with the infant under general anesthesia.

The procedure is the same as diagnostic tear duct probing in an adult; however, it is most important that the examiner observe the lacrimal probe under the inferior turbinate as it presents through the mucosa. It is very easy to create a false passage into the nose in an infant. This affords only temporary relief since it closes in a matter of days. The procedure is often conducted without such specific visualization, with subsequent irrigation possible through a false passage.

If the probe is not visible in the nose, the examiner grasps the protruding probe with forceps at the point of entry into the punctum and removes the probe. The distance from the forceps to the end of the probe can be measured, and the site of the atresia accurately located. If the probe was inserted less than 20 mm in the infant (or 35 mm in an adult), the nasolacrimal duct probably ends as a dead-end pouch. If the probe appears to have been within a few millimeters of the expected distance to the nose, the examiner reinserts it and forces it the remaining distance. Frequently, this opens the passage.

If the probe has been passed the normal 20 to 35 mm and is still not visible, the inferior turbinate should be inspected for abnormalities. An inferior turbinate lying tight against the lateral nasal wall frequently holds the valve of Hasner closed. If this is the situation, a Freer elevator can be used to fracture the inferior turbinate medially, which usually allows the mucosa to be broken by the probe and patency to be established. Occasionally, the probe is passed into the nose, and a bump is visible behind the mucosa under the inferior turbinate, although the probe cannot be made to perforate the mucosa. Under these circumstances, the tip of the probe may be exposed by cutting down onto the probe under the inferior turbinate.

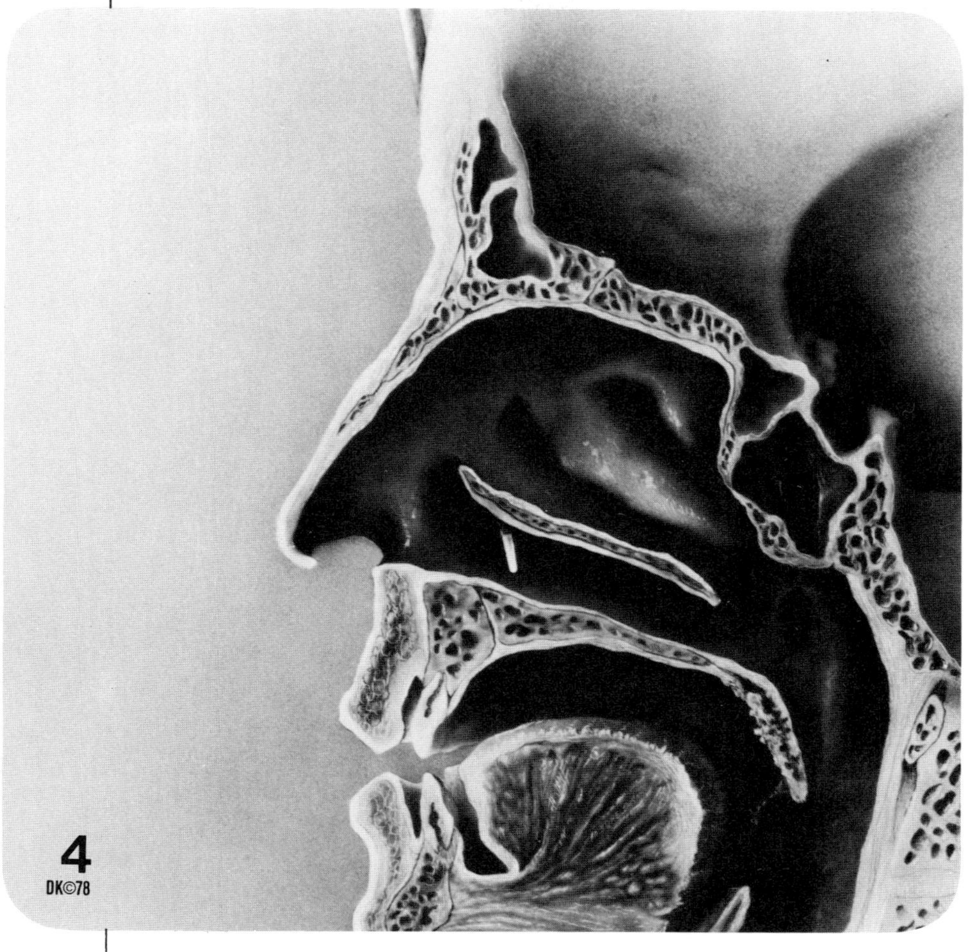

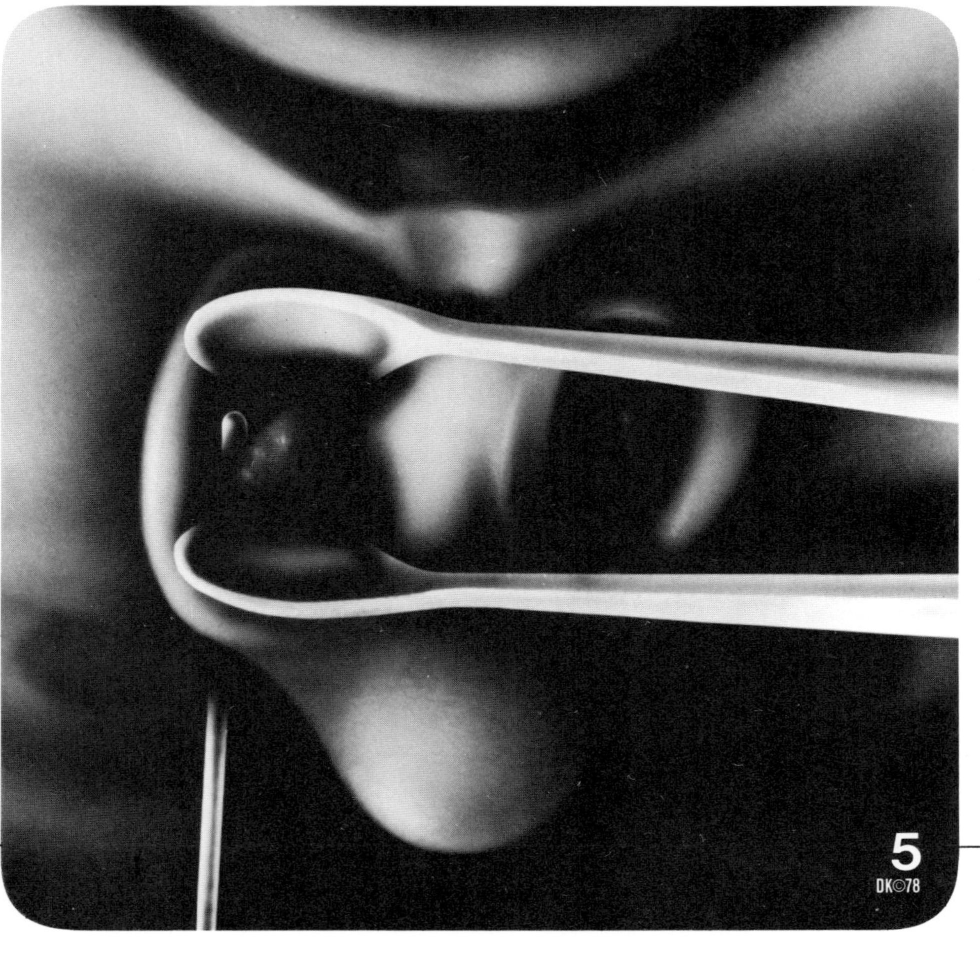

Donald F. Keller

PRIMARY DYE TESTING

John A. Burns, M.D.

The objective of the primary dye test (Jones No. 1) is to identify the site of physiologic obstruction in a patient who has been determined to have a partial obstruction by lacrimal irrigation and probing. It also differentiates patients in whom epiphora is due to hypersecretion from patients whose lacrimal excretory system is not functioning for a structural reason.

I recommend that this test be performed at a second appointment without preliminary manipulation of any portion of the lacrimal excretory system. It is a physiologic test, in which the lacrimal system is not manipulated; the punctum is not dilated and the nasal mucosa is not constricted.

The instruments necessary to perform the test are the same as those used for irrigation and probing. A nasal applicator is prepared by wrapping a small wisp of cotton around the round end of a Quickert probe, or if this is not available, a No. 1 Bowman probe may be used. The cotton should cover the distal 3 cm of the probe so that any part of the probe that encounters the entry of the nasolacrimal duct under the inferior turbinate is wrapped. Neophytes performing this test often wrap cotton too thickly on the probe tip, causing difficulty in placement of the probe under the inferior turbinate as well as increasing discomfort for the patient.

The patient should be seated upright, and the cornea is anesthetized. A nasal speculum opens the naris, and under direct visualization with an ENT headlight, the cotton-wrapped applicator is placed under the inferior turbinate along the lateral wall of the nose [1] [2] . The examiner instills fluorescein dye into the eye and, after three minutes, removes the probe from the nose and examines it for fluorescein.

The test is considered positive if dye appears on the cotton [3] . This indicates that the lacrimal excretory system is open, the lacrimal pump is functioning, and the cause of epiphora is hypersecretion. If no dye appears on the cotton, the test is recorded as negative. This negative result may be caused by constricted canaliculi [4] , constricted nasolacrimal duct [5] , lacrimal pump failure, or a combination of these factors. If the examiner had anticipated a positive test, the procedure is repeated to reduce the number of false-negative results.

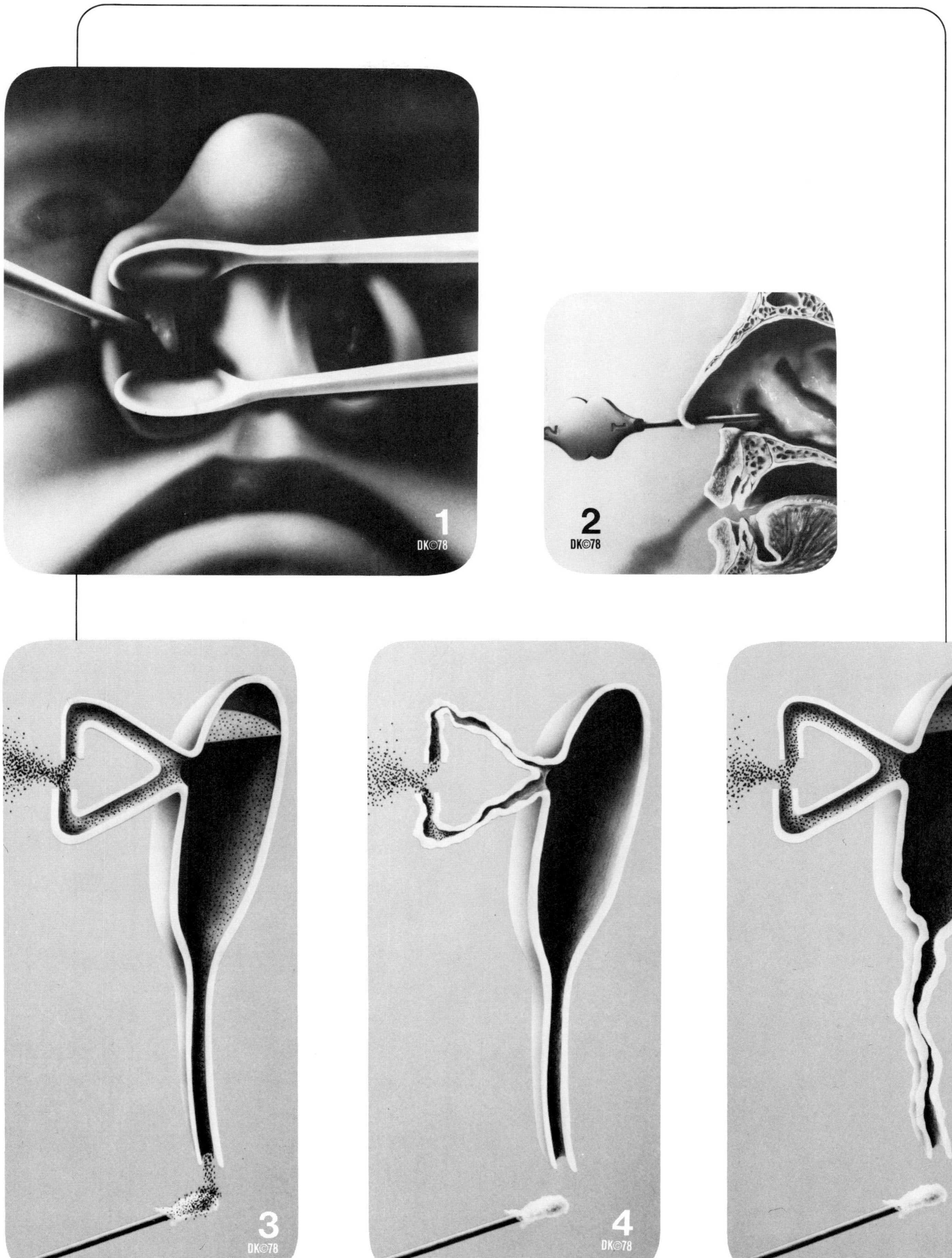

Donald A. Keller

SECONDARY DYE TESTING

John A. Burns, M.D.

A secondary dye test (Jones No. 2) is performed immediately after the negative primary dye test to determine whether the obstruction is above or below the neck of the lacrimal sac. The examiner irrigates any fluorescein dye remaining on the eye from the primary test and places a freshly prepared cotton-wrapped applicator under the inferior turbinate as in the primary dye test. A lacrimal cannula is inserted into the lacrimal sac. The sac is irrigated with saline, while the patient's head is tipped forward. The patient holds an emesis basin or towel to catch the saline as it drips from the nose.

If the test is positive, fluorescein stains the cotton probe [1]. If the test is negative, clear saline drips from the patient's nose, and no dye appears on the probe [2]. A positive test indicates a partial obstruction or lack of spontaneous drainage through the nasolacrimal duct. The usual treatment is dacryocystorhinostomy. A negative test, showing clear saline wetting the applicator and dripping from the nose, indicates that no dye reached the sac, and the probable cause of epiphora is either canalicular disease [3] or failure of the lacrimal pump. Previous probing and irrigation of the canalicular system will have excluded canalicular disease, thereby confirming the diagnosis as lacrimal pump failure, for which no cure currently exists.

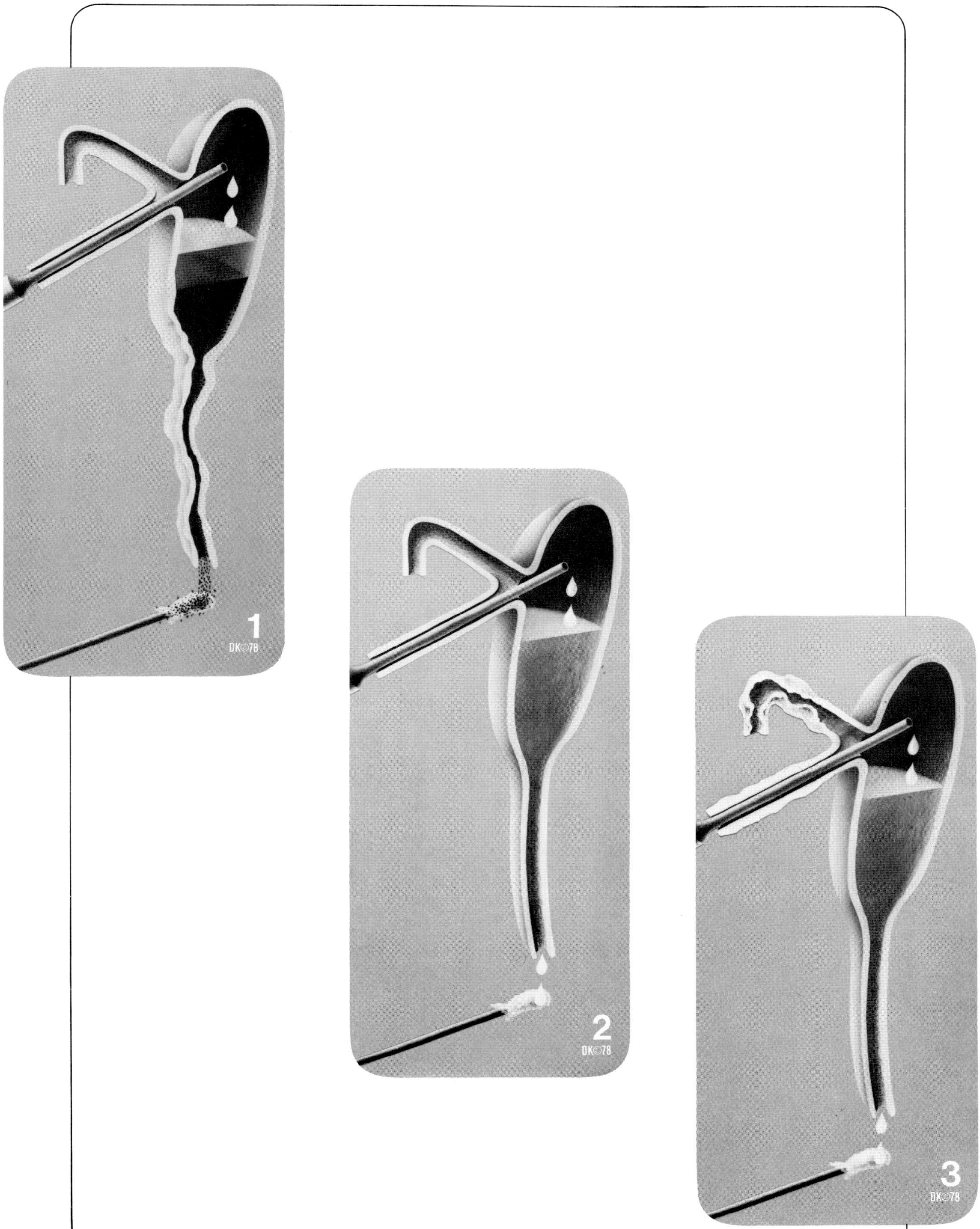
1
DK©78
2
DK©78
3
DK©78

INTUBATION OF THE LACRIMAL SYSTEM

John A. Burns, M.D.

Intubation of the nasolacrimal system is indicated in a number of situations. Among them are failure of tear duct probing, canalicular stenosis, canalicular lacerations, common punctoplasty, complicated dacryocystorhinostomy, partial nasolacrimal duct obstruction, and punctal stenosis. Quickert and Dryden's method of placing silicone elastomer (Silastic) tubing in the canalicular system has greatly improved the intubation procedure. Since the lacrimal system tolerates this material extremely well, it can be left almost indefinitely without irritation, migration, or rejection. We recommend use of the Guibor canalicular intubation set, which contains two stainless steel probes with a length of Silastic tubing permanently bonded between them.

Initially, if the punctum will not dilate, a one-snip procedure can be performed to open the punctum which facilitates passage of the probe and tubing into the canalicular system [1]. Before it is passed, the tube should be lubricated with mineral oil or ophthalmic ointment. The initial steps for passage of the probe are identical to those used in tear duct probing.

After the probe has been passed into the nose, it should be visualized under the inferior turbinate to confirm accurate placement [2]. To facilitate visualization, the nasal mucosa must be constricted with 1 percent phenylephrine hydrochloride or 4 percent cocaine hydrochloride.

A hemostat grasps the end of the probe and pulls it from the nose [3]. Care should be taken not to traumatize the nasal mucosa with the end of the probe since this may cause considerable bleeding, which complicates the passage of the second probe.

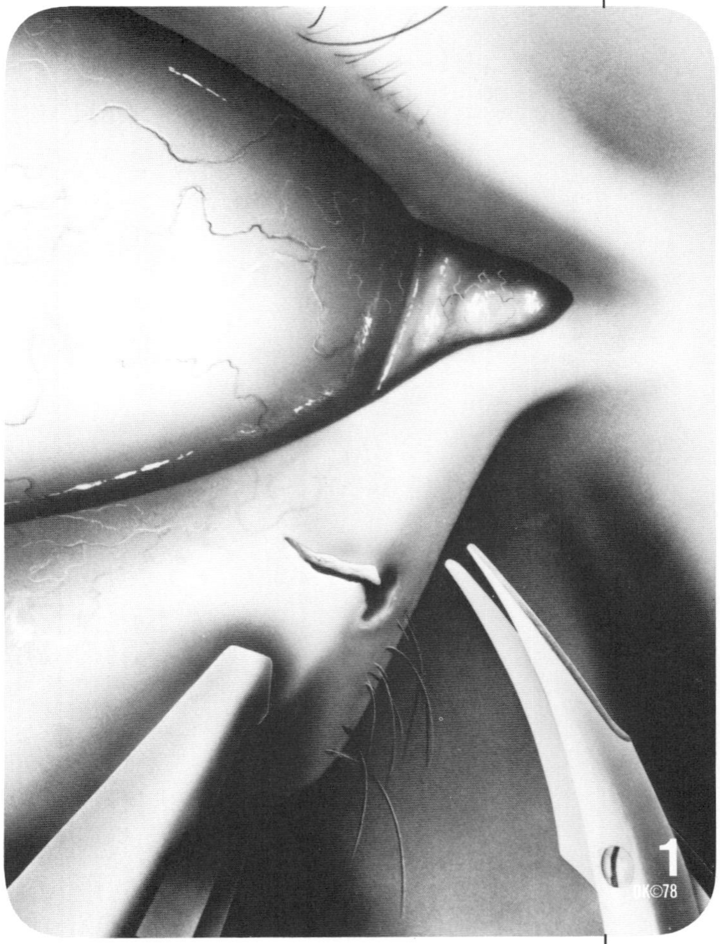

The surgeon passes the second probe with the attached Silastic tubing through the opposite canaliculus and into the nose [4]. Three to 4 mm of tubing should remain exposed which permits the eyelids to open and close normally. The tubing protruding from the nose is then tied with two square knots which are secured with 4.0 silk suture to prevent them from untying [5]. When the Silastic knot is reposited into the nasal ampulla, care should be taken not to create pressure on either the puncta or nasal mucosa as this will cut into the tissue.

The tubing is left in place for varying amounts of time. Generally it may be safely removed when the lacrimal system can be irrigated without resistance.

Donald A. Keller

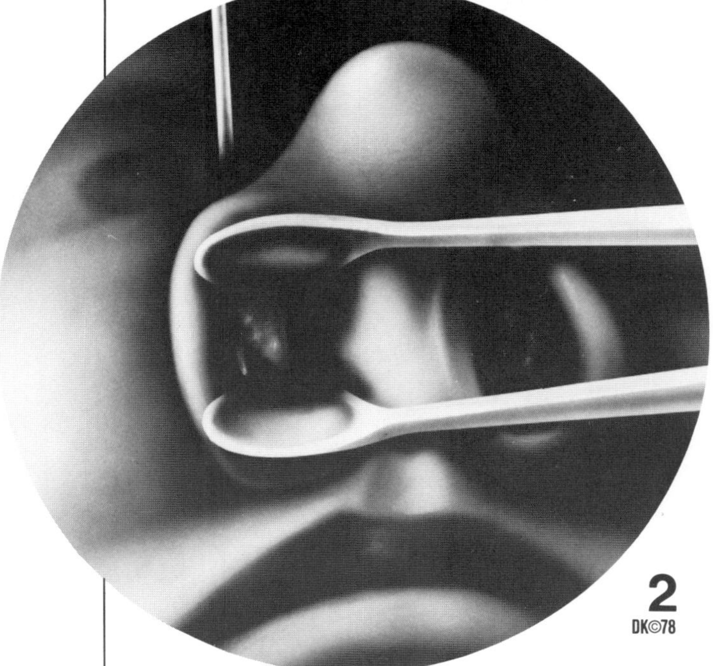

2
DK©78

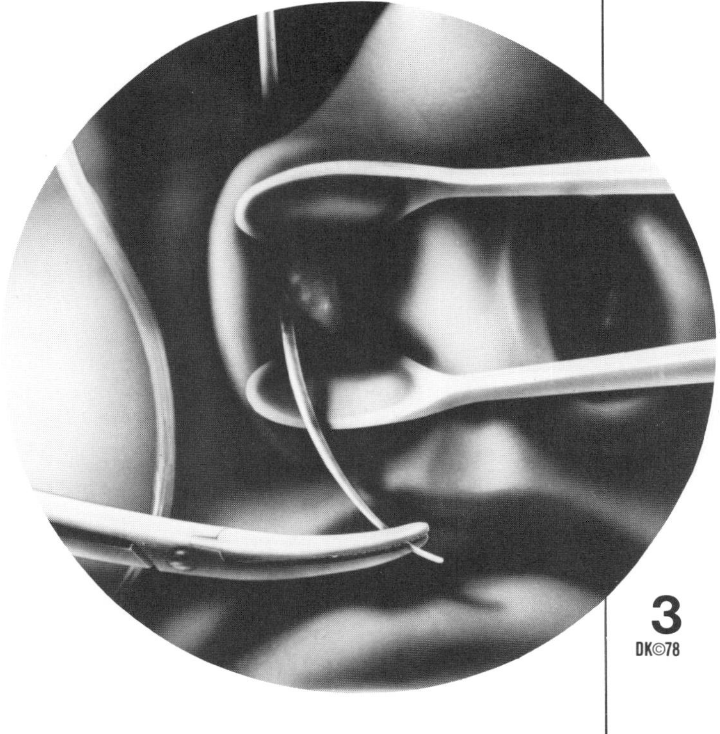

3
DK©78

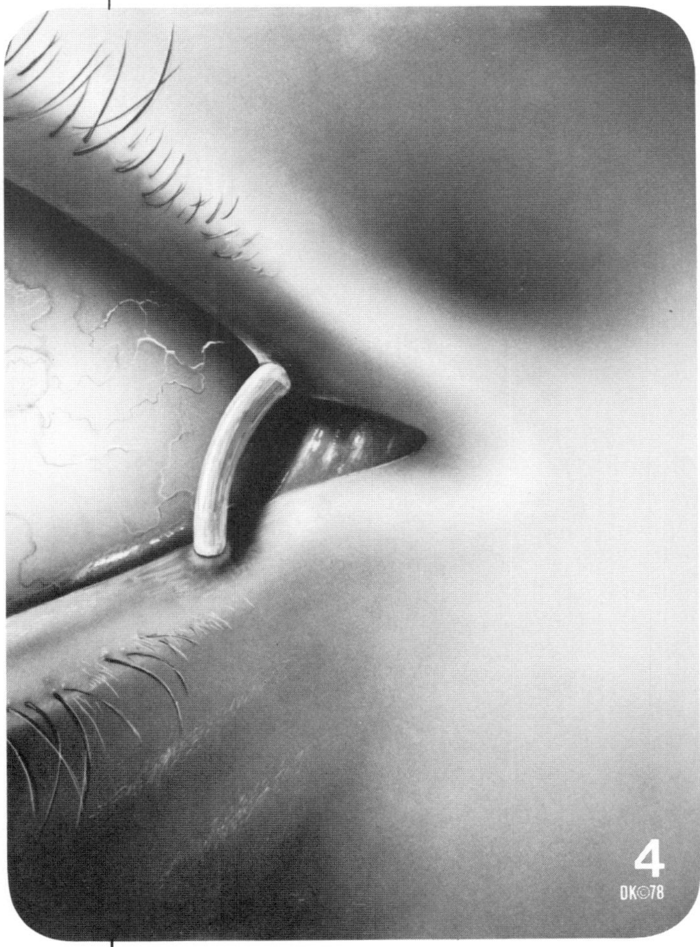

4
DK©78

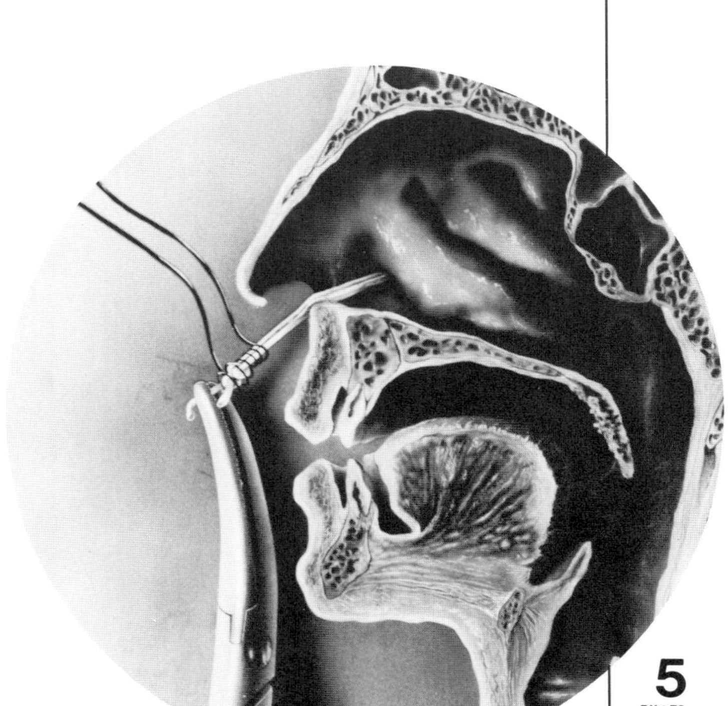

5
DK©78

Donald F. Keller

DACRYOCYSTORHINOSTOMY

John A. Burns, M.D.

In adults, the most common site of obstruction of the lacrimal excretory system is the nasolacrimal duct. Correction of this obstruction is best carried out by a dacryocystorhinostomy.

When performing a dacryocystorhinostomy, I use the procedure described here exclusively. I have rarely encountered failures of patency, although infrequent cases have required reopening the ostium. This procedure is simple to teach and eliminates a number of complicated maneuvers, as well as complicated instrumentation. It allows the surgeon a clear view of the common punctum. The common canaliculus and common punctum are unchanged in position in the lacrimal fossa, since the lateral and posterior sac walls are not moved. The ostium can be readily packed open to prevent stenosis. Traditionally, the flaps have been sutured posteriorly and anteriorly to prevent stenosis, although the reason the nasal wall does not regrow in a superior and inferior direction remains unexplained. Crimping the mucosal edges together around the circumference of the incision site helps to prevent the bony regrowth.

The instruments required to perform a dacryocystorhinostomy include those routinely available for tear duct probing and irrigation, as well as the standard instruments used for lid surgery. Special instruments include a lacrimal retractor, small and large Weiner frontal rasps, a Freer elevator, a size 0 Kerrison rongeur, a small bone chisel, and an orthopedic hammer.

A skin incision 1 mm medial to the anterior lacrimal crest and parallel to it extends from the inferior edge of the medial canthal tendon for 15 to 20 mm [1]. Most surgeons emphasize placement of the incision at one of three sites to avoid the angular vessels. On the contrary, the location of the lacrimal sac rather than this group of vessels dictates the incision site. If the incision exposes the angular vessels, they may be swept out of the way with a lacrimal speculum or, if inadvertently cut, may be easily closed with cautery. The angular vessels do not require ligation.

The initial incision penetrates to the orbicularis muscle only. The muscle layer is then opened by blunt dissection, which results in much less bleeding.

It is important to determine the size and location of the lacrimal sac before making an incision. This may be accomplished by irrigation. With saline irrigation of the lacrimal sac, a bulge is created that is easily palpable with the little finger if obstruction of the nasolacrimal duct is present. After the incision is made, saline irrigation enhances the visibility of the sac which can be seen along the rim of the anterior lacrimal crest.

After determination of the sac dimensions, the surgeon makes an incision 5 mm in length in the anterior wall of the lacrimal sac parallel to the anterior lacrimal crest and approximately 2 mm lateral to it [2]. The incision angles through the wall of the sac toward the middle of the medial wall of the fossa. The interior of the sac can be readily identified by its gray mucosal appearance. Confirmation that the sac has been opened is obtained by again irrigating the sac.

Traction sutures of 5-0 chromic catgut on both sides of the opening enhance exposure to the interior of the sac [3]. The sac should be inspected to insure that a tumor or

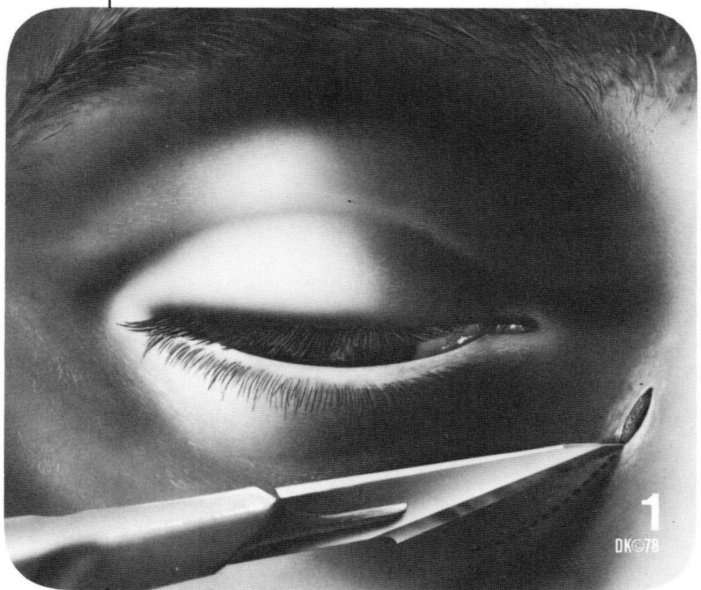

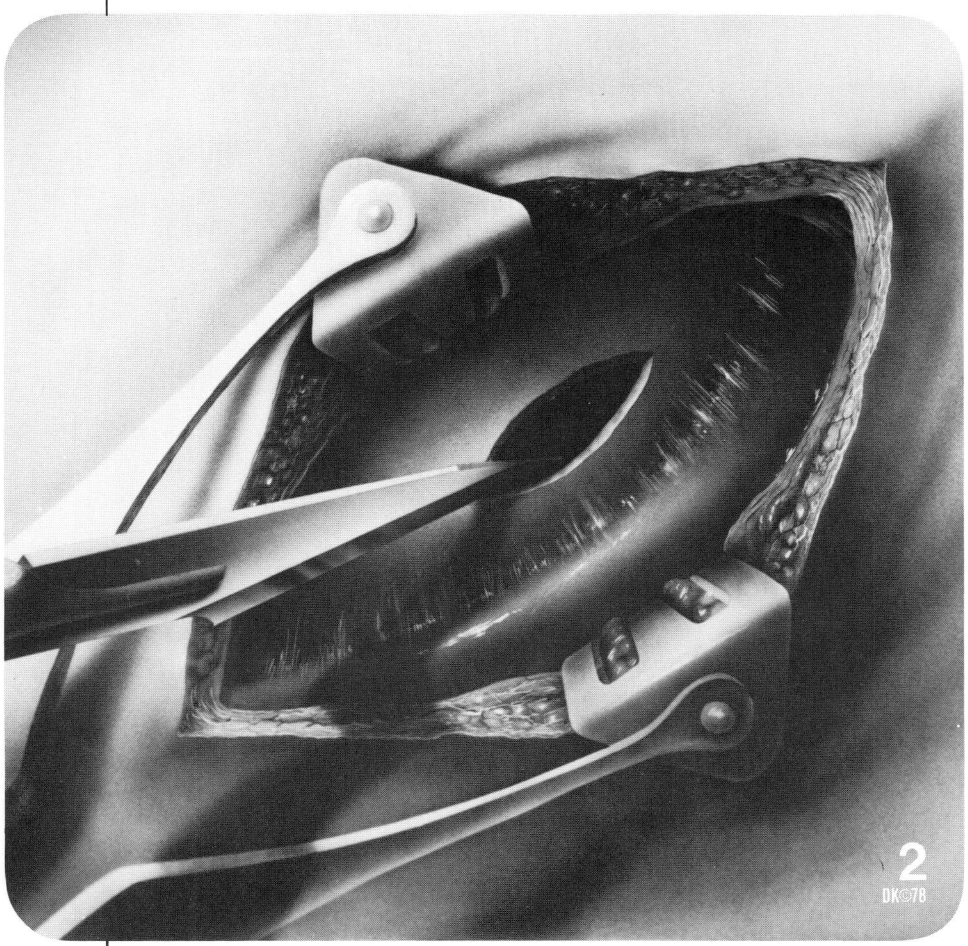

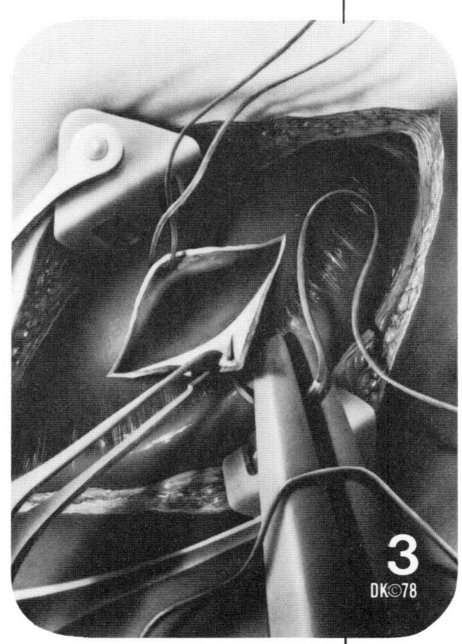

Donald F. Keller

dacryolith is not present. At this point, the surgeon inserts a probe through the common canaliculus and common punctum to insure their patency [4] .

After hemostasis has been obtained, a small Weiner rasp is placed in the most inferior and anterior aspect of the lacrimal fossa [5] , which is the location of the opening of the nasolacrimal duct. In most patients, gentle pressure with the frontal rasp against the medial wall of the lacrimal sac results in passage of the rasp through the medial wall of the sac and slightly into the nose [6] . The rasp is used to create the opening in the medial wall but is not used to enlarge it; the opening is enlarged with a larger Weiner rasp. A size 0 Kerrison punch is used to enlarge the opening in an anterior and inferior direction until the hole measures approximately 8 × 10 mm [7] . The biting action of the Kerrison punch presses the nasal mucosa

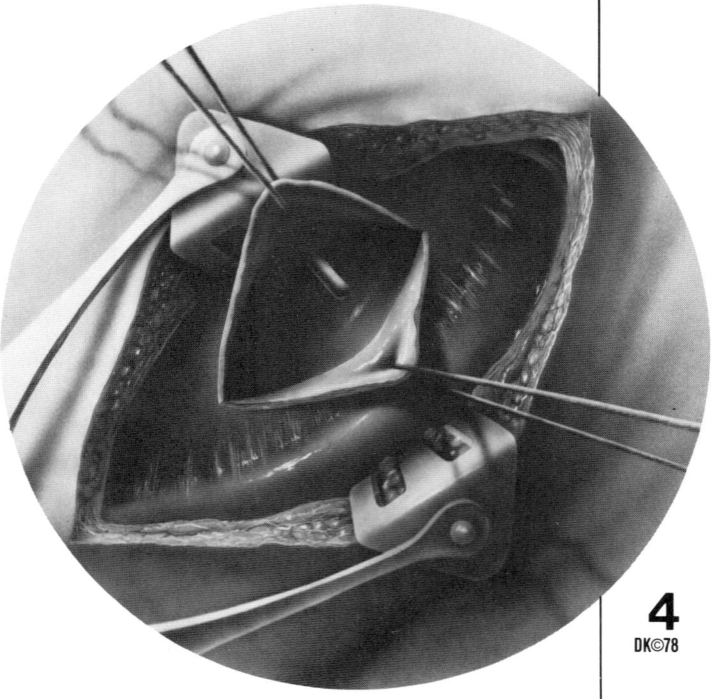

4
DK©78

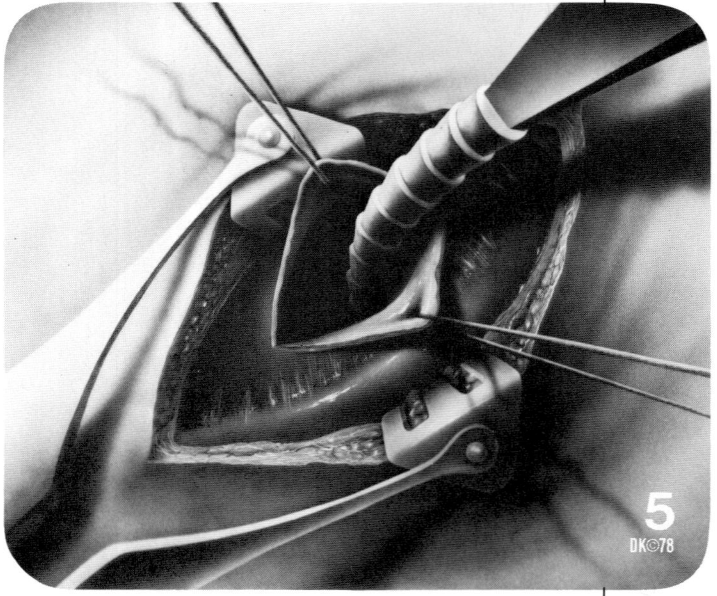

5
DK©78

Donald F. Keller

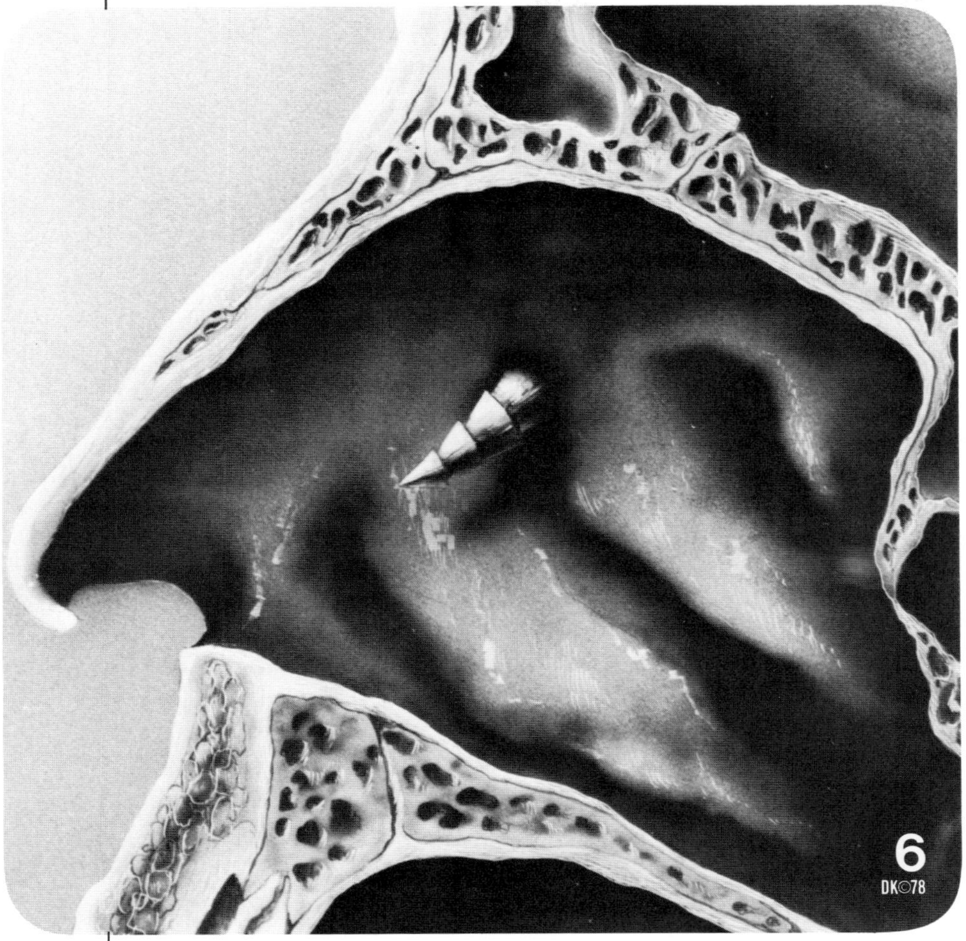
6
DK©78

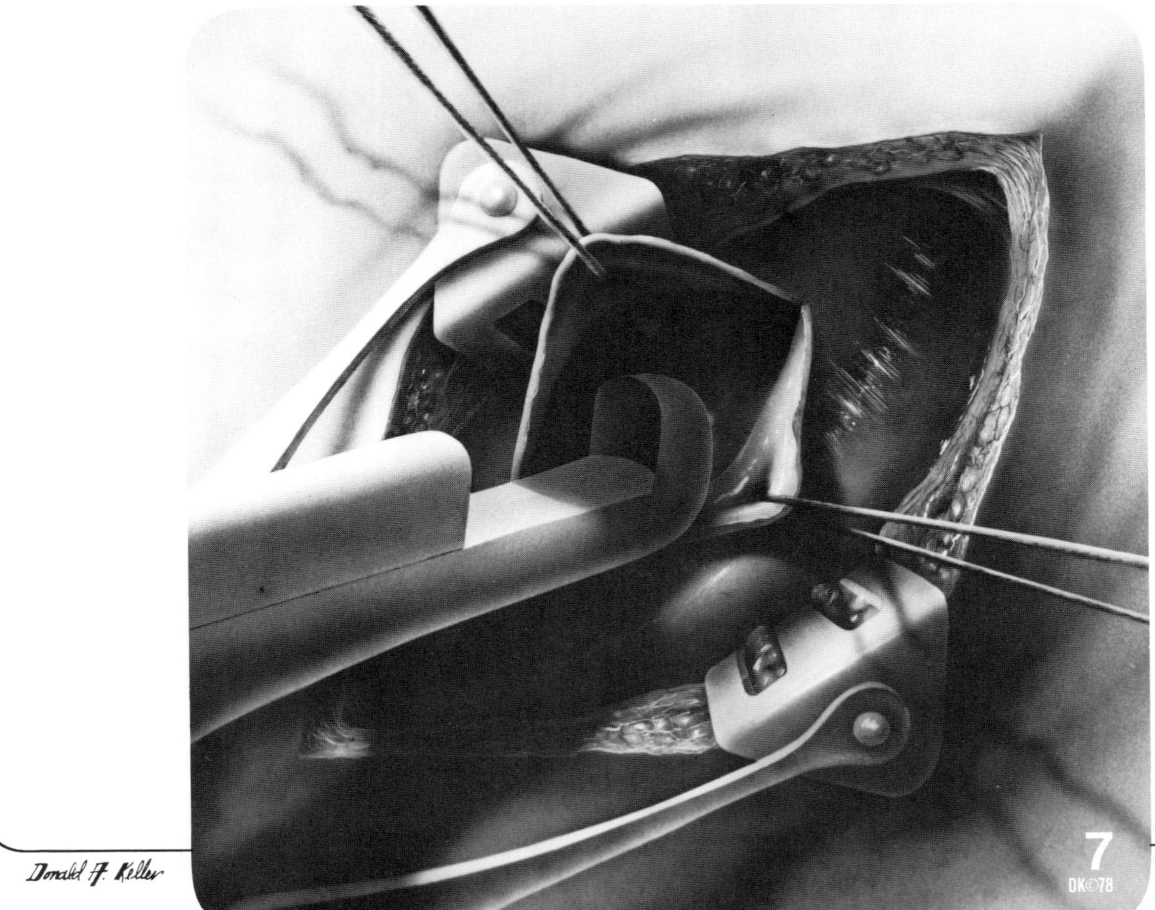
Donald A. Keller
7
DK©78

against the mucosa of the medial wall of the sac and fuses the two surfaces [8], thereby negating the need to suture the flaps together. If the surgeon is concerned about the patency of the canaliculus or common punctum, the canalicular system is intubated with silicone (Silastic) tubing and passed through the new ostium and into the nose where it is tied [9] [10].

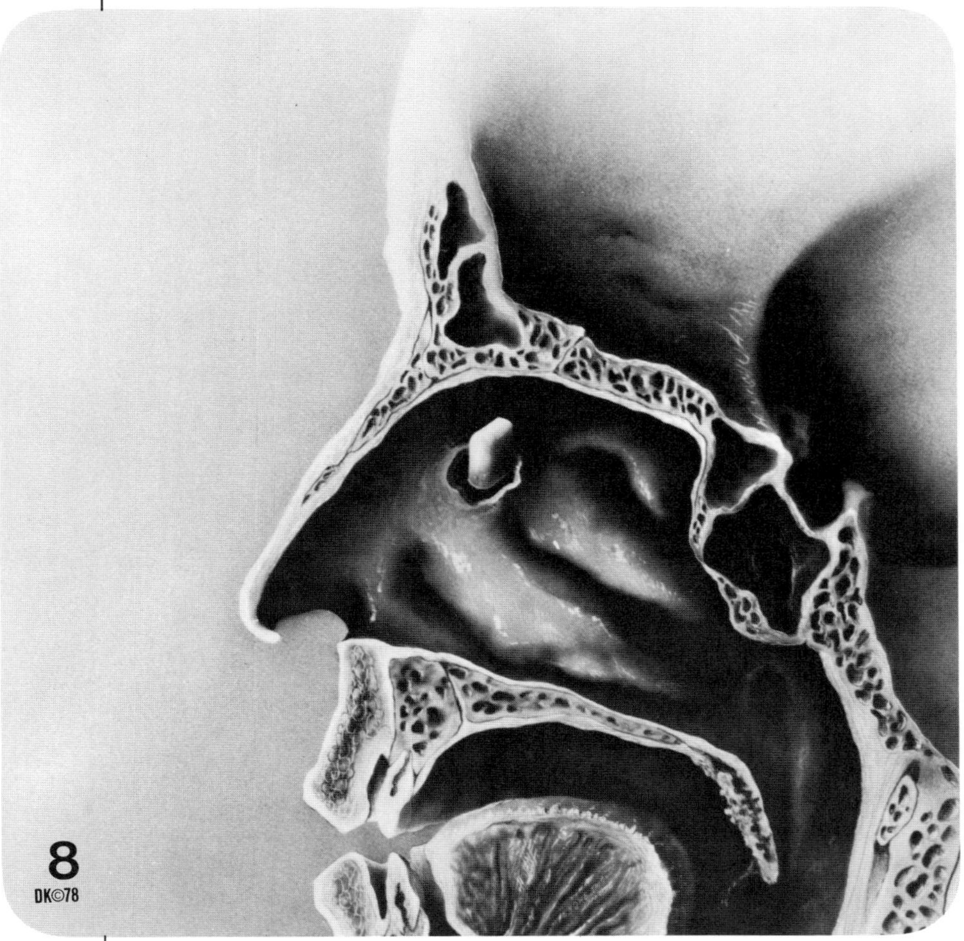

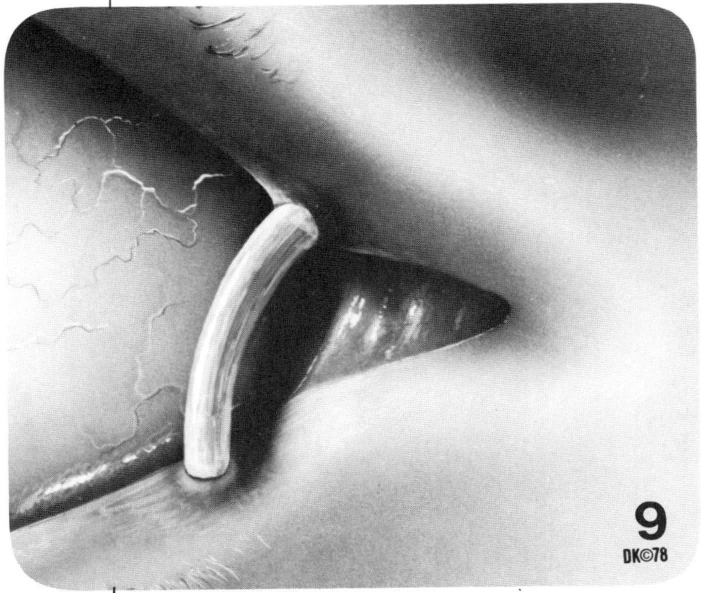

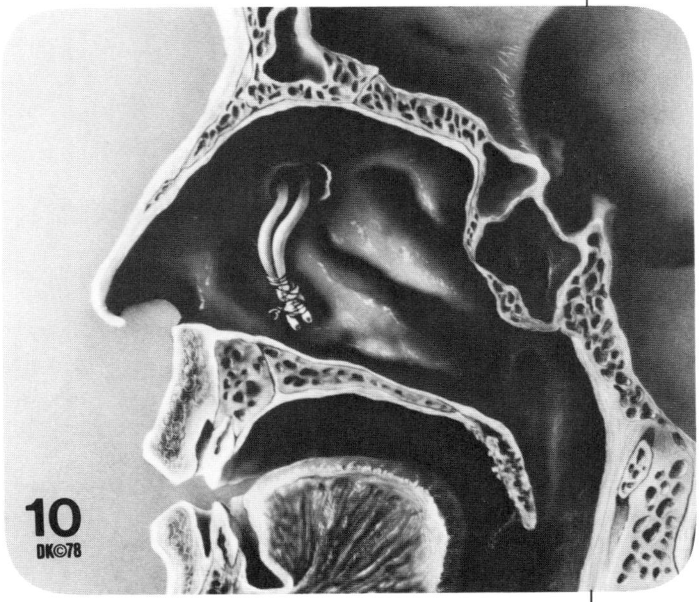

Donald A. Killer

After the creation of the ostium, the opening is maintained by packing both the sac and ostium with quarter-inch umbilical tape, impregnated with an antibiotic ointment. This is passed through the nose and into the sac [11]. The chronically dilated sac typically found in patients with chronic dacryocystitis holds approximately 10 cm of impregnated gauze.

Three 5-0 chromic catgut sutures close the anterior wall of the sac [12]. When suturing the anterior walls of the lacrimal sac, care must be taken not to include the packing in the suture bite.

Four sutures of 5-0 chromic catgut close the orbicularis muscle [13], and the skin incision is closed with 6-0 black silk sutures [14].

A nonadhering dressing and antibiotic ointment cover the incision site with light pressure. The pack is removed through the nostril between the fifth and seventh postoperative days. At this time the skin sutures are also removed. The lacrimal system should be irrigated immediately after removal of the pack. This is repeated every seven days for three weeks and then monthly for two additional postoperative visits.

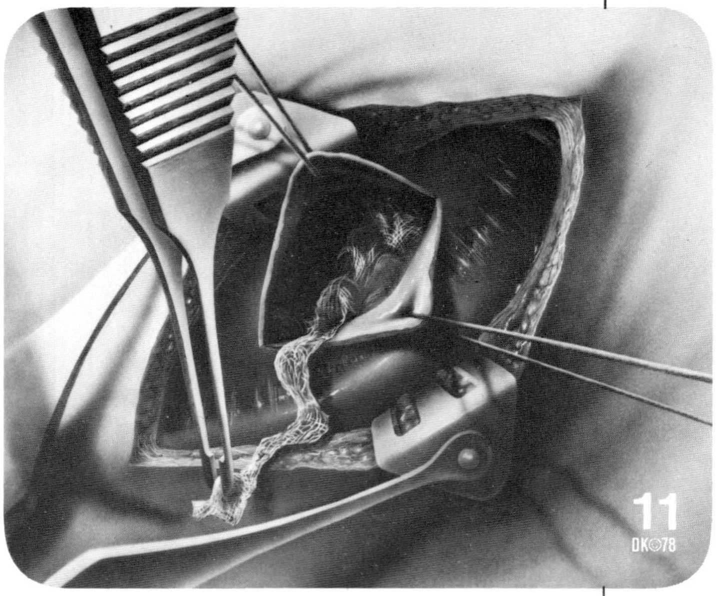

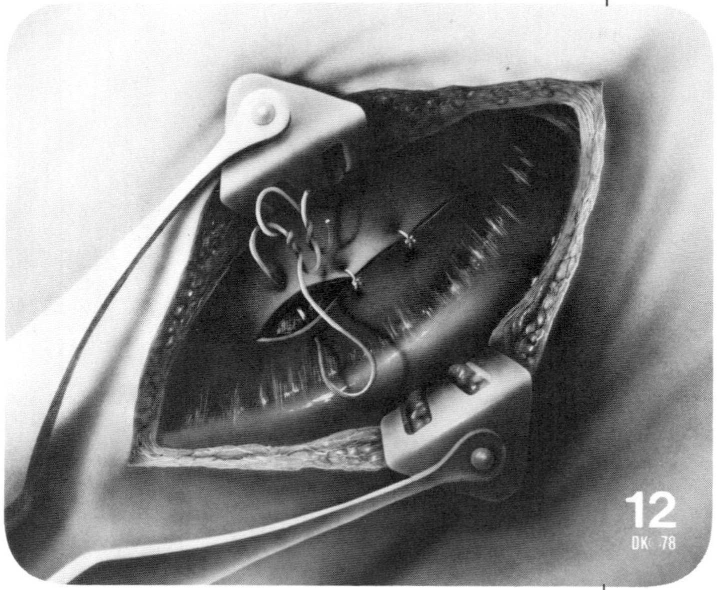

Donald F. Keller

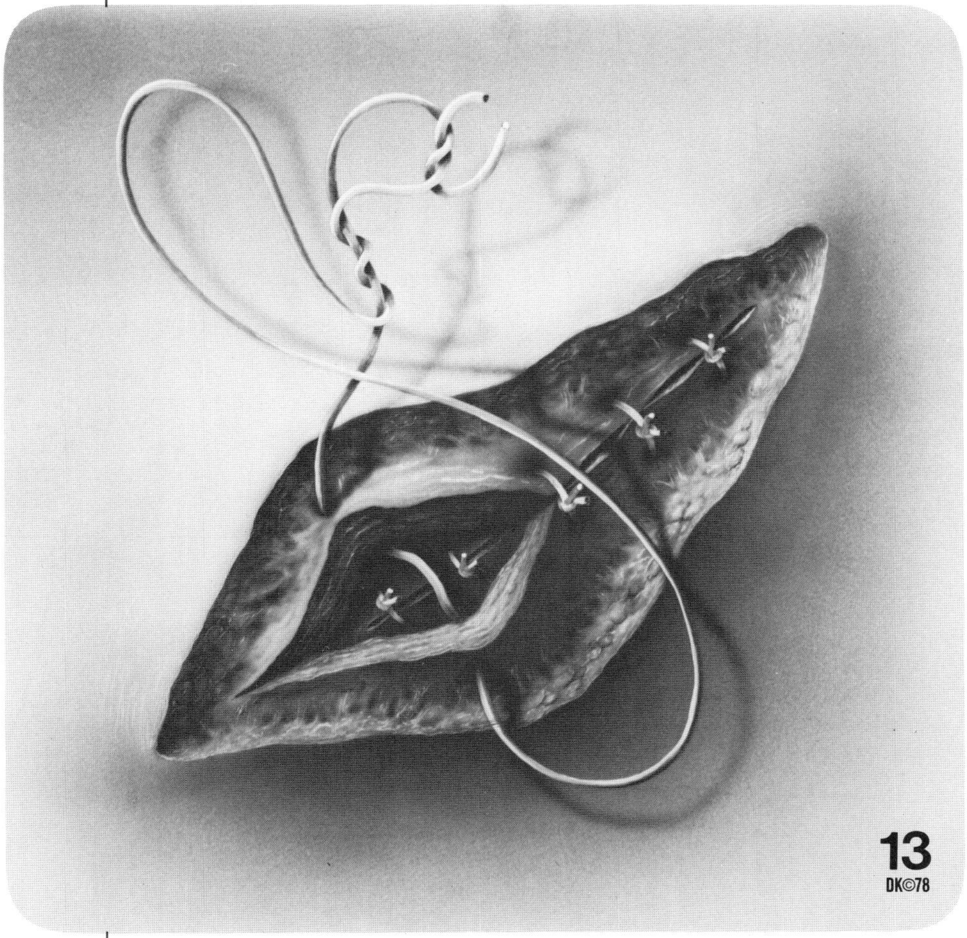

13

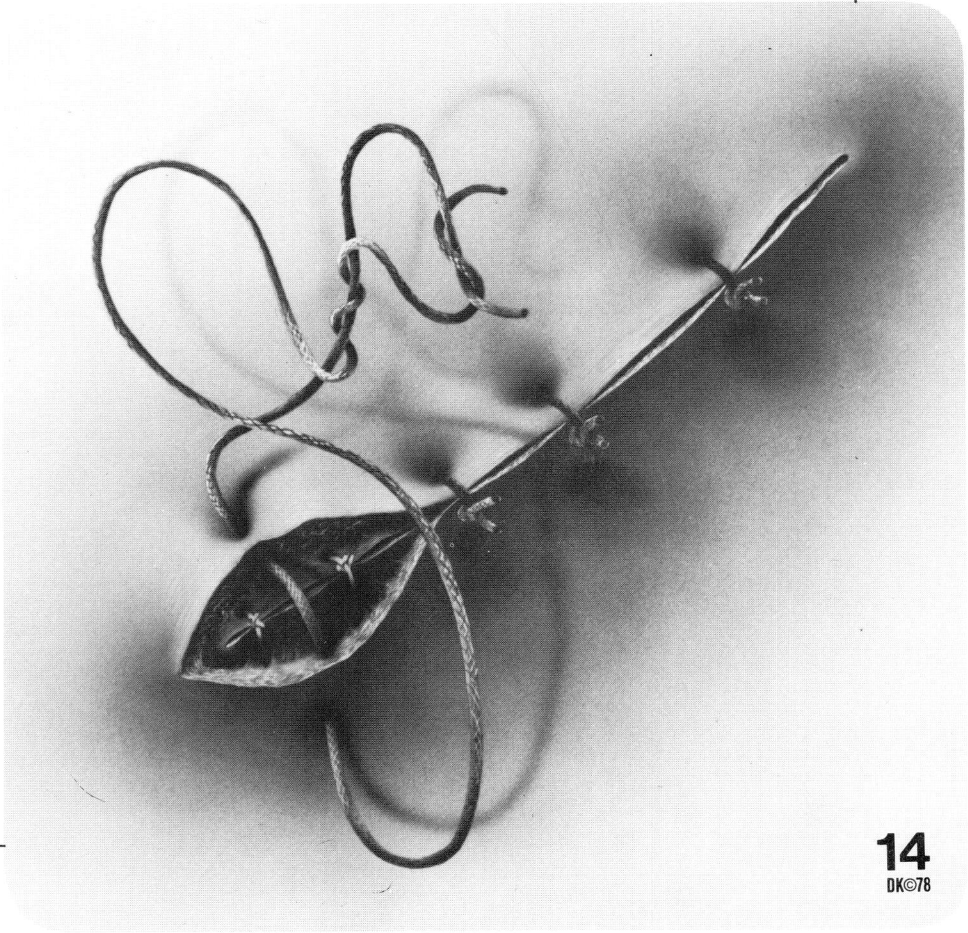

14

Donald H. Keller

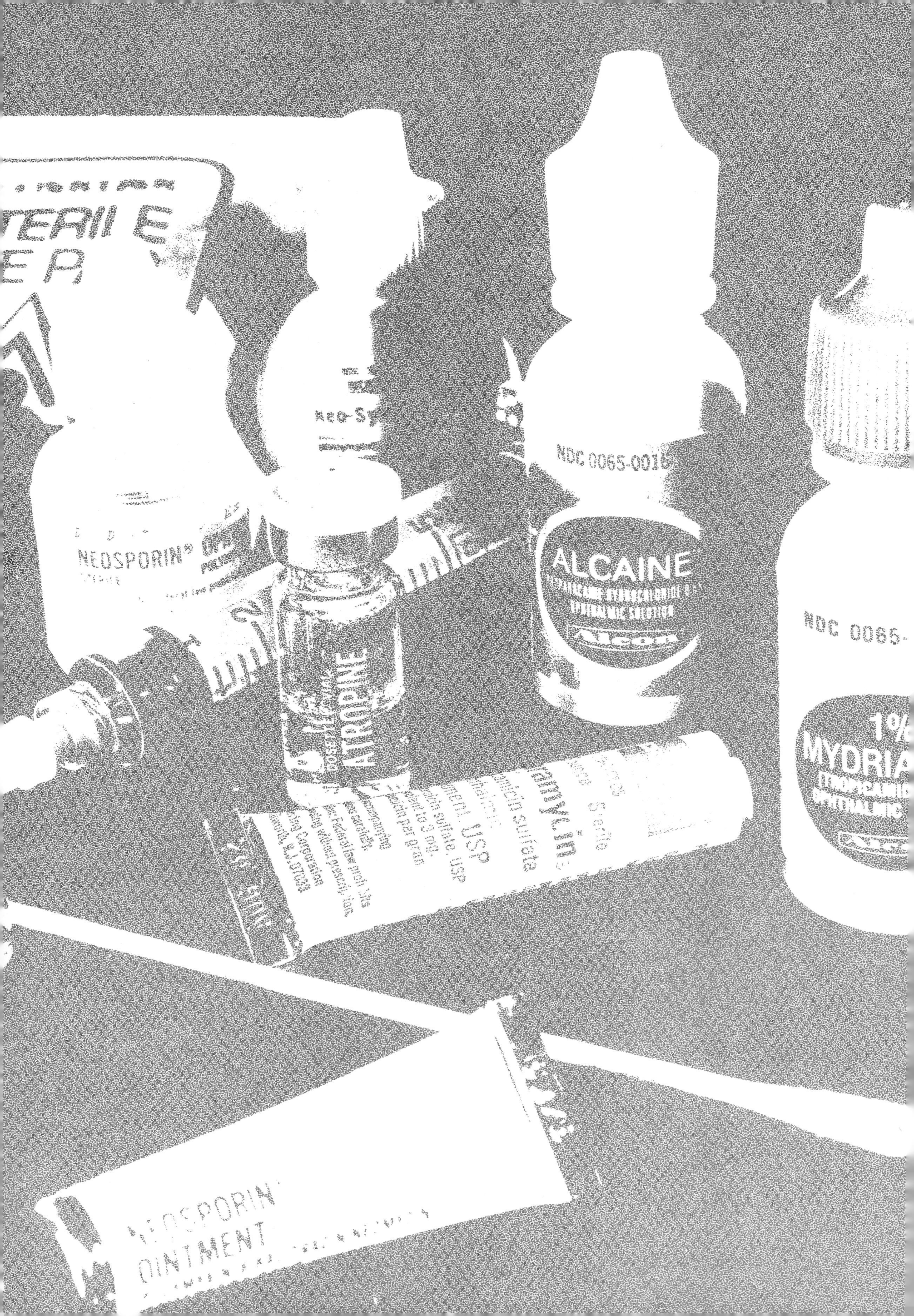
NEOSPORIN®
ALCAINE
OPHTHALMIC SOLUTION
Alcon
ATROPINE
1%
NEOSPORIN
OINTMENT

9
MEDICATIONS

MEDICATIONS

William H. Havener, M.D.

This chapter is not intended to be a condensed pharmacology book, nor does it repeat conventional wisdom. This discussion focuses on the use of medications rather than their pharmacologic properties in the hope of provoking the surgeon to reevaluate use of medications as adjuncts to surgery. In general, I believe that surgeons use too many drugs. Drugs are toxic and expensive, and a drug should not be used without concern for its specific effects.

PREVENTION OF INFECTION

PREOPERATIVE ANTIBIOTICS

Before and during every eye operation, the surgeon should constantly be alert to the sources of potential infection. Antibiotics and germicides may be of help in eliminating temporarily the normal flora surrounding the eye (to which the interior of the patient's eye has no more resistance than it does to other microorganisms). Traditionally, antibiotic eye drops are instilled the night and morning before surgery. This ritual probably does much more for the surgeon's peace of mind than for the eye. The studies on which use of preoperative ocular antibiotics are based are not ideal. Usually, a new antibiotic is used in a few hundred cases, and the results are contrasted to a comparable number of cases operated before introduction of the new antibiotic. Such a study is inadequately controlled and usually meaningless.

The microflora inhabiting the eyelids are difficult to eradicate, requiring days of antibiotic treatment rather than several instillations. Furthermore, the environment and the patient's body surface harbor innumerable microorganisms, which recontaminate the eyelids almost immediately. Quite possibly, the preoperative use of topical antibiotics does nothing more than to preselect resistant strains of organisms. The preoperative prophylactic use of antibiotics in a normal-appearing eye probably has little value in preventing infection (a culture from an antibiotic-treated eyelid will confirm this hypothesis).

GERMICIDES

Knowledge that microorganisms capable of destroying the eye reside on the eyelids, even after prophylactic antibiotic application, requires the surgeon to use effective germicides prior to incision. A variety of medications have been advocated. Quaternary ammonium compounds, such as benzalkonium chloride (Zephiran), are good detergents but are readily inactivated by adsorption to cotton fibers, such as those in the preparation sponges. In concentrations greater than 1:5000, benzalkonium is a cationic detergent and is neutralized by anionic detergents such as pHisoHex.

Considerably greater germicidal activity is achieved with pHisoHex. Unfortunately, it is also more toxic and can badly damage the corneal epithelium and stroma. Several cases have been reported in which the fellow eye was inadvertently contaminated with the pHisoHex preparation solution that contacted the cornea during surgery.

Povidone-iodine (Betadine) soap currently seems to be the best of the germicides. It kills microorganisms, yet causes only minimal and practically unnoticeable corneal epithelial damage. Betadine does not burn the skin, even if left on after rinsing.

PREPARATION TECHNIQUE

Cleaning of the eyelids is usually undertaken in a cursory and undisciplined manner. A good preparation is the best way to prevent infection and should result in sterile preoperative cultures. Most preparation leaves hundreds of microorganisms.

Several drops of 20 percent mild silver protein (Argyrol) in the cul-de-sac has limited germicidal qualities, but the purpose is to stain and render visible the mucus debris in the conjunctival sac. After good preparation, no trace of silver-protein staining remains.

Betadine-impregnated gauze balls are used to scrub the skin surrounding the eye, including nose, cheek, and forehead, with care taken to avoid the fellow eye. To cleanse the lid margins, which cannot be reached with gauze balls, applicator sticks with cotton-wrapped tips that have been dipped in Betadine may be used to scrub thoroughly the lid margins and eyelashes. Pulling on the skin of brow or cheek everts the lid margin to expose it to more complete scrubbing. No trace of crusting or debris may remain at the lash base. With special attention to the inner canthus, mucus threads can be wiped from the cul-de-sac; handling of the conjunctiva should be gentle. Normal saline can be used to irrigate the conjunctival sac, with both upper and lower lids everted for thorough access to the cul-de-sac. The skin surface is wiped with additional Betadine-soaked gauze balls, wiping from the center out, once with each ball. The center of the prepared area should not be rewiped with the same swab used on the contaminated periphery. A culture will confirm the quality of sterile preparation. The surgeon should not be satisfied with less than a sterile surface before opening an eye.

A good preparation is the most important step in the prevention of infection (assuming proper sterile technique and instrument sterilization).

POSTOPERATIVE ANTIBIOTICS

A variety of antibiotics have been advocated for routine subconjunctival injection after surgery. This irritates the eye unnecessarily and is irrational after clean and skillful surgery. Incisions should be closed tightly at the end of surgery, limiting the hazard of entry of surface contamination. Unless there is reason to believe the eye to be infected, such as known break in technique or penetrating injury, antibiotic injections are inappropriate.

Instillation of antibiotic ointments may have some merit. Bandaged eyelids tend to accumulate crusts and discharge adherent to the eyelashes. Such crusting is reduced by postoperative instillation of antibiotic ointment (for example, Neosporin ointment).

TREATMENT OF INFECTION

PREOPERATIVE TREATMENT

Elective eye surgery should never be undertaken in the presence of infection of the ocular surface. The absence of such infection, especially of the lacrimal sac, must be confirmed at the office visit before surgery and again before the operation begins.

If present, the infecting organism should be identified and treated with appropriate topical antibiotics. Surgery should be delayed until the infection is eradicated.

POSTOPERATIVE TREATMENT

The main reasons for postoperative inspection of the eye are to detect the presence of intraocular infection or wound disruption. Although the incidence of postoperative infection is quite low, principally because of the globe's rich vascular supply, all surgeons fear the signs that herald what may prove to be endophthalmitis. Differentiation between the normal response to surgery, aseptic iritis, and intraocular infection may be difficult initially. Unusual pain, redness, or haziness of the media is common to all three conditions. Hypopyon strongly suggests infection, but may result from iritis alone. Corneal opacity combined with hypopyon is almost surely an advanced sign of infection.

Prompt identification of the responsible microorganism is essential to institution of aggressive antibiotic therapy. Surface cultures do not necessarily identify the same organism that is inside the eye. If the surgeon is reasonably certain that intraocular infection is present, aspiration of intraocular fluid with a 27-gauge needle will provide material for culture and Gram stain. Such aspiration is unpleasant and presents a slight hazard, and is therefore inappropriate just because an eye is slightly red. If infection is obviously present, however, the surgeon must identify the organism and its antibiotic sensitivity.

Before specific identification of the organism, intravenous chloramphenicol, 2.0 gm to start, with 1.0 gm given every four hours, is effective. Chloramphenicol has 10,000 times the lipoid solubility of penicillin and penetrates the brain and eye barriers to achieve levels approximating half the plasma levels. Both gram-positive and gram-negative organisms are susceptible. The most effective antibiotic should be administered as soon as laboratory identification has been confirmed.

ANTI-INFLAMMATORY TREATMENT

CYCLOPLEGICS

Parasympatholytic drugs, such as atropine, reduce the abnormal permeability and protein leak of inflamed intraocular vessels. Except for duration of action, these drugs (atropine, homatropine, scopolamine, cyclopentolate, and tropicamide) have the same effect on the eye and are therapeutically interchangeable. All are potentially allergenic, although they are structurally dissimilar enough so that cross-allergic reactions do not occur. All are toxic and may be hallucinogenic.

Atropine is used almost routinely after major intraocular surgery and is usually continued for one to two weeks, or until aqueous flare is no longer visible on slit-lamp examination. Postoperative cycloplegic treatment is also appropriate in eyes with open-angle glaucoma, although many surgeons prefer a shorter-acting cycloplegic, such as scopolamine or cyclopentolate, if the eye is predisposed to pressure elevation.

CORTICOSTEROIDS

There is an almost universal conviction that routine postoperative use of corticosteroids makes eyes whiter, more comfortable, and generally better. Unfortunately, controlled studies indicate that this is a myth. Comfortable and relatively white eyes after surgery are the reward of meticulous and gentle technique, not the consequence of routine corticosteroid therapy.

A special place for corticosteroid therapy exists in corneal transplantation. Prolonged corticosteroid use may prevent graft rejection.

Corticosteroids render the eye immunologically incompetent, unable to resist invasion by microorganisms. They also cause cataract and make manifest the genetic tendency to open-angle glaucoma. Used intensively and early, they block wound healing.

PRESSURE CONTROL

Operation on hard eyes is undesirable. Vitreous loss occurs and creates problems, although attempts to lower pressure may also present difficulties.

Digital massage or pressure after retrobulbar anesthesia (1 percent lidocaine; 2 percent is unnecessary) results in marked hypotony, especially if hyaluronidase is included. Gentle and prolonged massage (up to five minutes) is probably the best way to achieve softness of the eye before surgery.

The relaxation of the extraocular muscles resulting from a good general anesthetic causes a substantial drop of intraocular pressure, though not so great as results from massage.

ACETAZOLAMIDE

Secretory inhibition reduces intraocular pressure somewhat, but not as much as results from digital massage. Preoperative acetazolamide is probably ineffectual.

OSMOTIC AGENTS

Absolutely dramatic softening of the eye may be obtained with intravenously administered mannitol (1.0 gm/kg) or orally administered glycerol. Since osmotherapy withdraws fluid across the blood-eye barrier, a functioning trabeculum is unnecessary, and hypotony can be achieved even in angle-closure glaucoma.

Because of unpleasant side effects (cerebral dehydration, cardiovascular overload, urinary distention, nausea, and vomiting), osmotherapy should be reserved for the unusual case, such as angle-closure glaucoma, or when vitreous problems are anticipated. Routine use of osmotherapy probably causes as many problems as it prevents, with no net gain.

MIOTICS

Eyes with glaucoma controlled preoperatively with miotic therapy should have the miotic discontinued before surgery. Miotics tend to increase protein leakage and promote the formation of posterior synechiae. Miotic use is not reinstituted until at least two weeks after surgery, or when the eye appears to be free of postoperative inflammation. Miotic therapy should not be resumed routinely, and then only if pressure rise requires treatment. (The misconception that miotic therapy causes retinal detachments is derived from the coincidence that old, glaucomatous, cataractous, or aphakic eyes are predisposed to develop other degenerative changes, such as retinal detachment.)

SEDATIVES AND ANESTHETIC AGENTS

The best tranquilizer is good rapport with the patient, who should have absolute confidence in the surgeon. After appropriate preoperative discussion and explanation, the awake patient, capable of carrying on an intelligent conversation, may undergo surgery without difficulty. Sedation and analgesia with 100 mg of pentobarbital sodium and 75 mg of meperidine are appropriate.

LOCAL ANESTHETIC AGENTS

The techniques of injection, described in previous chapters, are more important than the drugs used. Lidocaine is the most popular local anesthetic. A 1 percent concentration is optimal. Greater toxicity, with no additional anesthetic potency, is the only result of using 2 percent or 4 percent solutions. Lidocaine approaches toxic levels at 40 ml of 1 percent, 20 ml of 2 percent, and 10 ml of 4 percent. Epinephrine prolongs duration of anesthesia, especially if hyaluronidase is used. Hyaluronidase helps soften the eye, but shortens the duration of the anesthetic.

Toxicity from the injected medication is almost always due to epinephrine rather than to lidocaine. Tachycardia and apprehension are common responses to epinephrine. Dangerous hypertension is a remote possibility. Thyrotoxic patients and those with coronary artery insufficiency are at higher risk to epinephrine toxicity. On the other hand, the anesthetic effect dissipates more rapidly without the epinephrine, especially if hyaluronidase is included to promote softening of the eye.

Bupivacaine prolongs anesthesia for many hours, resulting in postoperative comfort. Unfortunately, its onset is erratic. For this reason, a mixture of lidocaine and bupivacaine may be more useful.

GENERAL ANESTHETIC AGENTS

General or stand-by anesthesia has become much more popular in recent years. It has the advantage of preventing the patient from distracting the surgeon during the procedure. Lengthy operations may be better tolerated under general anesthesia.

The surgeon might consider supplementing the general anesthetic with a retrobulbar injection. This may prevent rectus muscle contraction if the patient wakens during the procedure and squeezes his eyes in pain. Also, the anesthesiologist must be informed that succinylcholine causes a brief spasm of the rectus muscles.

Many patients fear general anesthesia as much as they fear surgery. The aftereffects of the anesthetic may linger for several weeks, just as it takes some time to recover from hepatitis or influenza.

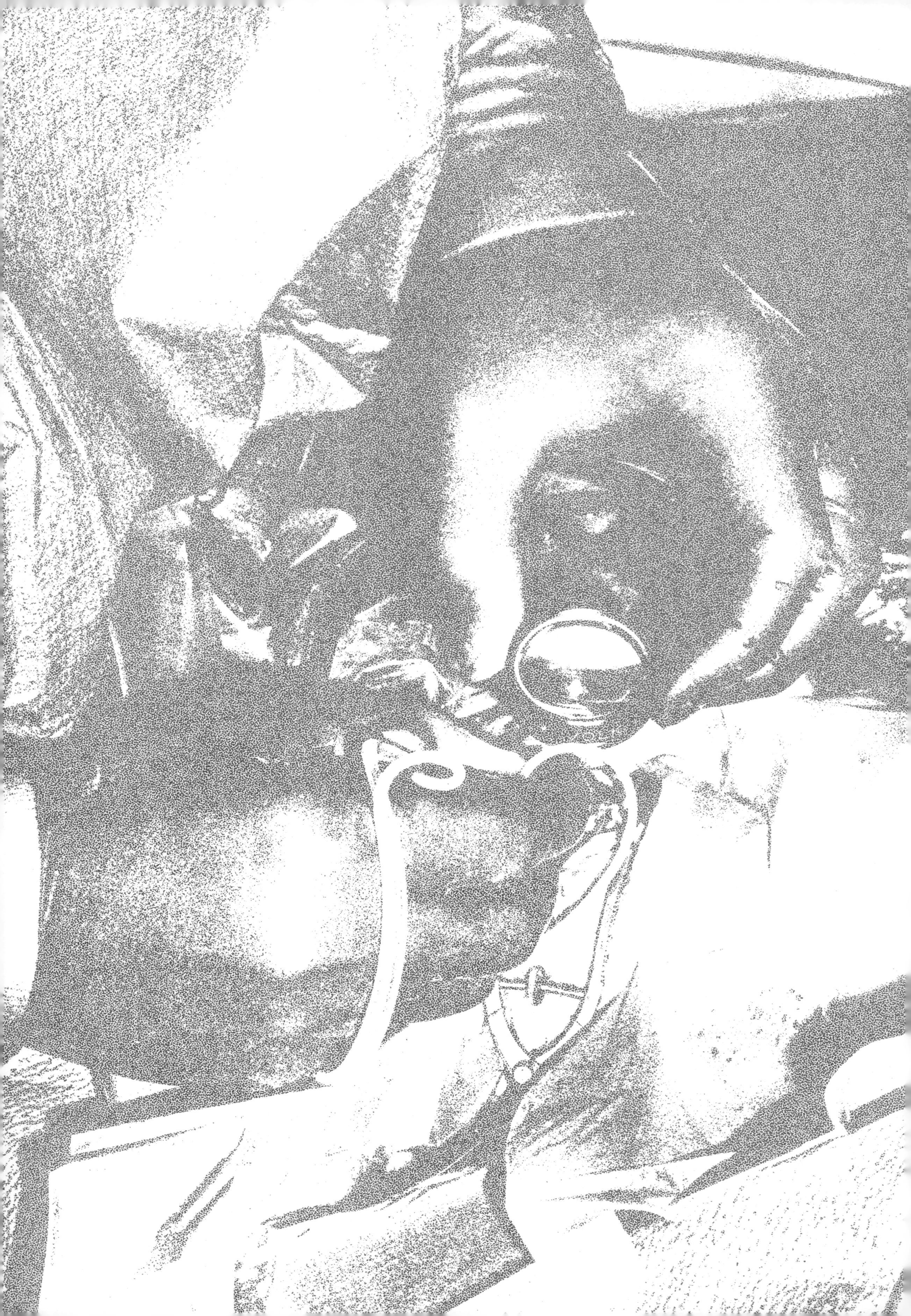

ANATOMIC INDEX

ANATOMIC INDEX

A

B

C

D

E

F

G

H

I

K

L

M

N

O

P

V

W

Z

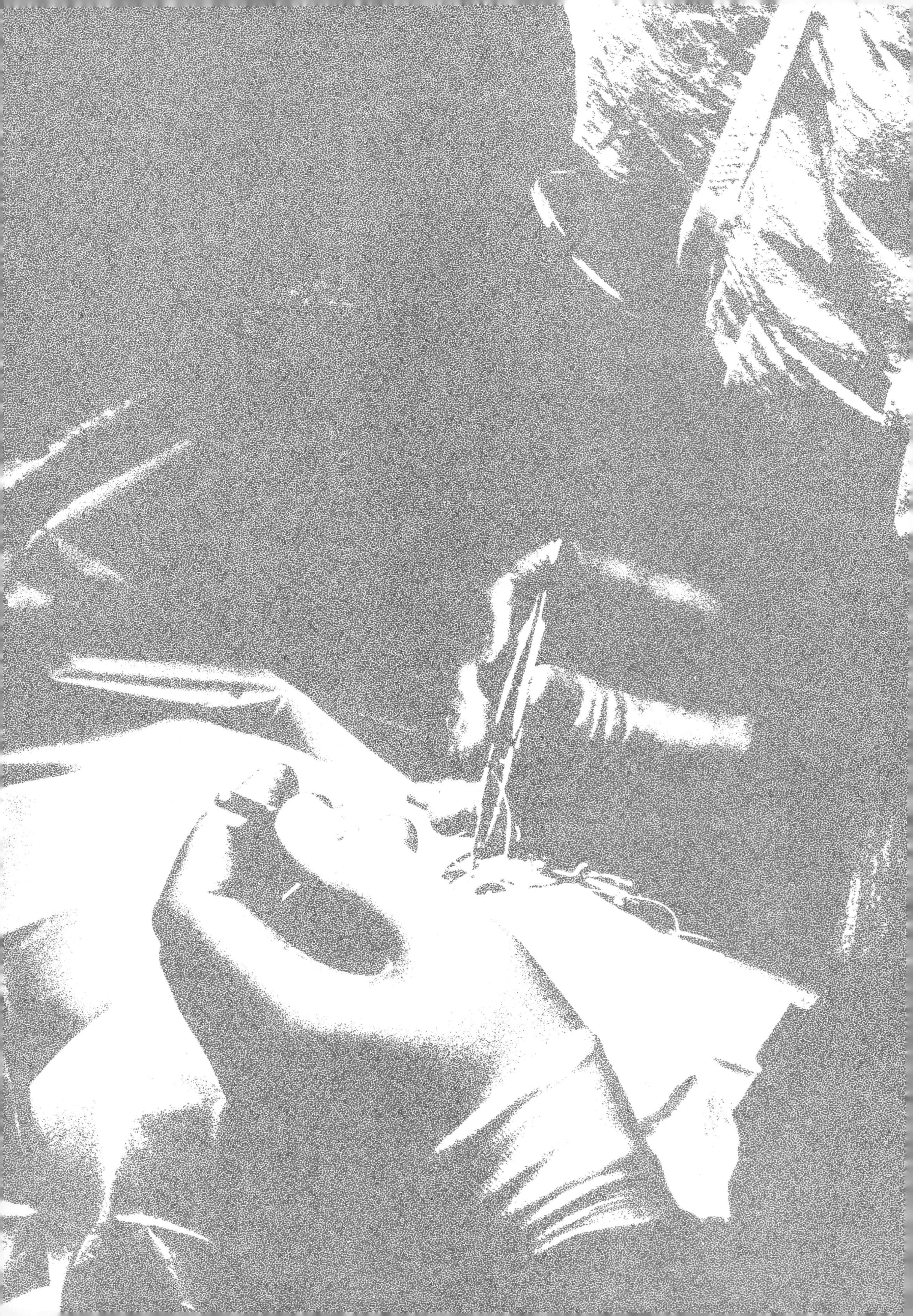

GENERAL INDEX

GENERAL INDEX

A

B

C

D

E

F

G

H

I

K

L

M

N

O

P

R

S

T

U

V

W

Z

Typesetting by
Capital Composition Company, Westerville, Ohio

Printed by
National Graphics Corporation, Columbus, Ohio

Bookbinding by
Nicholstone Book Bindery, Nashville, Tennessee